PRIMARY CARE OF THE ANTERIOR SEGMENT

Louis J. Catania, O.D.
Associate Professor and Consultant
Pennsylvania College of Optometry
Philadelphia, Pennsylvania

Chief of Primary Services
Vision Care Consultants, Inc.
Ardmore, Pennsylvania

APPLETON & LANGE
Norwalk, Connecticut/San Mateo, California

0-8385-7924-8

Notice: Our knowledge in clinical sciences is constantly changing. As new information becomes available, changes in treatment and in the use of drugs become necessary. The author(s) and the publisher of this volume have taken care to make certain that the doses of drugs and schedules of treatment are correct and compatible with the standards generally accepted at the time of publication. The reader is advised to consult carefully the instruction and information material included in the package insert of each drug or therapeutic agent before administration. This advice is especially important when using new or infrequently used drugs.

Copyright © 1988 By Appleton & Lange
A Publishing Division of Prentice-Hall

89 90 91 92 / 10 9 8 7 6 5 4

Prentice-Hall International (UK) Limited, *London*
Prentice-Hall of Australia Pty. Limited, *Sydney*
Prentice-Hall Canada, Inc., *Toronto*
Prentice-Hall Hispanoamericana, S.A., *Mexico*
Prentice-Hall of India Private Limited, *New Delhi*
Prentice-Hall of Japan, Inc., *Tokyo*
Simon & Schuster Asia Pte. Ltd., *Singapore*
Editora Prentice-Hall do Brasil Ltda., *Rio de Janeiro*
Prentice-Hall, *Englewood Cliffs, New Jersey*

Catania, Louis J.
    Primary care of the anterior segment / Louis J. Catania.
        p. cm.
    Includes bibliographical references and indexes.
    ISBN 0-8385-7924-8
    1. Anterior segment (Eye)—Diseases. I. Title.
    [DNLM: 1. Anterior Eye Segment. 2. Eye Diseases—diagnosis.
    3. Eye Diseases—therapy. 4. Primary Health Care. WW 210 C357p]
RE334.C37 1988
617.7—dc19
DNLM/DLC
for Library of Congress   88-16780
                                                    CIP

Acquisitions Editor: R. Craig Percy
Production Editor: Charles F. Evans
Interior Designer: M. Chandler Martylewski
Cover Designer: Kathleen Peters Ceconi

PRINTED IN THE UNITED STATES OF AMERICA

*With all my love
to my wife Stephanie
and the kids,
Russell,
Brian,
and
Lauren*

Contents

List of Tables

Preface and Acknowledgments

The most common word in this book is "usually." It is not a highly scientific term but one that accurately reflects the degree of certainty (or uncertainty) with which the clinician can "usually" rely on a written description of a disease condition. While scientific texts often tend toward the absolute, leaving the clinician wary of a potential range of variables that so often present, this text acknowledges and attempts to define the variables in hopes of comforting the clinician facing the atypical.

Addressing the "typical" is the purpose of this book, which reflects the clinical experiences of a busy doctor of optometry (and the outstanding professional and support staff, students, and residents with whom I have worked) responsible for the primary diagnosis and management of many thousands of patients over an 18-year period. I have had a long-time interest in, and concentration on, the primary diagnosis and management of common (typical) disease conditions of the anterior segment of the eye. Because of this interest, this book focuses on anterior segment eye diseases and the primary diagnosis and management of the most common presenting conditions of the anterior segment. If it's not covered within these pages, I haven't seen it, or "it just ain't common!"

This is a unique book in many ways. Although it does not claim to include pathophysiological or original research on each condition presented, it does include relevant clinical background information and many new clinical ideas, concepts, and methods of care used successfully over many years and not documented previously, either in the literature or in textbooks. Although the book does not claim to cover every condition of the anterior segment of the eye, those it does address are dealt with differently than in most texts: in a clinically systematic format consistent with an actual patient work-up and the practitioner's thinking and decision-making process. The book is truly by and for the busy primary eye care practitioner.

I invite you to read this book, reread it, use it, and refer to it often. Between its covers are contained a great deal of valuable information and practical tips meant for you, your practice, and especially your patients. The purpose of clinical educational materials should be to help you learn, help your practice grow, and when applied to your patients' needs, help them improve. The goal of this book is to help you meet each of those objectives by providing a straightforward approach to primary care of the anterior segment.

Louis J. Catania, O.D.

ACKNOWLEDGMENTS

It's really amazing how people are so extraordinary when they recognize their strengths and their opportunity to contribute to something worthwhile. Most of the folks on the following list will probably not even think they did anything very special for me or for this effort. None will ever fully know how much they actually did help and how much I will always appreciate them as special colleagues, professionals, and (mostly) friends.

Thanks don't come in alphabetical order, but this list does:

American Optometrists
Australian Optometrists
Randall Beatty
Linda Casser
Velia Catania (Mom)
Gilda and George Crozier
Murray Fingeret
Harold Gardner
Dolores and Lenny
  Genovese
Denise Guido
Eleanor Haight
Alden N. Haffner
Charles Hertz
Marita Krivda
Chauncey Levy
Tom Lewis
Mack Lipkin
Annette Marisi
John McGreal
Dennis Moss
Nancy Papapanu
Pennsylvania College of
  Optometry's faculty,
  students, and residents
R. Craig Percy
Philadelphia Health
  Associates
Max Presberg
Ron Reed
Melvin Remba
James Roberts
Jane Stein
Marie Taccone
Barry Thorne
Mervyn Weerasinghe
Barry Weismann
Wilson Health Center's
  professional and
  support staff
Mel Wolfberg
H. Ted Woodcome

A special thank you must also go to Dr. Janice Durham for her fine artwork throughout the book, to Randy Beatty for his physician's perspective in Chapters 5 and 6, to Scott Edmonds and Joe Shovlin for their contact lens expertise and contributions to Chapter 7, and to Olee Olsen for sharing interesting cases and clinical photographs with me over the years. Each of these people has had a direct influence on this book and deserves my special recognition and thanks.

Introduction

This book has been designed as a dynamic systematic text with a clinically oriented format for practical, easy use in multiple ways. It consists of five integrated parts for use by four different methods.

The five integrated parts of the book include the following:

- A Table of Contents.
- An in-depth narrative outline text of seven chapters, each constructed from five elements: (1) the universal SOAP (Subjective, Objective, Assessment, Plan) clinical format for each condition accompanied by Background Information where indicated, (2) 47 illustrations for understanding and clarity of certain clinical considerations and procedures, (3) 61 tables for synthesis and summaries of inter-related clinical information and facts, (4) 200 self-assessment questions and answers for pre-evaluation or postevaluation of your personal knowledge and understanding, and (5) references as footnote citations and annotated resources for expanded information.
- One hundred color plates of common conditions, each with a separate legend of description and associated case reports. (These color plates and their legends often provide information not found elsewhere in the text; I encourage you to use them when they are cited in the text.)
- Five appendices with cross-referenced page notations for quick review with the text: (1) commonly reported subjective symptoms with associated diagnostic considerations, (2) frequently noted objective signs with commonly associated diagnoses, (3) differential diagnostic considerations to "rule out" in frequently diagnosed conditions, (4) most common diagnoses by degree of presentation (i.e., mild, moderate, and severe) in a comparative chart format, and (5) a chart of post-operative aphakic and pseudophakic complications and management considerations.
- A standard book index.

The four methods of using this book are as follows:

- Read the complete text in its entirety for enjoyment and general familiarity with the overall content and formatting of information.
- Subsequently, when reading other technical literature or texts, refer to the narrative outline and tables for review or summary of practical, clinical information and considerations regarding specific diagnostic entities being discussed.
- Keep the book close to (or in) your examining room for quick-reference diagnostic and management information and tips when needed while your patient is "in the chair."
- Use the margin space provided throughout the text for note-keeping as a dynamic, ongoing method of incorporating recent applicable research and literature updates, changes (in thinking), new concepts, and so forth, into one reliable source. Also, bring the book along to appropriate lectures and seminars to record directly to a specific category any additional or new "clinical pearls" from the experts in the field.

It is hoped that this unique approach to a textbook will be able to serve your ongoing needs regarding primary care of the anterior segment. My attempt has not been to create something for everyone as much as to provide an easy-to-use, practical, comprehensive, dynamic, and ongoing up-to-date resource for those of us who must frequently diagnose and manage common anterior segment conditions in our day-to-day primary eye care practices.

Louis J. Catania, O.D.

1

General Therapeutic Considerations in Clinical Practice

I. Patient Care Considerations

A. SUBJECTIVE

1. Comprehensive history (Table 1–1)
2. Risk-factor analysis (Table 1–2)
3. Do not skip questions
4. Listen to, and learn from, each response

B. OBJECTIVE

1. Do not skip appropriate tests (Table 1–3)
2. Entering visual acuities (VAs), a medicolegal essential
3. Systematic approach most efficient
  a. Anatomical categories
    i. Eyelids and adnexa
    ii. Conjunctiva
    iii. Sclera and episclera
    iv. Cornea
    v. Anterior chamber and iris and ciliary body
    vi. Crystalline lens
  b. Pathophysiological etiologies
    i. Infectious
    ii. Inflammatory
    iii. Immunologic (allergic, hypersensitive, toxic)
    iv. Metaplasia (hypoplastic, hyperplastic)
    v. Neoplasia (primary, metastatic)
    vi. Dystrophy
    vii. Degeneration
    viii. Congenital (versus acquired)
    ix. Neurological
    x. Unknown etiology
4. Look, listen, and feel (palpate tissue structures)
5. Document findings thoroughly and accurately
  a. Photodocument if possible
  b. Use color coding when indicated[1] (Table 1–4)
  c. Use appropriate abbreviations (Table 1–5)

C. ASSESSMENT

1. Differential diagnosis most important clinical task
2. Rule out (R/O) other involvements (e.g., internal, extraocular muscles (EOM), systemic)
3. Consider laboratory workups (e.g., cultures, sensitivities, smears) versus clinical observation alone
  a. Newborns
  b. Chronic or unresponsive conditions
  c. Hyperacute conditions
  d. Postoperative involvement

TABLE 1–1. QUESTIONS TO INCLUDE IN PATIENT HISTORY

General considerations
- Observe and consider patient's general behavior
- Personalize your questioning
- Do not lead patient with loaded questions
- Let the patient talk and expand (within reason)
- Cross-question when indicated or necessary
- Listen

Specific questions
- Name
- Age
- Occupation
- Habitation
- Cohabitation
- Main statement of complaint (reason for visit?)
- Onset of symptoms (when did it begin?)
- Frequency (recurring, hourly, daily, weekly?)
- Intensity (constant, intermittent, quality, quantity)
- Duration (how long does it last?)
- Types of symptoms
  - Visual
  - Diplopia
  - Trauma (describe?)
  - Pain or irritation (where?)
- Ocular history
  - Prescription eyeglasses (how long and for what?)
  - Any previous injury, surgery, or diseases?
  - Any family history of eye disease?
- General health
  - Chronic disease
  - Present condition
  - Family history
  - Allergies, asthma
- Medication history
  - Taking any (ocular or other)
  - Allergies or idiosyncratic reactions
    - Topical
    - Systemic
- Nutritional habits
- Stress factors
  - Physical or environmental
  - Mental or psychological
  - Social or economic
- Risk factors (refer to Table 1–2)

TABLE 1–2. RISK FACTORS TO CONSIDER IN DIAGNOSIS

- History
- Age
- Sex
- Race
- Incidence or prevalence (frequency of disease: epidemiology)
- Demography (geographic distribution of disease)
- Common etiologies
- Genetic (hereditary) factors
- Predisposing conditions (e.g., systemic diseases, environmental hazards)
- Social, psychosocial, economic factors
- Neurogenic overlay (conversion syndromes)
- Psychogenic overlay (organic)

D. PLAN

1. Treatment plan should be response to diagnosis (Assessment)
2. Variable considerations in a treatment plan
   a. No treatment
   b. Observation (recheck) and monitoring
   c. Placebos if indicated and appropriate
   d. Consultation (another opinion)
   e. Referral (assistance with care)
      i. Technical or professional assistance
      ii. Alternative forms of care
      iii. Special forms of care
   f. Pharmaceutical agents
   g. Prescription writing (Fig.1–1) (Table 1–6)
3. Patient education, advice, counsel, and advocacy are essential with all forms of treatment

E. MANAGEMENT AND FOLLOW-UP

1. Decisions (i.e., when, where, how, and so forth) should be based on each individual case presentation
   a. Diagnosis
   b. Intensity of presentation
   c. Acute versus chronic onset
   d. Risk factors
   e. Prognosis (e.g., time frame, expected outcome)
   f. Psychological and emotional factors and needs
   g. Practical considerations
      i. Geographic (e.g., travel, weather) factors
      ii. Financial hardship
   h. Practitioner comfort and confidence in diagnosis
   i. Perceived patient compliance
2. Accessibility and availability of practitioner
   a. Office accessibility
   b. After-hours and weekend on-call availability
   c. Cross-coverage, answering services, and so forth
3. Patient care versus practitioner education or research
   a. Patients should pay for their doctor's care
   b. Patients should not have to pay for their doctor's ongoing educational or research interests

TABLE 1–3. OBJECTIVE TESTS IN ANTERIOR SEGMENT EXAMINATION[a]

- Observation (during patient interview)
  - Head position
  - Body posture
  - Scars (from injury or surgery)
  - Facial symmetry
  - Ocular and facial motilities
  - General complexion and skin quality
  - Quality and quantity of hair, eyebrows, eyelashes
  - Position of eyelids and lacrimal puncta
- Visual acuities
  - Distance (with and without correction)
  - Near (with and without correction)
  - Pinhole vision
  - Amsler grid
- Orbits and surrounding structures
  - Exophthalmometry
  - Palpation of bony margins
  - X-rays or ultrasound, if indicated
  - Upward gaze test for blowout fracture of orbital floor
  - Forced ductions test if indicated
  - Percussion of sinuses (bilateral comparisons)
  - Transillumination of sinuses
  - EOM evaluation for intraorbital causes of diplopia
  - Direct pressure (on globes) for unequal retrobulbar resistance
- Eyelids
  - Palpate for edema, masses, tenderness
  - Express ("milk") Zeiss, Moll, meibomian glands
  - Evert (single and double) upper eyelid
  - Evaluate blink function:
  - Rate
  - Magnitude (e.g., complete versus lagophthalmos)
  - Forced blink
  - Bell's phenomenon
  - Glabella tap test (in blepharospasm)
  - Fatigue lids with multiple forced blinks (rule out myasthenia)
  - Consider tensilon test if indicated
  - Measure lid apertures and motility (bilateral comparisons)
  - Examine eyelid margin quality
  - Evaluate eyelashes (quality, quantity, positioning)
- Lacrimal system
  - Palpate lacrimal gland (superior temporal aspect)
  - Examine lacrimal puncta (size, position, patency)
  - Regurgitation of lacrimal sac (nasalward)
  - Observe for epiphora or hyperlacrimation
  - Schirmer tear testing
  - Breakup time (BUT) with NaFl
  - Jones testing (#1 and 2)
  - Saccharin taste test
  - Diagnostic dilation and irrigation procedures
- Conjunctiva
  - Examine palpebral and bulbar portions under magnification
  - Check vascular patterns and surface characteristics
  - Move vessels and tissue with cotton-tip applicator
  - Vasoconstrict for differential diagnosis
  - Palpate preauricular lymph nodes
- Cornea and sclera
  - Gross observation (e.g., dimensions, curvature)
  - Transillumination (e.g., for defects, opacities)
  - Slit-lamp examination (with and without staining: NaFl and rose bengal)
  - Corneal sensitivity with cotton wisp (bilateral comparison)
  - Evaluate limbal juncture (e.g., vaculature, transition)
  - Examine scleral anatomy (surface, thickness, color, lesions)
- Anterior chamber
  - Measure intraocular pressure (digital and tonometry)
  - Examine aqueous humor for cells, flare, hypopyon, hyphema, foreign body
  - Estimate depth of chamber
  - Angle gonioscopy when indicated
  - Note iris coloration and/or heterochromias (unilateral or bilateral)
  - Evaluate iris surface and pupil border
  - Examine pupillary responses carefully
- Other tests
  - Blood pressure measurement
  - Pulse (radial)
  - Carotid bruit ascultation
  - Ophthalmodynamometry (ODM)
  - Blood glucose test
  - Cultures and sensitivities
  - Laboratory tests (if indicated)

[a]This list is comprehensive but not all-inclusive. Tests from such a list (and beyond) should be selected based on the examiner's judgment and diagnostic needs.

TABLE 1–4. COLOR CODE FOR OCULAR DIAGRAMMING

• Red	Hyperemia
	Hemorrhage
	Blood vessels
• Yellow	Exudate
	Casseous material
	Sebum
• Blue	Edema
• Green	Fluorescein staining
• Black	Opacities
• Brown	Pigmentation

F. OTHER CONSIDERATIONS

1. Tools needed
   a. Instruments and equipment (Table 1–7)
   b. Consumable supplies (Table 1–8)
   c. Pharmaceutical agents[2] (Table 1–9)
2. Accurate and thorough record keeping essential
   a. Neat and organized
   b. Record all positives
   c. Most important medicolegal consideration

TABLE 1–5. COMMON OPHTHALMIC ABBREVIATIONS

Abbreviation	Meaning
AC	Anterior chamber
c̄Rx	With spectacles
s̄Rx	Without spectacles
C/D	Cup–disc ratio
CF	Count fingers vision
D	Diopter (lens power)
dd	Disc diameter (for fundus measuring)
EOM	Extraocular muscles
E	Esophoria (at 20 ft or 6 m)
E'	Esophoria (at 14 in or 33 cm)
ET	Esotropia (distance) or Extraterrestrial
E(T)	Intermittent esotropia (distance)
ET'	Esotropia (near)
E(T)'	Intermittent esotropia (near)
HM	Hand motion vision
IOP	Intraocular pressure
KP	Keratitis precipitate
L	Left (e.g., LET)
LL	Lower eyelid
LP	Light perception
NLP	No light perception
NPC	Near point of convergence
OD	Right eye
OS	Left eye
OU	Both eyes
PD	Interpupillary distance
PERRLA	Pupils equal, round, reactive to light and accommodation
PH	Pinhole
R	Right (e.g., RET = right esotropia)
R/O	Rule out
RTC	Return check
SVP	Spontaneous venous pulsation
Ta	Applanation tonometry
UL	Upper eyelid
VA	Visual acuity
VF	Visual field
WNL	Within normal limits (or "We no lookie")
X	Exophoria (distance)
X'	Exophoria (near)
XT	Exotropia (distance)
X(T)	Intermittent exotropia
XT'	Exotropia (near)
X(T)'	Intermittent exotropia (near)
Δ	Prism diopters
(+)	Convex lens (for hyperopia)
(−)	Concave lens (for myopia)

TABLE 1–6. PRESCRIPTION (AND PHARMACEUTICAL) ABBREVIATIONS

Abbreviation	Meaning
a.c.	Before meals
ad lib	At pleasure
ASAP	As soon as possible
bid	Twice a day
Collyr., Coll.	Eyewash
Cum, c̄	With
Disp.	Dispense
gtt	One drop
gtts	Drops
h	An hour
hs	At bedtime
LE, L Eye	Left eye
No., #	Number
OD	Right eye
OS	Left eye
OU	Both eyes
P.C.	After meals
PO	By mouth
PRN	When necessary
q	Each, every (e.g., q4h)
qid	Four times a day
Q.S.	As much as needed
RE, R Eye	Right eye
Rx	Treatment, prescribe
Sig.	Label
Sine, s̄	Without
Sol.	Solution
STAT	Immediately
tid	Three times a day
Ung	Ointment
i	One
ii	Two
iii	Three

3. Appointment scheduling
   a. For problem-oriented care
      i. Brief office visit (BOV)
      ii. Office visit (OV)
      iii. Extended office visit (EOV)
   b. ASAP (as soon as possible)
   c. STAT (urgent or emergent)
4. Economic factors and third-party considerations
   a. Extensive business and practice management aspects must be understood and mastered regarding the financial aspects, economics, and proper management of a primary eye care practice
   b. The nature of such a discussion is beyond the scope of this book for three basic reasons:
      i. This book is primarily a clinical text
      ii. The author of this text is neither a business nor practice management authority
      iii. The nature of such material is temporal as compared with the content of this text, hence is best obtained through contemporary journal literature and lectures by experts in the field
5. A primary care philosophy (the "Seven C's")
   a. Compassion and communication
   b. Clinical competency
   c. Comfort and confidence
   d. Comprehensive care
   e. Coordination and continuity
   f. Counseling
   g. Cost consciousness

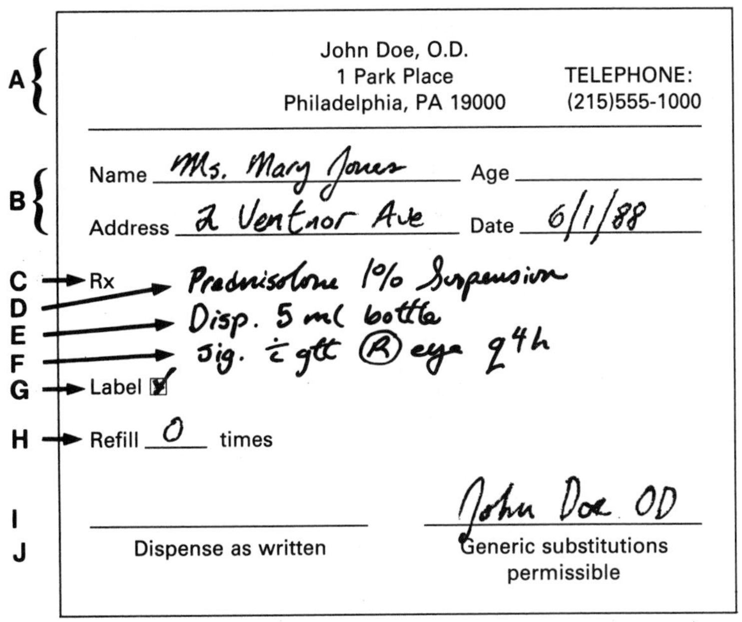

A { John Doe, O.D.
1 Park Place
Philadelphia, PA 19000

TELEPHONE:
(215)555-1000

B { Name Ms. Mary Jones Age
Address 2 Ventnor Ave Date 6/1/88

C → Rx → Prednisolone 1% Suspension
D → Disp. 5 ml bottle
E → Sig. c̄ gtt Ⓡ eye q4h
F
G → Label ☑
H → Refill 0 times

I
J Dispense as written

John Doe OD
Generic substitutions permissible

Elements of Prescription Writing

A. Doctor information: Name, address, telephone number (minimum); license number, DEA number, practice description, office hours (optional).

B. Patient information: Name, address, date (minimum); age, date of birth, male or female (optional).

C. Rx: Superscription (symbol only).

D. Inscription: Drug prescribed (brand or generic name); include description, concentration, vehicle.

E. Disp.: Amount, size to be dispensed.

F. Sig.: Precise directions to patient (how much, which eye, how often).

G. Label: Request for pharmacist to label container with instructions; the prescription form should include this (required in some states).

H. Refill: Indicate number of times patient allowed to refill (be conservative, do not allow a large number of refills).

I. Signature: Sign on appropriate line (substitution versus no substitution) semi-legibly!

J. Generic permission: Law in many states requires appropriate signature placement.

Tips from Pharmacist

- Write out or print legibly!
- Write out as much as you can in words or sentences.
- Do not abbreviate drug names (brand or generic).
- Write generics if you know your area pharmacists well.
- Know your area pharmacists well!

Figure 1–1.

TABLE 1–7. EQUIPMENT AND INSTRUMENTATION FOR ANTERIOR SEGMENT CARE

Item	Use	Item	Use
Essentials		*Nonessential Essentials*	
Snellen chart	Visual acuity (distance)	Binocular indirect ophthalmoscope and 20 D condensing lens	Fundus examination
Near point card	Visual acuity (near)		
Pinhole	Visual acuity		
Direct ophthalmoscope	Fundus examination	Burton (UV) lamp	Examination with NaFl
Tonometer	IOP measurement	Retinoscope	Refraction
Slit-lamp biomicroscope	For diagnosis	Trial lenses	Refraction
Transilluminator	Varied	External camera	Photodocumentation
Penlight	Varied	Goniolens (3-mirror)	Angle or fundus gonioscopy
Plus 20 diopter lens	Magnification		
Head Loope	Gross examination	Visual-field instrument	Peripheral fields
Millimeter rule	Measurement	Amsler grid	Central fields
Jeweler's forceps	Varied	Microscope	Cytology
Punctal dilator	In puncta	Color plates	Color vision
Lacrimal cannulus (needle)	For lacrimal irrigation	Ophthalmodynamometer (ODM)	Cerebrovascular diagnoses
3-cc syringe	For lacrimal irrigation	Exophthalmometer	Proptosis
Hypodermic needles 18-gauge (2 inches) 22-gauge (2 inches) 25-gauge (⅝ inches)	Varied (e.g. cyst drainage, FB removal)	Stainless steel tray	For instrument storage
		Eyelid evertor (Desmarre)	Eyelid eversion
Golf club spud	Foreign-body removal	Eyelid retractors (adult and pediatric size)	Eyelid retraction (for procedure)
Sphygmomanometer	Blood pressure	Toothed forceps	Grasping procedures
Stethoscope	Pressure and ascultation	Iris scissor	Varied
		Cautery	Varied
		Cilia forceps	Epilation
		Schirmer tear strips	Tear testing
		Foreign-body loop (Bailey)	Foreign-body removal
		Metal shield (Fox)	Eye protector

TABLE 1–8. CONSUMABLE SUPPLIES

Item	Use	Item	Use
Sodium fluorescein (NaFl) strips	Tissue staining	Cotton-tip applicators Sterile	Culturing
Rose bengal strips	Staining-devitalized cells and mucus	Nonsterile	Varied procedures
		Alcohol sponges	Antiseptic
Goniofluid or gel	Gonioscopy	Eyepads	Patching
2 × 2 gauze pads	Varied	Adhesive tape	Patching
Diagnostic agents (see Table 1–9)	Varied	Paper (Micropore)	Moderate adhesion
		Plastic (Dermiclear)	Good adhesion
Culture media (broth and/or agar)	For laboratory work	Cloth (Dermicel)	Good but expensive
		Adhesive remover	After taping
Microscope slides	Cytology	Zephiran HCl (1:750)	Antiseptic
pH paper	For chemical burns	PhisoHex	Antibacterial cleanser
Irrigating solution	Lavage (varied)	Cotton balls	For cleansing surface
		Therapeutic agents (see Table 1–10)	Varied
		Ammonia ampules	For vasovagal responses

TABLE 1-9. USEFUL IN-OFFICE PHARMACEUTICAL AGENTS

Name	Primary Purpose	Name	Primary Purpose
Drugs used primarily for ocular diagnosis		Polysporin	Ointment
Mydriacyl 0.5%, 1%	Pupil dilation	Sulfacetamide (15%)	Drops and ointment
Cyclogyl 0.5%, 1%, 2%	Cycloplegia	*Antiviral agents*	Initiating therapy
Neo-Synephrine 2.5%	Pupil dilation	Vira A	Ointment
Proparacaine 0.5%	Topical anesthesia	Viroptic	Drops
Fluress	Topical anesthesia with NaFl	*Anti-inflammatory agents*	Initiating steroid therapy
		Prednisolone 1%	For uveitis
Sodium fluorescein (NaFl)	Diagnostic stain	Dexamethasone 0.1%	For chemical burns
Rose bengal	Diagnostic stain (devitalized tissue)	FML	With glaucoma risk
		Hydrocortisone 0.5%, 1%	For allergic reactions
Drugs used for various purposes		*Antihistamine–decongestants*	Vasoconstriction and/or
Pilocarpine 2%, 4%	To reverse angle closure	Naphazoline HCl	allergy therapy
Diamox 250 mg caps	To reverse angle closure		(with antihistamine or
Glycerol 50% soln	To reverse angle closure		astringent)
Homatropine 2%, 5%	Pupil dilation (with uveitis)	*Lubricants (ointments and drops)*	Varied use
Scopolamine 0.25%	Pupil dilation (with uveitis)		
Adsorbonac 2%, 5%	Reduce diffuse edema	Mucomimetic drops	Daily use (ad lib)
Muro #128 ointment	Reduce dense edema	Ointments	Bedtime use
Antibiotic agents	Prophylaxis or initiating therapy	Hydrophilic soft lens	Bandage use
		Mast cell stabilizers	Mild to moderate allergic
Broad spectrum	Drops and ointments	Opticrom 4%	hypersensitivity
Combination drug (antibiotic/steroid)	Drops and ointments		responses
Gentamicin	Drops and ointments	Vitamin A (drops or ointments)	Dry eye syndromes
Tobramycin	Drops and ointments		

II. Pharmaceutical Considerations

A. MAJOR DRUG CATEGORIES

1. Autonomics (autonomic nervous system drugs)
   a. Antiglaucoma agents
      i. Miotics (cholinergic agonists)
      ii. "Epi" drugs (adrenergic agonists)
      iii. β-Blockers (adrenergic antagonists)
   b. Atropine group (cycloplegics and dilators)
      i. Atropine (0.5 percent and 1.0 percent)
         • Strongest cycloplegic drug
         • Duration up to 1 to 2 weeks
         • Prolonged immobilization of pupil may increase risk of posterior synechiae in anterior uveitis
      ii. Homatropine (2 percent and 5 percent)
         • Duration about 12 to 24 hours
         • Good dilator in treatment
      iii. Scopolamine (0.2 percent and 0.25 percent)
         • Duration about 24 to 48 hours

   • May work better than homatropine in darkly pigmented patients
      iv. Cyclopentolates (0.5 percent and 1 percent)
         • Short-acting cycloplegic
         • Popular diagnostic agent
      v. Tropicamide (0.5 percent and 1 percent)
         • Excellent short-acting dilator
         • Good for diagnosis and treatment
   c. Phenylephrine (2.5 percent and 10 percent)
      i. Short-acting dilator with no cycloplegia
      ii. Excellent sympathomimetic drug to combine with tropicamide (parasympatholytic drug) for maximal short-duration dilation
2. Anti-infective (antimicrobial) agents
   a. Antibiotics and antibacterials[3]*
      i. Aminoglycosides

---

*In alphabetical order.

- Widely used broad-spectrum topical agents[4]
- Drugs of choice for corneal infection
- Effective against gram-negative organisms and *Staphylococcus* (gram-positive)
- Oral forms highly toxic
- Popular topical ophthalmic forms
  Gentamicin
  Neomycin (approximately 5 percent risk of hypersensitivity reaction)[5]
  Tobramycin (most effective drug against *Pseudomonas*)[6]
- Other topical, oral, injectable forms
  Amikacin
  Kanamycin
  Netilmicin
  Streptomycin
  Vancomycin

ii. Bacitracin
- Effective against *Staphylococcus*
- Stable only in ointment form

iii. Cephalosporin agents (broad-spectrum oral)

iv. Chloramphenicol
- Excellent broad-spectrum topical
- Decreasing use due to increasing fear of fatal aplastic anemia risks

v. Erythromycin (topical and oral)
- Most effective against gram-positive organisms
  Staphylococcus
  Streptococcus
- Excellent alternative (backup) drug, except for antipseudomonal therapy

vi. Penicillins (oral forms only in eye care)
- Popular broad-spectrum oral agent
- Use penicillinase-resistant forms against *Staphylococcus*
  Cloxacillin
  Dicloxacillin
  Methicillin
  Nafcillin
  Oxacillin
- Beware of allergic patients
- Alternative drugs
  Cephalosporins
  Erythromycin

vii. Polymyxin B
- Effective *Pseudomonas* inhibitor
- Popular in bacitracin combination (e.g., Polysporin)

viii. Sulfacetamide (10 percent, 15 percent, and 30 percent)
- Popular broad-spectrum topical agent
- Increasing resistant staphylococcal strains to 10 percent concentration[7]
- Popular in steroid combinations (e.g., Blephamide, Vasocidin)

ix. Tetracycline
- Useful oral and topical broad-spectrum antibacterial action as well as actions against other pathogenic microbial agents (e.g., *Chlamydia*)
- Also acts as anticollagenolytic agent in corneal disease[8]
- Can cause depression and discoloration of developing bone and teeth
  Avoid in children under 12 to 15 years of age
  Avoid in pregnancy (and even in females of childbearing age)
- Also risk of phototoxic (sun) response
- Good alternative drug: erythromycin

x. Combinations of the compatible drugs common

b. Antifungal agents
  i. Highly toxic drugs
  ii. Nonocular drugs are occasionally used (e.g., Amphotericin B, Nystatin)
  iii. Only specific ocular drug: Natamycin

c. Antiviral agents
  i. 5-Idoxyuridine (IDU) (e.g., Stoxil)
  - Increasing resistant strains
  ii. Vidarabine (e.g., Vira A)
  - Ointment only
  iii. Trifluridine (e.g., Viroptic)
  - Drops only
  - Broadest spectrum
  - Toxic with prolonged use
  iv. Acyclovir (e.g., Zovirax)[9,10]
  - Least toxic antiviral
  - Not approved for use in the eye

d. Pesticidals (antiparasitic agents)

i. Eserine ointment for pediculosis (lice)
ii. Kwell shampoo for pediculosis
iii. Mercuric oxide for demodex (mite)
iv. Pyrethrin ointments
3. Anti-inflammatory agents (steroids)
   a. Actions
      i. Inhibit adverse tissue changes
      ii. Reduce scarring potential
      iii. *Steroids do not cure disease*
   b. Indications
      i. Inflammatory reactions
      ii. Toxic, hypersensitive (allergic) reactions
      iii. Associated inflammatory pain
   c. Contraindications
      i. Infections (without significant inflammatory component)
      ii. Herpes simplex epithelial keratitis
      iii. Active ulcerative process
   d. Adverse reactions
      i. Problems with prolonged use (topical and systemic)
      ii. Reduces mitotic healing (deep corneal abrasions)
      iii. Can raise intraocular pressure
      iv. "Masking effect"
         • Artificially whitens inflamed eye without treating underlying disease
   e. Drug selection
      i. Consider relative strengths (Table 1–10)
      ii. Fluorination increases steroid strength by 30 to 50 times
      iii. Prednisolone penetrates cornea most effectively
      iv. Always taper steroids when terminating

TABLE 1–10. RELATIVE STRENGTHS OF TOPICAL OPHTHALMIC STEROIDS[a]

Steroid	Relative Potency
Cortisone	0.8
Hydrocortisone	1.0
Medrysone (e.g., HMS)	1.0
Prednisolone (e.g., Pred Forte)	4.0
Methylprednisolone	5.0
Triamcinolone (e.g., Kenalog)	5.0
Fluorocortisone	10.0
Betamethasone	25.0
Dexamethasone (e.g., Decadron)	25.0
Fluorometholone (e.g., FML)	40.0

[a]Fluorinated steroids are usually about 30 to 50 times the strength of primary steroids.

• Reduce gradually over 3 to 5 days
• qid to tid to bid to 1 X and off
   f. Personal feeling: All eye practitioners should coordinate use of oral steroids through medical practitioners with in-depth experience in their use (e.g., dosages, adverse reactions)
4. Mast cell stabilizers (e.g., Opticrom 4%)[11,12]
   a. Most effective in chronic and subacute allergic presentations
   b. Relieves symptoms only
5. Topical anesthetic agents
   a. 0.5 percent proparacaine (many brands)
   b. Benoxinate plus NaFl (e.g., Fluress)
   c. For office use only: *Do not prescribe or dispense*
      i. Retards healing
      ii. Multiple in-office use during examination procedures is no problem
6. Antihistamines and decongestants (vasoconstrictors)
   a. Topical and oral agents useful in eye care
   b. Prescription and over-the-counter drugs of relatively equal value[13]
   c. Avoid overuse of topicals (too frequent, too strong, too long)
      i. Risk of "rebound" vasodilation
   d. Frequently in combination forms
7. Lubricants and tear substitutes
   a. Effective dosage: 6 to 10 instillations per day
   b. Mucomimetic drops
   c. Ointments
   d. Vitamin A (drops and ointments)[14]
   e. Hydrophilic contact lenses (acting as bandage)
8. Hypertonic saline agents
   a. For reduction of epithelial and mild anterior stromal edema
   b. Two percent and 5 percent drops (e.g., Adsorbonac)
      i. Refrigerate 5 percent to reduce stinging
      ii. Frequent (q1–2h) or ad lib dosages acceptable
   c. Five percent ointments at bedtime or in dense edemas
   d. Corneal epithelial surface must be intact (i.e., no deep or large abrasions)
   e. Can be used in conjunction with contact lenses

9. Miscellaneous agents
   a. Aspirin, ibuprofen, and flurbiprofen
      i. Non-narcotic analgesics
      ii. Nonsteroidal anti-inflammatories (NSAIDs)
         • Aspirin dose should be minimum of 3 g/day (10 5-gr tablets) to reach effective blood level within 24 to 48 hours
         • Ibuprofen dose range of 800 to 2400 mg, producing effective blood level within 3 to 4 hours
      iii. Rule out contraindications
         • Gastrointestinal disorders
         • Anticoagulant (bleeding) disorders
         • Serious kidney disease history
      iv. Acetaminophen (Tylenol) is not quite as effective for anti-inflammatory use
   b. Topical flurbiprofen (Ocufen) being used as NSAID for multiple purposes
      i. Pre- and postoperative control of miosis
      ii. Cystoid macula edema control
      iii. Surface inflammation therapy
   c. Compresses (hot and cold)
      i. Hot for conditions needing vasodilation
         • Infection and inflammation
         • Nonallergic (e.g., traumatic) edema
      ii. Hot-air (hair) blow dryers also an effective source of heat for variable causes of edema
      iii. Cold for conditions needing vasoconstriction
         • Allergic and hypersensitivity reactions
         • Intracellular bleeding
   d. Heavy metals as astringents and as anti-infectives
   e. Irrigating solutions
   f. Pressure patching
   g. Sodium fluorescein (NaFl) stains any epithelial cellular disruption
   h. Rose bengal stains devitalized (dead) cells
   i. Hydrophilic soft contact lenses
      i. As lubricators (e.g., dry eye syndromes)
      ii. As reservoir for drug delivery
      iii. As protective shield (e.g., entropion)
      iv. As bandage in corneal epithelial diseases
   j. Spectacle lenses
      i. As protection in hazardous situations
      ii. As protection for monocular patients
      iii. For ultraviolet protection (UV coatings)

B. PRACTICAL CONSIDERATIONS

1. Determine dosage, concentration, and duration of drug use by diagnosis and degree of presentation
2. Vehicles
   a. Use drops (solutions or suspensions) for ocular surface conditions
   b. Use ointments for superficial lid conditions and prolonged effect on ocular surface
   c. Creams and lotions provide increased skin penetration for allergic lid reactions
3. HCl versus acetate versus sulfate salts may affect penetration rates in varying disease states (clinically insignificant)
4. Buffering of ophthalmic solutions dictates initial comfort but not a major factor in drug use
5. Sterility required in ophthalmic drugs, but realities of use relate more to aseptic, contamination-free drug and container conditions
6. Drug instillation (for topical ophthalmic agents)
   a. Standard methods are fine but are usually a problem for patients, especially the elderly (Figs. 1–2 and 1–3)
   b. Reservoir technique useful for lids and mild ocular surface conditions
   c. One drop is better than two (reduces hyperlacrimation dilution)
   d. If you think you (or the patient) missed first drop, drop again (and again if necessary)
      i. You cannot overdose an eye very easily
      ii. Cul-de-sacs hold only 1 drop
   e. Topical anesthetic instilled first increases drug absorption
   f. Separate instillation of drops or ointments (same or different) by at least 1 minute
   g. Block puncta if drug has systemic implications[16]
   h. Ask pharmacist to help instruct patient

Instillation of Eyedrops: Patient Instruction Sheet

1. Wash your hands before and after using eye medications.
2. Tilt your head back and look up at the ceiling. You may want to lay down on your back if it is easier.
3. Place a finger on your cheek just under your lower eyelid and gently pull down until a "V" pocket is formed between your eyeball and your lower lid.
4. Put 1 to 2 drops into the eye. Do not let the dropper tip touch the eye or eyelashes. This may contaminate the medication.
5. Do not blink your eyes, simply close them very lightly and leave them closed for approximately one minute. Blinking and closing your eyes hard pushes the drop out of the eye and onto your cheek. We want the drop *in* the eye.
6. If you still have difficulty getting the drops into your eyes, tilt your head back and with your eyes closed, place 1 to 2 drops in the corner of your eye. With your head still tilted backward, open your eyes and look up at the ceiling. This will then allow the medication to get into the eye.

Figure 1–2.

7. Run topical antibiotics a minimum of 5 to 7 days
8. Always consider a nondrug approach if clinically reasonable

C. COMPLICATIONS AND ADVERSE REACTIONS

1. Hypersensitivity reactions (common and superficial)[16]
   a. Erythema or hyperemia
   b. Itching and irritation
   c. Treatment
      i. Eliminate source
      ii. Cold, decongestants, steroids (if severe)

Instillation of Eye Ointments: Patient Instruction Sheet

1. Wash your hands before and after using eye medications.
2. Tilt your head back and look up at the ceiling—you may want to lay down on your back if it is easier.
3. Place a finger on your cheek just under your lower eyelid and gently pull down until a V pocket is formed between your eyeball and your lower lid.
4. Place a small amount (about ¼ inch) in the V pocket: Do not let the tip of the tube touch the eye or eyelashes—this may contaminate the medication.

Figure 1–3.

2. Vasovagal (syncope) responses
   a. Pale, clammy, short blackout
   b. Blood pressure decreases rapidly
   c. Treatment
      i. Position head below the level of the heart (between the knees)
      ii. Ammonia (smelling) salts
3. Prolonged-use reactions
   a. Delayed hypersensitivities (type IV reactions)
   b. Reduced healing rate (steroids and topical anesthetics)
   c. Medicamentosa (any medicine, any time)
   d. Steroid responses (short and long term)
4. Cardiopulmonary reactions
   a. Hyperventilation
   b. Cardiac arrest
   c. Treatment: cardiopulmonary resuscitation (CPR)
5. Anaphylaxis
   a. Rare
   b. Treatment: Call for help immediately
6. Iatrogenic considerations (not you!)

III. Basic Guidelines

A. TEN SIMPLE PHILOSOPHIES FOR SAFE AND EFFICIENT PATIENT CARE

1. "F–I–D approach"
   a. Frequency–intensity–duration (of a condition)
   b. Consider each aspect in the history and your instructions to the patient
2. "Diagnose things by the company they keep!"
   a. A single clinical finding by itself means very little diagnostically
   b. A single clinical finding in the com-

pany of others becomes a differential clue

3. "If you hear hoofs and see stripes, think zebras!"
   a. Do not overlook the obvious
4. "It ain't rare if it's in your chair!"
5. "Pharmacists are not just 'counters and pourers'!"
   a. They are perhaps the most accessible, educated, and up-to-date resources available regarding drugs, pharmacology, and toxicology
   b. Available to health professionals and patients
   c. Grossly underused by all
6. "When you're a hammer, everything starts looking like the head of a nail!"
   a. An important consideration (especially to your patient) when referring or seeking consultation
   b. The nonsurgical primary eye care provider should counsel their patients carefully on all levels of care and their alternatives
7. "Never be the last to see an eye before it goes blind!"

   a. Sullin's referral law
   b. No explanation required
8. "The 'You can't win' theory!"
   a. You prescribe correctly, but they never do it! (Expect a high rate of noncompliance)
   b. You prescribe and they do it, but who's to say it helped? (Post hoc, ergo propter hoc: "after this, therefore because of this")
   c. You do not prescribe, and they get better anyway!
9. "If an undocumented clinical variable could occur, it will occur the first time you manage a condition (probably on a Friday afternoon!)"
   a. Murphy's Law: primary care corollary #13
   b. Do not panic or accuse yourself too quickly
10. "Crawl, walk, and then run!"
    a. Go from the simple to the complex
    b. Go from the early to the advanced
    c. Go from the chronic to the acute
    d. Go from the lids to the conjunctiva to the cornea

IV. Self-assessment Questions

1. The patient requiring short-term pupil dilation therapy with no cycloplegia is best treated with:
   a. Homatropine
   b. Scopolamine
   c. Tropicamide
   d. Phenylephrine
2. All of the following are aminoglycosides *except:*
   a. Erythromycin
   b. Gentamicin
   c. Tobramycin
   d. Neomycin
3. The topical agent of choice for corneal infection is:
   a. A penicillin
   b. A sulfacetamide
   c. An aminoglycoside
   d. Chloramphenicol
4. Erythromycin is a good alternative drug to each of the following *except:*
   a. Tetracycline
   b. Tobramycin

   c. Penicillin
   d. Cephalosporins
5. Developing bone depression and discoloration of teeth is a documented risk with:
   a. Bacitracin
   b. Tetracycline
   c. Erythromycin
   d. Cephalosporins
6. What antiviral agent is experiencing increasing numbers of resistant strains of herpes simplex?
   a. Zovirax
   b. Viroptic
   c. Vira-A
   d. Stoxil
7. The antiviral agent available only as an ointment is:
   a. Vidarabine
   b. 5-Idoxyuridine
   c. Acyclovir
   d. Trifluridine
8. Short-term adverse effects of topical ste-

roids may include any of the following *except:*
   a. Reduced mitotic healing
   b. Posterior subcapsular cataracts
   c. Increased intraocular pressure
   d. "Masking" effect
9. The actions of steroids include all of the following *except:*
   a. Anti-inflammatory action
   b. Resolution of primary disease process
   c. Inhibition of adverse tissue changes
   d. Reduction of scarring potential
10. Which steroid penetrates intact cornea best?
   a. Prednisolone
   b. Hydrocortisone
   c. Dexamethasone
   d. Fluorometholone
11. The contraindications for steroid use include all of the following *except:*
   a. Infection
   b. Herpes simplex epithelial keratitis
   c. Active ulcerative process
   d. Toxic, hypersensitivity reaction
12. Which of the following is a mast cell stabilizer?
   a. Naphozoline
   b. Phenylephrine
   c. Cromolyn sodium
   d. Pseudoephedrine
13. Mast cell stabilizers are clinically most effective at what level of presentation?
   a. All levels
   b. Acute symptoms
   c. Advanced physical signs
   d. Subacute or chronic presentations
14. Decongestants achieve their clinical effect through:
   a. Vasodilation
   b. Vasoconstriction
   c. Histamine inhibition
   d. Histamine release
15. A potential adverse effect from overuse of topical antihistamine and decongestants is:
   a. Infection
   b. Vasoconstrictive reaction
   c. "Rebound" vasodilation
   d. Ciliary spasms
16. Which of the following is *not* effective antiedema therapy?
   a. Heat
   b. Hypertonic saline
   c. High-water soft lenses
   d. Lubricants
17. Hypertonic saline agents are effective antiedema agents at which level of the cornea?
   a. All levels
   b. Epithelium
   c. Full-thickness stroma
   d. Endothelium
18. The best amount of eyedrops instilled at one time is:
   a. One drop
   b. Two drops
   c. Three drops
   d. "Squirt" technique
19. A minimum duration of antibiotic therapy should be no less than:
   a. 24 to 48 hours
   b. 5 to 7 days
   c. 2 to 4 weeks
   d. 1 month
20. The most common systemic-related reaction to topical ophthalmic medications is:
   a. Grand mal seizures
   b. Cardiac arrest
   c. Anaphylactic shock
   d. Vasovagal response (syncope)

For answers, refer to Appendix 6.

REFERENCES

1. John T, Saini JS, Rao GN, et al: Schematic documentation of cornea and anterior segment problems in clinical practice. Cornea 4:220, 1985–1986
2. Stram, BL: Generic drug substitution revisited. N Engl J Med 316:1456, 1987
3. Leopold IM: Update on antibiotic in ocular infections. Am J Ophthalmol 100:134, 1985
4. Mehta NJ, Webb RM, Kohel GB, et al: Clinical inefficiency of tobramycin and gentamicin sulfate in the treatment of ocular infections. Cornea 3:228, 1984–1985
5. Baldinger MD, Weiter JJ: Diffuse cutaneous hypersensitivity reaction after dexamethasone/polymyxin B/neomycin combination eyedrops. Ann Ophthalmol 18:95, 1986
6. Turgeon PW, Kowalski RP, Roat MI: Bacterial sensitivity to gentamicin and tobramycin. Association of Research in Vision and Ophthalmology 1:193, 1987 (abst)
7. Dougherty JM, McCulley JP: Comparative bacteriology of chronic blepharitis. Br J Ophthalmol 68:524, 1984
8. Perry MD, Golub LM: Systemic tetracyclines in the treatment of noninfected corneal ulcers: A case report and proposed new mechanism of action. Ann Ophthalmol 17:742, 1985

9. Grant DM: Acyclovir ("Zovirax") ophthalmic ointment: A review of clinical tolerance. Curr Eye Res 6:231, 1987
10. Nesburn AB, Willey DE, Trousdale MD: Effects of Acyclovir therapy during artificial reactivation of latent herpes simplex virus. Exp Biomed J 172:36, 1983
11. Allansmith MR, Ross RN: Ocular allergy and mast cell stabilizers. Surv Ophthalmol 30:229, 1986
12. Goen TM, Sieboldt K, Terry JE: Cromolyn sodium in ocular allergic diseases. J Am Optom Assoc 57:526, 1986
13. Abelson MB, Yamamoto GK, Allansmith MR: Effects of topically applied ocular decongestant and antihistamine. Am J Ophthalmol 90:254, 1980
14. Tseng SC, Maumenee AE, Stark WJ, et al: Topical retinoid treatment for various dry eye disorders. Ophthalmology 92:717, 1985
15. Zimmerman TJ, Koener KS, Kandarakis AJ, et al: Improving the therapeutic index of topically applied ocular drugs. Arch Ophthalmol 102:551, 1984
16. Wilson FM: Adverse external ocular effects of topical ophthalmic medications. Surv Ophthalmol 24:57, 1979

ANNOTATED REFERENCES

Bartlett JD, Jannus SD (ed): Clinical Ocular Pharmacology. Boston, Butterworths, 1984
Two major sections, one on pharmacology and one on clinical care. Section on pharmacology has some excellent chapters on fundamental concepts regarding categories of ocular drugs.

Boyd JR (ed): Drug Facts and Comparisons. Philadelphia, JB Lippincott, 1987
Comprehensive analysis and comparisons of all prescriptions and OTC drugs in all systemic, topical and ocular categories. Published annually and updated monthly.

Fraunfelder FT: Drug Induced Ocular Side Effects and Drug Interactions, ed 2. Philadelphia, Lea & Lebiger, 1982
Outline text of reported adverse reactions and interactions of ocular and systemic drugs. Details systemic manifestations from ocular drugs and ocular effects of systemic drugs and topically applied ocular medications.

Fraunfelder FT, Roy FH (ed): Current Ocular Therapy, Vol 2. Philadelphia, WB Saunders, 1985
Short descriptions of all major ocular diseases and brief summaries of standard therapeutic regimens, including drugs, dosages, and prognosis.

Physician's Desk Reference for Ophthalmology. Oradell, NJ, Medical Economics, 1987
Annual compilation of all ophthalmic drug (prescription and OTC) products. Includes package insert information on each drug. Front section on standard and ocular drug categories.

2

Diagnoses (by SOAP) of the Eyelids and Adnexa

Chapter Outline

I. Some Common Disorders*

A. BLEPHAROPTOSIS (DROOPING OF UPPER EYELID)

---

*In alphabetical order.

Subjective

- Most important consideration in history is to establish congenital versus acquired nature
- If congenital

   1. Confirm with photos (old straight-on portrait views)
   2. Check for familial tendencies
- If acquired
   1. Careful medical history
   2. Evaluate diurnal patterns (for myasthenia gravis)
   3. Check for associated neurological signs
   4. Medications?
   5. Check for mechanical causes (e.g., lid masses)
- Question closely regarding associated diplopia
- Cosmetic concern

Objective

- Varies from subtle difference between lid apertures, to noticeable drooping (unilateral or bilateral), to total unilateral or (less common) bilateral closure
- Congenital
   1. More frequent bilateral presentations
   2. Superior tarsal fold usually absent or poorly developed
   3. May show backward torticollis (head tilt)
   4. Brow wrinkling common
- Acquired
   1. Usually unilateral (with exceptions)
   2. Diurnal variations with drooping greater in PM
   3. Increases with stress factors (e.g., fatigue)

Assessment*

- Congenital versus acquired (most important)
- Most common possibilities if acquired
   1. Neurological or neuromuscular causes
   2. Multiple sclerosis
   3. Myasthenia gravis
   4. Graves' (thyroid) disease
   5. Syndromes
- Consider anatomical asymetry in ptosis with normal function
- Photograph, if possible and monitor aperture sizes

Plan

- For congenital
   1. Reassure
   2. Consider ptosis crutch
   3. Consider conservative cosmetic surgical approach
   4. If vision obscured in newborn, early surgical intervention becomes indicated to reduce risks of amblyopia ex anopsia
- For acquired
   1. Establish possible cause at first visit
   2. Refer ASAP to appropriate specialist

Follow-up

- Recheck congenital or anatomical cases annually
   1. Compare measurements to previous findings
   2. Recheck neurofunction, and other systems

---

*See also Appendix 2.

- Confirm care on referred acquired ptosis patients
- Provide or suggest genetic counseling in severe congenital cases

B. BLEPHAROSPASM (MYOKYMIA, CLONUS, ESSENTIAL BLEPHAROSPASM)

Subjective

- Unilateral or bilateral
- No pain involved
- Usually "twitching" sensation
- Less common: spastic forced closures (essential)[1]
- Intermittent or constant
- Onset and duration variable

Objective

- Most lid tics not observable
- Check blood pressure
- Palpate lids for masses
- Do glabella tap (reflex test) for Parkinson's
- Examine CV and CVII (cranial nerves V and VII)
- Check refractive error

Assessment*

- Rule out disease or foreign-body reactions
   1. Lids (e.g., trichiasis)
   2. Conjunctiva (e.g., foreign matter on tarsus)
   3. Cornea (e.g., keratitis)
- Rule out raised IOP
- Rule out possible neuromuscular diseases
   1. MS (Utoff and LaHermit signs)
   2. Myasthenia (lid-fatigue test or biceps test)
- Consider other common etiologies
   1. Emotional status (neurogenic or psychogenic conversion syndrome)
   2. Physical stress and habits
   3. Dietary patterns (when, where, how)
- Consider neurosis or psychosis

Plan

- Refer (if appropriate) for cause
- Reassure patient
- With children, instruct parents against negative reinforcement
- Counsel patients on possible causes
- Oral and topical antihistamines and decongestants suggested for relief (questionable: placebo?)
- Quinine reported helpful
- Biofeedback therapy used occasionally
- Botulism toxin used in severe (essential) cases[2]

Follow-up

- If no diagnosis, call or recheck in 2 to 4 weeks or PRN
- Also nice to call referred patients in 4 to 6 weeks
- Counseled patients should be rechecked in 4 to 6 weeks

C. BURNS

Subjective

- History of chemical splash, radiation or thermal burn
- Pain ranges from mild discomfort to severe

Objective

- First-degree burn (most common)
  1. Superficial chemicals, sunburn, and so forth
  2. Superficial dry erythema
  3. Mild to moderate edema
- Second-degree burn
  1. Thermal burns and so forth
  2. Blistering of skin
  3. Tissue "weeping"
- Third-degree burn
  1. Deeper tissue brown, white, or charred
  2. Extensive erythema and edema

Assessment

- Determine specific causative agent
- Nature of accident
- Duration of contact
- Degree of burn
- Check carefully for eyeball involvement

Plan

- Refer third-degree burns for secondary (specialist) or tertiary (hospital) care
- For first- and second-degree burns
  1. Mild tissue reactions may require only cleansing of surface with or without topical antibacterial ointment (q4h for 3- to 5-day minimum)
  2. Careful cleansing of area with cold, sterile sponging (e.g., gauze pads) using saline or Burrows solution
  3. Debride loose burned tissue
  4. Remove any foreign matter
  5. Open blister formations and let them drain
  6. Frequent cold compress applications
  7. Heavy ointment coverage of area
     a. Antibacterial agents (e.g., Polysporin)
     b. Also Butesin Picrate ointment as a mild anesthetic (optional)
  8. Loose gauze dressing over ointments
- Oral analgesic if necessary (e.g., aspirin)

Follow-up

- Dressing should be changed daily (in office or by patient) first 3 to 5 days, depending on degree of burn
- Upon scab formation, dressing can be discontinued and thinner layers of antibacterial ointments should be continued for 7 to 10 days

D. CHLOASMA (LARGE BROWN HYPERPIGMENTED AREAS)

Subjective

- Cosmetic concern
- Found mostly in pregnant females
- More pronounced in darker races

Objective

- Large brownish spots around lid and brow areas
- Irregular shapes and sizes
- Ill-defined fading borders
- Healthy-looking tissue surfaces

Assessment

- Rule out melanoma (irregular surfaces and changes in tissue characteristics)
- Differentials include nevi or raised lesions

Plan

- No therapy indicated
- Reassure patient
- Sometimes fades

E. COLOBOMA (NOTCH OR CLEFT ON EYELID MARGIN)

Subjective

- Congenital abnormality (nonhereditary)
- Unilateral (more common) or bilateral
- Greater in superior lid
- Patient may report dry eye symptoms
- Frequently detected during routine examination
- Occasionally large enough to produce cosmetic concern
- Associated notching may also occur in eyebrow

Objective

- Most often found in medial portion of superior lid
- Least frequent in lateral aspect of lower lid
- Other congenital deformities frequently associated
  1. Especially with lower lid involvement
  2. Usually cranial boney changes or dermoids
- Notches are usually small, triangular shaped, full thickness in lid margin
- Rounded edges and no lashes
- Occasionally, cleft may be large enough to cause corneal exposure and drying

Assessment

- Examine for associated findings or syndromes, such as dermoids, FLKs ("funny-looking kids")
- Check cornea for secondary effects

Plan

- Reassurance
- Patient education
- If cornea involved (i.e., exposure keratitis) lubricate
- In syndrome-related cases, suggest genetic counseling

Follow-up

- Necessary in complicated cases only
- Photodocument for long-term management

F. CONTUSION (BLUNT) INJURIES[3] (Color Plate 1)

Subjective

- History of blunt blow to orbital region
- Variable pain on palpation

Objective

- Variable degree of "pitting type" lid edema
- Ecchymosis ("black eye" or purplish-red blood color)
  1. Blood accumulation greater in lower lid
  2. Loose blood may seep across bridge of nose
  3. Blood occasionally forms organized hematoma (firm purplish–black palpable mass, usually lower lid)
- Bony orbital rim tenderness (general or focal)
- Conjunctival hemorrhages may be present as well

Assessment

- Rule out ocular injury
  1. Hyphema
  2. Iridodialysis
  3. Retinal detachment
  4. Anything
- Check inferior rectus for entrapment
- Examine with careful palpation for "crepitation" (emphysema or air in the tissue)
  1. Means sinus fracture
  2. May be blowout (orbital floor), but much more common is ethmoidal (medial wall) fracture
  3. Refer for radiological evaluation and diagnosis
- Palpate bony tissue for fractures
  1. Simple, comminuted, etc.
  2. Check associated numbness at nerve distributions

Plan*

- For uncomplicated edema secondary to contusion injury

---

*See also Appendix 4.

  1. Alternate hot and cold compresses
  2. Oral decongestants (e.g., Benadryl) if indicated
- For ecchymosis without crepitus or fractures
  1. Cold packs for first 24 hours (to reduce bleeding)
  2. Follow with hot packs for 3 to 5 days
  3. Oral decongestants if desired to reduce edema
- For ecchymosis with crepitus or fractures
  1. Cold packs for first 24 hours
  2. Hot packs for 5 to 7 days
  3. Oral antibiotic for 7 to 10 days (broad spectrum)
  4. Oral decongestant
  5. If substantial fracture or blowout entrapment, refer for ophthalmological consult

Follow-up

- For ecchymosis without crepitus
  1. Recheck in 3 to 5 days or PRN
- For ecchymosis with crepitus
  1. Recheck in 2 to 3 days (rule out cellulitis, and so forth)
  2. Return check (RTC) 7 to 10 days (rule out secondary complications)
  3. Recheck PRN

G. DERMATOCHALASIS (SUPERIOR EYELID OVERHANG)

Subjective

- Middle to older age groups
- Usually bilateral
- Familial tendency
- Often produces cosmetic concerns

Objective

- Draping of superior lid tissue over septum or lid margin
- Loose and redundant tissue fold
- May show puffiness due to fatty tissue herniation
- Produces pseudoptosis

Assessment

- Rule out causes of true blepharoptosis
- Rule out causes of secondary lid edema
- Similar condition (far less common), called blepharochalasis, in younger age ranges caused by edema or inflammatory swelling of unknown etiology

Plan

- Reassurance
- Blepharoplasty if indicated for functional vision (i.e., loss of superior field: uncommon) or cosmetic relief

H. ECTROPION (EYELID TURNS OUTWARD)

Subjective

- Chronic epiphora (typical "wet eye" presentation)
- May have no complaints

Objective

- Inferior lid margin or lacrimal puncta (punctal ectropion) not in contact with globe or lacrimal lake
- Epiphora
- Usually lid atonia due to aging

Assessment

- Rule out cicatricial (scarring) causes
- Rule out mechanical causes

Plan

- Nothing indicated for asymptomatic patients
- Surgical repair necessary for problem cases
- "Taping" methods both temporary and questionable

I. ENTROPION (EYELID TURNS INWARD) (Color Plate 2)

Subjective

- Corneal foreign body sensation
- Hyperlacrimation or lid spasms
- Infrequently congenital or a problem in children secondary to an epiblepharon (medial lid infolding)

Objective

- Inferior lid and lashes turn inward and rub against corneal surface
- Inferior irregular to vertically oriented foreign body tracking on cornea
- Commonly caused by spastic response upon forced closure of lids (spastic entropion)

Assessment

- Rule out simple trichiasis
- Rule out corneal foreign body
- Check for signs of other infectious and inflammatory lid disorders (e.g., chronic staphylococcal blepharitis)

Plan

- Surgical procedure usually indicated
- If surgery contraindicated or refused
  1. Complete epilation (lash removal) indicated
  2. Low water hydrophilic bandage lenses may help
  3. Ongoing lubrication therapy indicated for corneal protection and comfort
- Taping methods may offer temporary relief

Follow-up

- Manage secondary corneal complications closely

J. EPICANTHUS (INNER CANTHAL NASAL FOLDS)

Subjective

- Almost always bilateral
- Very common in oriental races
- Common in Caucasian infants
- Associated with flat bridges (e.g., Down's syndrome)
- Pseudostrabismic appearance (frequent peds referral)

Objective

- Folds start in upper medial lid and "dissolve" into lower lid (reversed in many syndromes)
- Folds vary in degree (e.g., width, prominence)
- Occasionally may be tight enough to push lashes inward and cause corneal irritation
  1. Especially in cases of dense lashes
  2. With epiblepharon (congenital infolding of lid)
- May present with blepharoptosis (congenital)
  1. Usually hereditary
  2. Greater in males

Assessment*

- Rule out congenital syndromes (check for stigmata)
- Rule out true strabismus
  1. Cover testing
  2. Hirshberg reflexes
  3. Motilities (EOMs)
  4. Pseudostrabismic "pinch test"

Plan

- Reassurance and patient (or caretaker) education
- Infrequently, cosmetic surgery (in adults only!)

Follow-up

- Recheck pseudostrabismus every 3 months for 12 months
- After 12 months, go to every 6 months

K. FOREIGN BODIES ON TARSUS

Subjective

- Contributory history of foreign matter (e.g., sand, fiberglass)
- Foreign-body (corneal) sensation

---

*See also Appendix 3.

Objective

- Corneal foreign-body tracking (FBT)
- Localization of embedded material (with slit lamp or loop)
  1. Single or double lid eversion necessary
  2. May be difficult to accomplish due to lid spasms secondary to corneal irritation

Assessment

- Fiberglass difficult to visualize
- Rule out primary corneal lesions (e.g., dendrite)
- Check corneal epithelium for foreign matter

Plan

- Remove foreign matter (with lid everted)
  1. Lavage (strong irrigation)
  2. Wetted cotton-tipped applicator
  3. Swab tissue with cotton tip (valuable in dislodging poorly visualized materials)
- Use instruments for removal if necessary
  1. Spuds ("golf club" type)
  2. Forceps (jeweler's type)
- Prophylactic antibiosis (optional) 1×

Follow-up

- PRN

L. INSECT BITES OR STINGS

Subjective

- Contributory history (e.g., mosquito, bee, small carnivore!)
- Itching
- Stinging sensation
- Occasionally throbbing pain
- Rarely (but very possibly) systemic reactions

Objective

- Pinpoint lesion (with stinger possibly embedded)
- Usually focal edema around site (may be diffuse)
  1. Erythema possible
  2. Bleeding possible

Assessment

- Rule out any severe allergic, asthmatic, or atopic history
- Do not worry about identifying (or catching) the culprit

Plan

- If stinger in situ, "flick" it out with fingers
  1. Do not use grasping instruments
  2. Do not pinch or grasp stinger with fingers; at risk of injecting additional toxin

- Cold packs
- Oral decongestant (e.g., Benadryl) if indicated
- Topical hydrocortisone (0.5 to 1 percent) ointments or creams if needed for subjective relief
- If severe systemic reaction developing or history of significant allergic tendencies, consult physician

Follow-up

- PRN

M. LACERATING INJURIES

Subjective

- Contributory history of lacerating injury

Objective

- Consider superficial dermis versus deeper fascia or muscle layer wound
- Parallel (along normal fold) versus vertically oriented wound (probable scar formation)
- Consider wound edges
  1. Straight edges falling together in apposition
  2. Jagged, gaping, irregular (probable scarring)
- Lid lacerations greater than 5 to 10 mm are potential risks

Assessment

- Rule out eyeball involvement
- Evaluate risks of scar formation (keloids)
  1. Depth
  2. Orientation (along folds versus vertical)
  3. Edges
  4. Length
  5. Keloid formation greater in black races
- Rule out damage to surrounding or underlying tissues and structures
  1. Lacrimal system
  2. Orbicularis muscle
  3. Lid margin

Plan

- Problem lacerations or secondary tissue damage should be referred for appropriate suturing and surgical care
- For simple lacerations
  1. Clean wound thoroughly (e.g., hydrogen peroxide, Zephiran HCl 1:750)
  2. Remove any foreign matter
  3. Antibacterial ointments (e.g., Polysporin)
  4. Standard dressing

Follow-up

- Redress wound in 3 days
- Remove dressing in about 1 week
- PRN

N. LAGOPHTHALMOS (INCOMPLETE EYELID CLOSURE)

Subjective

- Exposure keratitis symptoms (i.e., foreign body (FB) sensation)
- Chronic AM corneal irritation
- Dry eye syndrome

Objective

- Usually about 2- to 5-mm opening on normal lid closure
- Patient usually able to force complete closure
- Secondary corneal involvement
  1. Superficial punctate keratitis (SPK) in band region (exposed corneal area)
  2. Possible corneal anesthesia
  3. Epithelial erosion (greater in AM)

Assessment

- Rule out tear dysfunction
- Rule out epithelial basement membrane disorder
- Check for weak or absent Bell's phenomenon
- Lid cicatrix
- Assess closure with head tilted back (chin up)
- Measure lid separation on closure

Plan

- Lubricate cornea (daytime: drops; bedtime: ointments)
- Extended-wear soft lenses as bandage
- Tap lids shut for sleeping
- Consider tarsorrhaphy in cases in which corneal protection is inadequate

Follow-up

- Manage secondary corneal involvements closely (every 3 months)
- Reassess measurements intermittently

O. MADAROSIS (LOSS OF EYELASHES) (Color Plate 3)

Subjective

- Congenital (ocular alopecia) versus acquired
- Unilateral or bilateral
- Usually cosmetic concern

Objective

- Patchy loss or filamentation of lashes
- Occasionally complete loss
- Eyebrows generally not involved (only in congenital alopecia)

Assessment*

- Most frequent cause is *Staphylococcus*
  1. Toxic response
  2. May or may not see other signs of lid involvement
- Rule out systemic relationships (e.g., medications, hair loss elsewhere on body)
- Rule out trichotillomania

Plan †

- Antistaphylococcal lid therapy (every 6 to 12 weeks) (Table 2–1)
- Photodocument if possible
- Refer for medical evaluation if suspicious

Follow-up

- Recheck postantistaphylococcal therapy
- If onset less than 3 months, prognosis guarded to good
- If onset greater than 3 months, prognosis poor

P. POLIOSIS (WHITENING OF EYELASHES)

Subjective

- Congenital (ocular albinism) versus acquired
- May be unilateral or bilateral on upper or lower lids
- Cosmetic concern

Objective

- Patchy or complete whitening (loss of pigmentation) of eyelashes

Assessment

- Most frequent cause is *Staphylococcus*
  1. Toxic response
  2. May or may not see other signs of lid involvement
- Rule out vitiligo[4]

Plan †

- Antistaphylococcal lid therapy (every 6 to 12 weeks) (Table 2–1)
- Photodocument if possible

Follow-up

- Recheck postantistaphylococcal therapy
- If onset less than 3 months, prognosis guarded to good
- If onset greater than 3 months, prognosis poor

---

*See also Appendix 2.
†See also Appendix 4.

TABLE 2–1. STAPHYLOCOCCAL RISK-REDUCTION PROGRAM

Treatment steps	Dosage/Duration		
	Subclinical	Chronic	Acute
1. Skin/scalp hygiene	Daily/ongoing	Daily/ongoing	Daily/ongoing
2. Hot compresses	HS/2–4 wk	HS/3–6 wk	q4h/24–28
3. Lid massage	Optional	HS/3–6 wk	Not indicated
4. Lid scrubs	1–2 ×/wk/6 mo and RTC	HS/3 mo and RTC	HS/1–2 wk (after pain resolves)
5. Antistaphylococcal lid ointment	Optional	HS/2–4 wk (e.g., Bacitracin)	q4h/5–7 days (e.g., gentamicin)

tid = 3 × per day; q ___ h, every ___ hour(s); HS, at bedtime; RTC, return check.

Q. SUBCUTANEOUS CILIA (INGROWN EYELASH)

Subjective

- Occasional localized irritation of lid margin
- May produce corneal foreign-body sensation
- Occasionally cosmetic awareness of irregular lash

Objective

- Eyelash misdirected into epidermis of lid (Fig. 2–1)

- May enter lid tissue at one site and exit in close proximity or terminate within tissue
- Occasionally a foreign-body granuloma (small spongy vascularized tissue mass) may develop around ingrown lash
- Infrequently secondary infection or inflammation at site
- Frequently lash will irritate corneal surface

Assessment

- Common cause is chronic toxic *Staphylococcus*
- Rule out multiple sites
- Rule out cicatricial causes

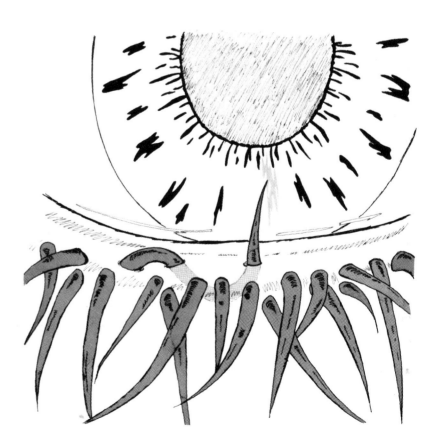

Figure 2–1.
Subcutaneous cilia

Plan*

- Cut loop of lash midway between hair follicle orifice and subcutaneous portion
- Remove distal portion of lash by "threading" it through epithelialized channel
  1. Use cilia or jeweler's forceps
  2. Pull firmly and steadily
- Epilate proximal lash portion from follicle
- Prophylax 1× with antibacterial ointment at site

Follow-up

- PRN

R. TRICHIASIS (INTURNING LASH OR LASHES) (Color Plate 4)

Subjective

- Congenital (e.g., epiblepharon) versus acquired
- Corneal foreign-body sensation
- Frequently hyperlacrimation and epiphora
- Normal lid position (not entropic)

Objective

- Inferior lid involved more frequently than superior
- Fine filamentary lashes or complete lash(es) turn inward and rub against inferior corneal surface
- Inferior vertical or irregular foreign-body tracking

Assessment

- Frequently caused by chronic staphylococcal reaction
- Rule out cicatricial causes
- Rule out districhiasis (rare): additional row of lashes posterior to the mucocutaneous lid margin

Plan*

- Epilation with cilia forceps (or tweezer)
  1. Re-emergence very possible
     a. 2 to 4 weeks in youth
     b. 4 to 8 weeks in adults
  2. Repeated epilations not dangerous
- Cauterization of follicle of limited value
- Electrolysis may work, but very uncomfortable
- Low water soft lens bandages of some value
- Treat any active or chronic marginal lid disorders
- Treat secondary corneal involvement with lubrication

Follow-up

- Patient can self-manage condition if handled steadily and properly instructed
- PRN or recurrence of corneal irritation

S. TRICHOTILLOMANIA (NEUROTIC TWISTING, TWIRLING OF HAIRS)

Subjective

- Usually perfectly normal-acting person
- May express stressful life conditions
- Generally unaware of any neurotic tendencies

Objective

- Unconscious habitual tendency to repeatedly twirl, twist or pull at a lock of hair
  1. Common in males and females with long hair
  2. Common in men (and some women!) with beards and mustaches
  3. Eyelashes and eyebrows potential sites
- Tendency produces ultimate loss of hair at site
  1. Potential causes of madarosis
  2. Can result in patchy eyebrows with resultant cosmetic concern

Assessment

- Rule out other causes of patchy hair loss
- Check for alternate sites (beyond lashes and brows)
- Confirm habit by asking patient about tendency

Plan

- Reassure regarding eyelid involvement
- Advise on tendency
- Suggest attempt to eliminate habit (not easy!)

T. VITILIGO (HYPOPIGMENTATION OR DEPIGMENTATION)[4]

Subjective

- Usually a bilateral presentation on lids (and any other body surfaces)
- Usually presents before age 20
- Frequent family history (greater than 50 percent of time)
- Slowly progressive with increasing age (depigmented areas enlarge)
- Condition totally asymptomatic

Objective

- Well-defined bilateral patches of depigmented skin
- Generally symmetric appearance
- Any overlying hair (including eyelashes and eyebrows) that also loses pigmentation
  1. Cause of secondary poliosis
- More prominent in dark races and blacks

*See also Appendix 4.

Assessment*

- Determine autosomal-dominant family history (greater than 50 percent of family carry trait)
- Rule out associated syndromes (e.g., Vogt–Kayanagi–Harada, albinism)
- Check for associated systemic causes
  1. Thyroid disease
  2. Anemias
  3. Pituitary disorders

Plan

- Education and reassurance
- Cosmetic camouflage (e.g., makeup)

*See also Appendix 3.

- Skin protection from sun
- Dermatologic referral if patient desires
  1. Certain oral preparations in combination with ultraviolet therapy yield some cosmetic benefits
  2. Some topical dermatologic agents have proved effective in certain cases
- Photodocument if possible

Follow-up

- Reassess ocular (eyelid) involvement annually
- PRN

II. Acute and Chronic Blepharitis (Color Plates 5, 6, and 7)

A. MARGINAL (BACTERIAL) FORMS

Background Information

1. Generally staphylococcal in origin (especially chronic forms)
   a. *Streptococcus* and gram-negative bacteria tend to produce hyperacute forms (e.g., heavy discharge, preseptal cellulitis)
2. Some general considerations about *Staphylococcus*
   a. Most common bacteria in and around the eyes
      i. On the lid margin 100 percent of the time (normal flora)
      ii. On the conjunctiva 75 percent of the time[5]
   b. Gram-positive noncapsulated spheroidal bacteria
   c. Most common strains associated with eye care
      i. *Staph. aureus* (hemolytic)
      ii. *Staph. epidermidis* (nonhemolytic)
   d. *Staphylococcus* produces 32 exotoxins that can affect the eye
      i. α-Toxin (dermonecrotic) significant irritant to ocular membranes
      ii. Produced by *Staph. aureus*
   e. Leading cause of marginal infiltrative keratitis
   f. Can cause central corneal ulceration, but slower proliferating and less in-

flammatory organism than *Streptococcus* (gram-positive) and the gram-negative bacteria
   g. Bacteriocidal (cell wall active) antibiotics (or higher concentration bacteriostatic agents) are most effective treatment drugs
      i. Bacteriocidals
         • Penicillins (oral use only)
         • Cephalosporins
         • Aminoglycosides
         • Bacitracin (topical ointments only)
      ii. Bacteriostatics (in high concentration)
         • Erythromycin (ophthalmic and oral forms)
         • Sulfonamides (15 percent concentration)
   h. About 65 percent of staphylococci are resistant to 10 percent sulfonamides[6]
   i. About 85 percent of staphylococci produce penicillinase or β-lactamase enzymes, which neutralize penicillin
      i. Penicillinase-resistant penicillins (or cephalosporins) should be used for *Staphylococcus*
         • Methicillin
         • Oxacillin
         • Dicloxacillin
         • Keflex (cephalosporin)
      ii. Rule out penicillin allergies before using any penicillins
         • About 10 to 12 percent cross-

sensitivity between penicillin and cephalosporins
  - Alternative oral agent (erythromycin)
3. Frequently combined seborrheic and staphylococcal origin in young adults
4. Most common form is nonpurulent (squamous) type
   a. Increased marginal hyperemia
   b. Marginal telangiectasia (red vascularized sites)
5. Squamous types may have significant nonbacterial immunological (hypersensitivity) etiologic component[7]
6. All types may be caused by noninfectious factors
   a. Makeup
   b. Pollutants
   c. Ametropias
   d. Soaps, preservatives
7. Synonyms
   a. Chronic marginal blepharitis
   b. Staphylococcal blepharitis
   c. Ulcerative blepharitis
   d. Seborrheic blepharitis

Subjective

For Acute Forms
- Moderate to severe pain (especially on palpation)
- Rapid onset, worsening over 24- to 48-hour period
- May be associated with prodromal history
  1. Trauma (often streptococcal or gram-negative)
  2. Systemic illness (e.g., sore throat, ear infection)

For Chronic Forms
- History of months to years duration
- No distinct symptoms
- Mild irritation
- Chronicity usually annoyance to patient
- Often reports of "eyes stuck shut on waking"
- May report family history of condition
- History of recurrent hordeolii or chalazia
- May show poor hygiene tendencies or problems with chronic dry dermatitis and dandruff (seborrhea)
- Cosmetic concern

Objective

For Acute Forms
- Usually unilateral: bilateral forms strongly suggest systemic cause
- Moderate to dramatic lid edema and erythema
- Generally entire lid margin (360°) affected
- Mild to moderate crustations
- Frequently associated with ocular surface involvement (e.g., conjunctivitis, keratitis)

- Frequently presents with (or leads to) preseptal cellulitis (Color Plate 7)
  1. Edema and erythema spread beyond orbital rims
  2. Pain (on palpation) spreads beyond orbital rims

For Chronic Forms
- Almost always bilateral
- Thickened, rounded, ill-defined, hypertrophic lid margins (tylosis)
- Moderate to abundant flat yellowish crustations around base of lashes (rosettes)
- Varying degrees of associated eyelash involvement
  1. Madarosis
  2. Poliosis
  3. Trichiasis
- Hordeolii or chalazia (or residual signs)
- Occasional shallow ulcerations at lid margins
- May produce superficial, cracking, and "weeping" eruptions (eczematoid) at skin fold sites
  1. Particularly at outer canthal lid fold

Assessment*

For Acute Forms
- Consider causative agent
  1. From clinical presentation (history and physical findings) if possible
  2. Culture if hyperacute or nonresponsive
- Rule out impetigo
  1. Staphylococcal or streptococcal infection
  2. Young adults or children with poor hygiene
  3. Usually warm-weather incidence
  4. Soft yellowish pustules
  5. Silvery or gold crustation forms over days to weeks
  6. Vesicle formations found on surrounding skin
  7. Requires broad-spectrum topical and oral agents
- Rule out other causes of blepharitis
  1. Viral
  2. Pediculosis
  3. Allergic
- Rule out preseptal (and orbital) cellulitis
- Rule out acute dacryocystitis
  1. Localized inferior nasal involvement
  2. Associated wet eye syndrome (epiphora)
- Rule out acne rosacea

For Chronic Forms
- Differentiate dry-seborrheic (squamous) type from pure infectious staph type (with heavy crustations) from combined presentations (common)
- Rule out meibomianitis
- Rule out demodicosis
- Rule out lingering acute or subacute forms
  1. Streptococcal and gram-negative bacteria

---

*See also Appendix 3.

    2. Impetigo
    3. Viral forms
    4. Pediculosis
- Rule out acne rosacea

Plan*[8]

- Antistaphylococcal (Table 2–1)

Follow-up

For Acute Forms
- Should be stable or improving in 48 to 72 hours
- Continue treatment for at least 5 to 7 days
- If condition is worsening
    1. Reconfirm diagnosis
    2. Check on patient compliance and reinstruct
    3. Re-evaluate for preseptal cellulitis development
    4. Consider adding broad-spectrum oral antibiotic
- Upon resolution, instruct on preventive measures

For Chronic Forms
- Improvement usually significant in 4 to 6 weeks
- Gradually reduce dosages to maintenance levels
- If no improvement
    1. Reconfirm diagnosis
    2. Check on patient compliance and reinstruct
    3. Continue treatment plan
    4. Discontinue ointments in squamous forms
- Advise patient on potential chronicity
- Reduce fatty foods in all seborrheic types
- Instruct on ongoing preventive and maintenance therapy

Prevention and Maintenance

- Refer to Figure 2–2.

B. MEIBOMIANITIS

Background Information

    1. Believed to be congestion of meibomian glands
    2. Buildup of meibum (fatty esters) in glands
    3. Frequently associated with seborrhea
    4. May have staphylococcal or immunological etiology[7]
        a. Probably combination of both

Subjective

- Nonspecific irritation (greater in morning)
- May report burning sensation
- Cosmetic concern

- Often associated with personal and family atopic (dermatological) history and seborrhea
- Commonly presents with ocular surface involvement and associated corneal symptoms (i.e., FB sensation)

Objective

- Usually bilateral
- Mild to moderate inflammatory appearance to posterior lid margin and palpebral conjunctiva
    1. Papillary blepharoconjunctivitis appearance
    2. "Velvety" soft hyperemic palpebral surface
- Congested orifices of multiple meibomian glands
    1. A line of whitish-yellow plugs along lid margin (milia)
    2. Usually greater on inferior lid margin
- Soft, edematous, rounded margins without crustations
- Frequent ocular surface involvements
    1. Almost always a blepharoconjunctivitis (greater inferiorly)
    2. Blepharokeratoconjunctivitis (inferior to diffuse)
    3. Tear film disturbances, including quick tear breakup time (BUT) and "froathy" tear meniscus

Assessment †

- Rule out marginal blepharitis types
- Rule out acne rosacea
- Often associated with chronic alcoholism

Plan

- Hot packs bid to qid
- Lid massage bid to qid[9]
- Oral tetracycline in unresponsive or severe cases
    1. Loading dose of 500 mg (1×) for acute cases
    2. 250 mg qid for 10 to 30 days
- Topical combination antibiotic and steroid suspension, tid
    1. Administer after lid massage
    2. Do not use ointments in meibomianitis
    3. Drop suspension on fingertip and apply to lid
    4. If ocular surface involved, drop 1 qtt on eye

Follow-up

- Should be stable or improving in 1 to 2 weeks
- Reduce medications slowly (2 to 4 weeks)
- If condition not responding to maximal therapy
    1. Reconfirm diagnosis
    2. Check for compliance and reinstruct patient
    3. Recheck history for alcoholism or acne rosacea
- Advise patient on potential chronicity

---

*See also Appendix 4.

†See also Appendix 3.

PREVENTIVE CARE OF THE EYELIDS

PATIENT INSTRUCTION SHEET

AFFIX PROFESSIONAL CARD
OR STAMP HERE

RECOMMENDED FOR: _____   DATE: _____

FOLLOWUP APPOINTMENT: DATE, _____   TIME, _____

STEP #	EXPLANATION/INSTRUCTION	INITIAL FREQUENCY	ONGOING SCHEDULE

1	General hygiene
	
	  a. Face cleaning (with soap and/or water)
	  b. Scalp cleaning (with anti-dandruff shampoo)
	  c. Lid cleaning (eyelids, eyebrows, etc.)		

2	Warm compresses
	
	  a. Heat washcloth under tap water for about 1 minute
	  b. Apply cloth to closed lids for about 1 to 2 minutes
	  c. Reheat, reapply and cycle for 5 to 10 minutes		

3	Lid massage
	
	  a. Place fingertip under margin (edge) of lower lid
	  b. Press fingertip firmly inward against eyelid
	  c. Replace fingertip at inner, middle and outer lid margins		

4	Lid scrubs
	
	  a. Wrap a washcloth around 1 or 2 fingers
	  b. Heat the cloth with tap water and add baby shampoo
	  c. Close lids and scrub lid margins (edges) with washcloth
	  d. Rinse lids with warm water		

5	Ointment application (Optional)
	
	  a. Squeeze 1/4 inch of ointment onto fingertip and discard it
	  b. Squeeze 1/2 inch of ointment onto fingertip and wipe it onto the closed lid margins
	  c. Dab extra ointment at the outer corner of the lid margins
	  d. Wait 3 to 5 minutes and gently wipe the closed lids dry		

These eyelid procedures are NOT A CURE for your condition. However, done
properly as recommended by your doctor, these simple procedures can help control
your problem and prevent more serious complications to your eyes.

Your next followup appointment (if indicated):
DATE: _____   TIME: _____

PRIMARY EYECARE INC.
EDUCATIONAL SERVICES

Copyright 1985, Primary Eyecare, Inc.
1414 Malcolm Drive, Dresher, PA 19025

Figure 2–2.
Patient instruction sheet

C. HERPES SIMPLEX VIRUS (Color Plate 9)

Background Information[10]

1. Most common virus in humans (only natural host)
2. Two forms of virus: herpes simplex virus type 1 (HSV-1) (oral) and herpes simplex virus type 2 (HSV-2) (genital)
3. Sources of HSV infection
   a. Primary infection
   b. Recurrent infection (after primary attack)
   c. Transmission from symptomatic or asymptomatic carrier
4. Transmission is through direct contact
   a. Mostly saliva and mouth contact
   b. Also contact with active skin lesions (vesicles)
   c. Incubation period approximately 1 week
5. Primary HSV attacks uncommon but dramatic
   a. Mostly in children and young adults
   b. Older age ranges protected by immunity
6. Greatest risk for primary infection from age 6 months to 5 to 10 years old (as immunity begins to develop)
   a. Approximately 70 percent of children infected by 5 years of age

b. Approximately 90 percent of these infections remain subclinical
c. Approximately 70 percent immune to HSV by 15 to 25 years of age
d. Approximately 90 percent immune to HSV by 60 years of age
7. Recurrence will occur in 25 percent of HSV infections
8. Aggravating or inciting factors for recurrence
   a. Sunlight (UV)
   b. Trauma (especially localized to ocular area)
   c. Extreme heat or cold
   d. Fever
   e. Steroids
   f. Infectious disease (systemic or ocular)
   g. Surgery
   h. Epilation

Subjective

- Mild to moderate discomfort (moderate to severe in primary attacks)
- Patient frequently reports history of recurrences or fever blisters at mucocutaneous border of lip
- Rule out genital HSV infection

Objective

- Usually unilateral but could spread across midline
- Lower lid involved more frequently than upper
- Diffuse patches of small, sometimes pinpoint size vesicles on a mild to moderately edematous (swollen) erythematous base
- Clear fluid vesicles change to yellowish pustules within a 3- to 5-day period
- Yellowish pustules harden into crusts over a 7- to 10-day period and shed without scar formation
- Occasionally vesicles or pustules may break down into shallow ulcers that heal within about 2 weeks
- Mild to moderate lymphadenopathy may be present (can be severe in primary infection)

Assessment*

- Differentiate primary from recurrent attack
- Rule out herpes zoster virus
- Rule out bacterial infection
- Rule out other eyelid dermatoses

Plan

- Treatment optional in mild cases (HSV blepharitis is a self-limiting condition)
- Acyclovir topical cream tid to q4h
  1. Other topical antivirals not effective on skin
  2. Add oral acyclovir in more severe presentations
- Prophylactic topical antibiotics optional

---

*See also Appendix 3.

- Supportive therapies
  1. Cold packs
  2. Domeboro packs
  3. Alcohol wipes
- Regarding ocular surface
  1. Not involved: do not treat
  2. Hyperemia without keratitis (SPK): optional
     a. Lubricants
     b. Prophylactic broad-spectrum antibiotic
  3. Keratitis (SPK): Viroptic tid to qid
  4. Dendrite(s): Viroptic q2h

Follow-up

- Recheck skin and ocular surface at 3- to 5-day intervals
- Consider medical or dermatological referral if lesions not remitting within 7 to 10 days
- Advise patient on recurrent nature of disease and ''triggering'' factors
- Recheck eyes and lids annually or PRN

D. HERPES ZOSTER VIRUS (Color Plate 93)

Background Information[11]

1. Varicella-type virus infecting dorsal root ganglion
   a. Virus called ''chickenpox'' in children
   b. Virus called ''shingles'' in adults
2. Usually affects first division of trigeminal nerve
3. When herpes zoster virus (HZV) affects the nasociliary branch[12]
   a. Vesicle at tip of nose (Hutchinson's sign)
   b. Approximately 75 percent risk of ocular involvement (ophthalmicus)
   c. Approximately 25 percent risk of ophthalmicus without Hutchinson's sign

Subjective

- Acute attack usually preceded by a tingling sensation in the scalp region on affected side
  1. Often noted early with hair combing or brushing
  2. Precedes observable clinical signs
- Prodromal itching and mild irritation around eye
- May report history of shingles elsewhere on body
- Upon clinical manifestation, pain becomes quite severe

Objective

- Always unilateral with lesions up to midline
- Diffuse inflammatory erythema spreads from forehead down to upper (and sometimes lower) lid

- Fluid-filled vesicles form first
  1. Follow nerve fiber linear patterns (dermatomes)
  2. Varying levels of surrounding edema
- Within 3 to 5 days, vesicles erupt into ulcerations
  1. HZV ulcers will produce permanent scarring
  2. Scars may produce ectropion, ptosis
  3. Certainly, scarring remains cosmetically apparent
- Lymphadenopathy may be present during acute phase
- Postherpetic neuralgia results in chronic ongoing pain of moderate to severe degree

Assessment*

- Rule out herpes simplex virus
- Rule out bacterial infection
- Rule out other eyelid dermatoses
- Rule out systemic neoplastic disease
  1. Often associated with HZV infections in adults
  2. Medical evaluation indicated in primary attacks
- Rule out eyeball involvement (common)

Plan

- Medical or dermatological consultation indicated
- Topical and oral steroids valuable
- Oral acyclovir valuable in first 3 to 5 days
- Vitamin B reported as helpful
- Supportive therapies
  1. Warm and cold packs
  2. Domeboro packs
  3. Alcohol wipes
  4. Non-narcotic and if necessary narcotic analgesics
- Topical prophylactic antibiotic ointments (and steroid combinations) often used in healing phase
- Regarding ocular involvement (common and variable)
  1. No involvement: do not treat
  2. Variable findings: treat accordingly

Follow-up

- Advise patient carefully
  1. Regarding postherpetic neuralgia
  2. Regarding permanent scarring
  3. Regarding ongoing ocular risks (highly variable)
  4. Recurrent attacks
- Recheck eyeball annually or PRN

E. ALLERGIC FORMS (Color Plate 10)

Background Information

1. Immediate (type I) allergic response associated with antigen–antibody reaction and histamine release by mast cells

*See also Appendix 3.

  a. Responsive to antihistamines and mast cell stabilizers [i.e., cromolyn sodium (Opticrom)]
  b. Most common clinical presentations
    i. Urticaria responses (erythematous patches)
    ii. Hay fever, atopic dermatitis
2. Delayed (type IV) allergic response associated with cell-mediated (lymphocyte) reactions
  a. Responsive to steroids
  b. Contact dermatitis, medicamentosa

Subjective

- Sudden (immediate-type) onset or slowly increasing (delayed type) signs and symptoms
- Personal or family history of allergies or asthma
- History of previous skin eruptions or dermatites
- Distinct symptom of "itching"
- Constant rubbing or desire to rub eye(s)
- History of allergen (usually difficult to ascertain)
  1. Contactants
    a. Plants
    b. Chemicals
    c. Cosmetics
    d. Soaps
    e. Sprays
  2. Ingestants
    a. Foods
    b. Drugs
- Possible systemic disease relationship
  1. Vascular (angioedema)
  2. Nephritic (kidney disease)

Objective

- Unilateral (contact) or bilateral (contact or endogenous-systemic) presentations
- Localized patches of edema and erythema (with frequent ocular surface involvement)
  1. Variable degrees from mild to dramatic
  2. Variable types
    a. Soft "pitting" edema
    b. Induration (thickening and hardened)
    c. "Brawny" edema (brownish tissue coloration)
- Erythema or eczematoid (dry, scaly) reactions
- Occasional cracking and "weeping" skin folds
  1. Called excoriation
  2. Beware of secondary infection
- Occasional vesicular or pustular formations

Assessment

- Determine offending allergen if possible
- Rule out systemic causes
- Rule out primary or secondary (toxic) infection
  1. Bacterial (especially staph and its exotoxins)
  2. Viral

Plan*

- Remove allergen (only actual cure)
- Frequent cold packs
- Domeboro packs (optional)
- Oral antihistamines and decongestants (e.g., Benadryl)
- If patient has specific prescription for other allergic reactions suffered, institute its use
- Topical astringent or anti-inflammatory creams
  1. Zinc preparations
  2. Hydrocortisone (0.5 to 1 percent) qid for 3 to 7 days
  3. Stronger steroids in severe reactions
  4. Base topical dosages on degree of presentation
- In very severe conditions, a short course of oral steroids may be indicated (co-manage with physician)

Follow-up

- Based on degree of initial presentation
  1. Mild: recheck in 3 to 5 days or PRN
  2. Moderate: recheck in 2 to 3 days
  3. Severe: recheck in 24 to 48 hours
- Check IOP with any steroid use
- Adjust treatment regimen, dosage, duration based on returning signs and symptoms
- If condition is not responsive or worsens in 3 to 5 days, consult patient's primary physician or allergist
- If allergen not determined, advise as to recurrent risk

F. DEMODICOSIS

Background Information[13]

1. Demodex folliculorum (causative organism) is a mite found almost universally in adults over age 50
2. Mite lives in hair follicles and sebaceous glands
   a. Most abundant in hair follicles on tip of nose and eyelid margins
3. Usually subclinical but if excessive in amount can produce toxic or hypersensitive marginal-type reaction

Subjective

- Often, patient is symptom free (in for routine care)
- Older patients frequently report the "itchy-burnies"

Objective

- Bilateral, indurated (thickened by chronic edema and inflammation) lid margins
- Inflammation ranges from subclinical to moderate

- Collarettes attach around base of each lash
  1. Vary in degree from thin rings to full length of cilia
  2. Differ from staphylococcal rosettes (flat crusts at base of lash) in length of lash involvement
- Hair follicle assume raised pyramid shape with lash emanating from apex of pyramid
- Can be observed in advanced cases by epilation and microscope (oil emersion slide) examination[14]

Assessment

- Rule out other marginal blepharitis (especially staphylococcal)
- Rule out pediculosis

Plan

- Light lid scrubs hs for 10 days
- Warm packs hs for 10 days
- One percent meruric oxide ointment hs for 10 days
  1. Plain Vaseline can be used if mercuric oxide contraindicated
  2. Avoid Eserine ointment (as some recommend) due adverse secondary prolonged miosis and ciliary spasms
- Vigorous cleansing of lid margins in morning during 10 days of treatment and ongoing, tid

Follow-up

- Recheck after 10-day treatment plan
- If no improvement
  1. Recheck diagnosis
  2. Confirm compliance and reinstruct
  3. Reinstitute treatment plan for additional 10-day period
- Advise patient on chronicity
- Ongoing light lid scrubs weekly
- Recheck lids in 6 months or PRN

G. PEDICULOSIS

Background Information

1. Infrequent (fortunately!) infestation of eyelid margins by body lice (*Pediculus corporis*), head lice (*Pediculus capitis*), or pubic lice (*Phthirus pubis*)
2. Transmitted by contact with carrier, heavy scalp infestation, contaminated garments, bedsheets or by sexual contact
3. Most common in children and young adults

Subjective

- Usually a subacute presentation with symptoms of mild to moderate itching and irritation of eyelids (usually bilateral)
- History may include exposure to known carrier(s) (as in a classroom situation)

---

*See also Appendix 4.

Objective

- Gross observation of lids reveals crusty marginal appearance, sometimes with brownish discoloration
- Slit lamp examination reveals nits (eggs) and actual organisms adherent to lashes and skin of lid
- In more severe infestation, shallow ulcerations may develop, as well as secondary keratoconjunctivitis

Assessment

- Rule out other forms of marginal blepharitis
- Attempt to determine source of infestation

Plan

- Coordinate appropriate management of source of infestation
- Remove (as best as possible) nits and lice from lid
  1. Toothed or jeweler's forceps work well

  2. Careful debridement with alcohol-saturated cotton-tip applicator may be effective
- Numerous agents are recommended for treatment at a bid to tid frequency for approximately 5 to 7 days. However, some must be used very carefully on the lid margins due to potential irritative (toxic) effects of pediculocides to the ocular surface
  1. One percent mercuric oxide ointment
  2. Eserine ointment (not recommended due to miosis)
  3. Plain petroleum jelly or any bland ointment base
  4. Pyrethrin ointments (pediculocide)
  5. Kwell shampoo (pediculocide)
  6. RID shampoo (pediculocide)
- If nits persist after 1-week treatment
  1. Recheck diagnosis
  2. Confirm compliance and reinstruct
  3. Retreat for additional week
  4. Consider reinfestation from untreated primary source

III. Some Common "Lumps and Bumps"*

A. BASAL CELL CARCINOMA (Color Plates 11 and 12)

Subjective

- Most common malignant tumor (neoplasia) of eyelid[15]
- History of slow developing, nonresolving lesion
- Usually a positive history of extensive UV exposure to sunlight
- Increasing frequency in older patients
- More frequent in fair-complected patients
- Often, previous history of skin cancer
- Frequently present as multiple sites[16]

Objective

- More prevalent on the lower lid
- Very early forms look like vascularized nodules, with loss of surrounding skin texture
- Varying degrees of central umbilicated ulceration
- Borders tend to be "pearly" or hardened (to both appearance and palpation) and slightly raised
- Variable amounts of pigmentation noted centrally
  1. May be absent in early lesions
  2. More prominent in darker races and patients
- Transillumination (with slit-lamp or bright light source) of involved skin surface may reveal a dark periphery and brighter central zone to lesion
- Occasionally, surface of lesions may become either secondarily infected or inflamed, or both

  1. Overlying purulent discharge and crustation
  2. Surrounding erythema or ulceration

Assessment[†]

- Metastasis almost nonexistent in basal cell
- Inner canthal lesions require more rapid attention due to potential deeper tissue extention
- If lesion secondarily infected or inflamed, run short (1- to 2-week) course of antibiotic–steroid combination
  1. Resolution of lesion indicates no cancer
  2. No response to treatment suggests possible neoplasia
- Most appropriate differential diagnostic test for highly suspicious clinical lesions is tissue biopsy[17]
- Basal cell is a slow-growing neoplasia and need not be considered a STAT referral
  1. Referral within weeks to months is adequate
  2. Highly questionable lesions may be monitored

Plan

- Advise patient of possible nature of lesion, but reassure as to the low-risk nature of this type of cancerous lesion
- Refer for biopsy and pathological diagnosis
- Surgical excision and repair (i.e., skin grafting if indicated) is standard treatment
- Photodocument if possible

---

*In alphabetical order.

†See also Appendix 2.

Follow-up

- If surgical referral deferred for any reason (e.g., patient reluctance, fear)
  1. Document and record reasons carefully
  2. Monitor lesion closely (every 3 months)
  3. Recommend biopsy and excision at each visit
- After surgery, recheck patient annually or PRN

B. CHALAZION (GRANULOMA OF MEIBOMIAN OR ZEISS GLAND) (Color Plate 13)

Subjective

- Very common lid lump
- External chalazion is granuloma of Zeiss gland
- Internal chalazion is granuloma of meibomian gland
- Acute chalazion is a synonym for hordeolum
- Frequently associated with chronic blepharitis
- Painless unless inflamed (acute chalazion)
- May remain stationary in size or progress (slowly)
- Occasionally present after hordeolum (secondary chalazion)

Objective

- Hard, firm, round or elongated mass inside lid
- External form (Zeiss) extend or evulse outward (frequently located at lid margin)
- Internal form (meibomian) remain internalized or point inward toward palpebral conjunctiva
- Both types can become superficially infected or inflamed

Assessment*

- Rule out neoplastic lumps and bumps
- Rule out systemic possibilities in chronic recurring chalazia (i.e., granulomatous diseases)
- Rule out lid infectious causes
- Rule out acute rosacea in recurrent forms

Plan

- If chalazion measures less than 8 to 10 mm
  1. Hot compresses as frequently as possible
  2. No less than qid for additive effect
- Do not massage mass
- If chalazion greater than 8 to 10 mm, surgical excision indicated
- Direct steroidal injections occasionally used[18]
- Treat any superficial infections or inflammations before surgical excision

Follow-up

- If heat therapy employed, recheck in 2 weeks
  1. If reducing, continue to resolution

---

*See also Appendix 3.

2. If no improvement (and patient compliant), consider additional 2 weeks or surgery
- Advise patient on possible recurrences and instruct on weekly lid palpations for early detection

C. DERMOID (BENIGN, DEVELOPMENTAL OUTPOCKETINGS OF TISSUE)

Subjective

- Usually noted at birth or in early years
- Found at numerous sites on body
- More common in syndromes (e.g., Hallerman–Streif)
- Most common ocular sites are superior temporal brow region and outer canthus, usually under lid angle
- Multiple embryological and histological origins
- May change in size through life
  1. Changes frequently produce first awareness (and resulting concern) in later years
  2. Cosmetic concern
- Always painless

Objective

- Solid, firm collagenous-like surfaces
- Smooth surface masses with overlying skin sliding easily over buried surfaces
- Exposed surfaces may contain hair follicles, fatty tissue, sebaceous glands
- Mass usually stationary or slightly movable

Assessment

- Differentiate from very movable subcutaneous sebaceous cyst
- Rule out neoplastic potential
- Check for syndromes (associated stigmata)

Plan

- Reassurance and patient education
- Refer for cosmetic removal if patient desires
- Measure and diagram dermoids reported as changing

Follow-up

- Recheck changing size potential every 6 months
- General recheck annually or PRN

D. HEMANGIOMA (BENIGN VASCULAR TUMOR)

Subjective

- Present congenitally or shortly after birth
- May enlarge during first 6 months, followed by regression
- Sometimes associated with other congenital abnormalities or syndromes

- Painless
- Cosmetic concern

Objective

- Vascular anomalies (tumors) of superficial blood vessels causing flat or slightly elevated, circumscribed, colored lesions on skin surface
- Varying types
  1. Capillary (strawberry) hemangioma is flat, superficial, and rapidly growing during infancy with usual (but unpredictable) regression by adolescence
  2. Cavernous type is a raised deeper mass
  3. "Spider" angioma (vascular spiders) are non-congenital types that occur during pregnancy, and in other conditions, generally resolving spontaneously
  4. Port-wine stains (nevus flammeus) are deep purple-red skin discolorations (common in Sturge–Weber syndrome; a phakomatotic disease (Color Plate 96)
  5. Racemose aneurysm is a grapelike vessel cluster
  6. Mixed forms
- Superficial capillary type most common
- Colors vary from faint pink, purple, blue to red
- Straining and crying can cause dramatic changes in size, elevation, and coloration of lesions
- Variable sizes from pinpoint to entire lid (e.g., port-wine stain in Sturge–Weber syndrome)
  1. When superior lid involved in port-wine stain, glaucoma risk substantially increased
- Superficial lesions may blanch on pressure (good differential for nevus or melanoma)

Assessment

- Examine the patient carefully for other congenital anomalies
  1. Colobomas
  2. Syndrome stigmata
  3. Choriodal hemangioma
- Determine type of hemangioma and prognosis
- Rule out pigmented lesions
  1. Benign or malignant
  2. Nevus or melanoma

Plan

- If other congenital abnormalities or signs of any syndromes noted, refer for pediatric or medical workup
- Reassure, educate, and advise patient (or caretaker) as to prognosis
- Some laser therapies are used for hemangiomas but should be discouraged during early stages
- Photodocument and measure

Follow-up

- Recheck children annually and compare photos and measurements

- When likelihood of spontaneous regression unlikely (adolescence or beyond), advise regarding cosmetic options

E. HORDEOLUM (STAPHYLOCOCCAL INFECTION OF ZEISS, MOLL, OR MEIBOMIAN) (Color Plates 15, 16, and 17)

Subjective

- Synonym: acute chalazion
- Staphylococcal infection to single of multiple glands
  1. External type involves Zeiss or Moll glands
  2. Internal type involves meibomian gland(s)
- Acute presentation, usually within 24 to 48 hours
- Moderate to dramatic generalized lid tenderness with distinct tenderness on focal palpation of affected gland
- Frequently associated with chronic blepharitis

Objective

- External type (often called "stye") most common
  1. Presents at lid margin
  2. External suppuration (exudate points outward)
  3. May suppurate through gland orifice or break through skin surface
  4. Mild to moderate edema and erythematous ring limited to immediate surrounding area
- Internal type less common but more frequently seen in the office setting due to increased pain and clinical signs
  1. Deeper response (internal lid tissue)
  2. Sometimes lump may point inward toward palpebral conjunctiva or out meibomian orifice
  3. Lid edema and erythema is moderate to severe, often diffusing throughout the involved (upper or lower) lid, sometimes burying the localized swollen gland
- Occasionally, a virulent organism (with or without treatment) may progress, enlarge and encapsulate into a lid abscess

Assessment*

- Carefully palpate edematous and erythematous lids for area of focal tenderness
- Rule out other causes of painful lid edema
  1. Acute blepharitis (diffuse)
  2. Acute dacryocystitis (inferior nasal tenderness with secondary hyperlacrimation)
- Beware of secondary preseptal cellulitis
  1. Common complication with internal hordeolum
  2. May be present on first visit or within 48 hours after initiating topical therapies
  3. Cellulitis will not respond to topical therapy
- Differentiate clinical degree to determine appropriate therapeutic approach

---

*See also Appendix 3.

1. External type (therapeutics optional)
2. Internal without preseptal cellulitis (topicals)
3. Internal with preseptal cellulitis (topicals and orals)
4. Lid abscess (surgical drainage plus orals)

Plan*

- For external hordeolum
  1. Hot packs qid
  2. Topical bacitracin ointment (e.g., Polysporin) bid to qid (optional)
- For internal hordeolum:
  1. Hot packs qid
  2. Topical gentamicin ointment qid
  3. With preseptal cellulitis, add oral agents 250 mg qid
     a. Penicillinase-resistant penicillin
     b. Cephalosporin (e.g., Keflex)
     c. Erythromycin
- For lid abscess (encapsulated infection)
  1. Surgical incision and drainage
  2. Oral antistaphylococcal drug
- Significant pointing or suppuration of external or internal type may be optionally drained by superficial needling and gentle milking of gland (it will be painful)

Follow-up

- Recheck all internal hordeolii within 48 to 72 hours
  1. If stable or improving, continue treatment for 5 to 7 days (minimum) and recheck
  2. If worsening, consider preseptal cellulitis or abscess and adjust treatment accordingly
- Upon resolution, instruct patient on ongoing staph preventive–maintenance program

F. KERATOSES (HYPERKERATINIZED PLAQUES IN ELDERLY)

Subjective

- Most common in adults beyond age 40 to 50
- Distribution over entire body with increased prevalence to exposed skin areas (i.e., face)
- Changes are slow and insidious
- Some forms regarded as precancerous (nonmetastatic)

Objective

- Flat or slightly elevated
- Dry scaly lesions on atrophic patch of skin
- Usually has a light gray-brown coloration
- Well circumscribed lesions with distinct borders
- Appears as plaque "floating" on skin surface

---

*See also Appendix 4.

Assessment

- Rule out neoplastic changes
- Rule out keratoacanthoma (rapid-growing, large mass)
- Rule out melanomas, nevi, verrucae, papilloma
- Increased suspicion in younger age ranges

Plan

- In early stages, greasy ointment base coverage may abort or arrest advancement
- Chronic erosion of edges, recurrent infection, or inflammation should be biopsied
- Excision for cosmetic reasons or suspicion best accomplished by dermatologist
- Photodocument if possible

Follow-up

- Ongoing management should include periodic monitoring of any changes
  1. Size, shape, pigmentation
  2. Surface quality and edge erosion
- Recheck large, prominent lesions every 6 to 12 months

G. MOLLUSCUM CONTAGIOSUM (VIRAL WART)

Subjective

- All age groups but most frequent in children
- Occasionally presents as mildly irritating lump on eyelid
- When on lid margin, may cause transient ocular surface irritation (keratoconjunctivitis) of viral etiology
- May be mildly contagious with autoinoculation most common
- Occasional cosmetic concern

Objective

- Small (3- to 6-mm) umbilicated nodule(s) with yellow "cheesy" material (or dry when inactive) central core
- May be multiple on lid and elsewhere on body
- Activity (central discharge) remits and exacerbates spontaneously
- Occasionally lesion may enlarge dramatically but will always resolve without scarring

Assessment

- Rule out basal cell carcinoma
- Differentiate other lumps and bumps

Plan

- When lesion quiet (dry central core), leave alone
- When center discharging cheesy or waxy material
  1. Clean surface with alcohol wipe

2. Loosen central core material with sharp curetting instrument (e.g., spud, needle)

3. Squeeze out contents with fingers or cotton swabs (appositional pressure)

4. Reclean surface with alcohol wipes

Follow-up

- Recheck in 1 week or PRN
- Same lesion may require multiple treatments (three to five) with eventual resolution

H. NEOPLASTIC CONSIDERATIONS (BEYOND BASAL CELL)

Subjective

- Lesion does not act or respond as anticipated
- Lesion is not common for patient's age, sex, race, demography
- History of other skin lesions elsewhere on the body
- History of other neoplasias or systemic disease
- Older patients
- Patients with history of excessive UV skin exposure
- Family history of skin cancers
- Fair-complected patients
- Pain and or irritation associated with suspicious lesion
- Acute versus chronic onset and duration
- Rapid or irregular growth patterns

Objective

- Quality of the tissue looks irregular
- Surface integrity and quality questionable
- Changes in lesion not consistent or predictable
- Neovascular patterns around or within lesion
- Recurrent infections or inflammations at site
- Bleeding or ulceration of lesion
- Uncharacteristically large lumps or bumps
- Associated tearing or conjunctival hyperemia
- Erosion of the margins or surface of a lesion

Assessment (Malignant Lesions of the Eyelid and Adnexa)

- Carcinomas
  1. Basal cell epithelioma (most common)
  2. Squamous cell[19]
  3. Intraepithelial (Bowen's disease)
  4. Adenocarcinoma of the meibomian glands
- Sarcomas
  1. Lymphosarcoma
  2. Reticulum cell
  3. Giant follicular lymphoma
  4. Burkitt lymphoma
  5. Hodgkin's disease
  6. Kaposi's sarcoma, frequently found in acquired immune deficiency syndrome (AIDS)

- Nervous tissue tumors
  1. Neurofibromatosis
  2. Mucousal neuroma
  3. Neurilemoma
  4. Schwannoma of Abrikossoff
  5. Ganglioneuroma
- Pigmented tumors: malignant melanoma
- Metastatic tumors (secondary to primary tumor)[20]

Plan

- With serious doubt or suspicion regarding any lump or bump of the lid, recommend excision and biopsy[21]
- If referral deferred or refused for any reason, document rationale thoroughly and monitor closely
  1. Photodocument if possible
  2. Diagram and measure accurately

Follow-up

- Recheck suspicious lesions frequently (every 3 months)
- Photodocument all changes and progressions and remeasure and diagram at each visit
- Continue to advocate for referral and biopsy

I. NEVUS (PIGMENTED SPOT)

Subjective

- Usually congenital or early onset
- Occasionally changes in size or pigmentation
  1. Hormonally related
  2. Pregnancy, puberty
- May be history of other nevi on body
- Cosmetic concern

Objective

- Three types
  1. Dermal
    a. Most common
    b. Deep form
    c. May be raised or flat
    d. Hardly ever becomes malignant
  2. Junctional
    a. Superficial form
    b. Usually flat
    c. May convert to melanoma
  3. Transitional: mixed dermal and junctional form
- Pigmented (usually brownish) or amelanotic (white or clear) spots on skin surface
- Commonly found at lid margins
- Well-defined borders
- Usually less than 8- to 10-mm diameter
- May increase in size with aging (beware of malignant changes, especially in junctional forms)
- May also decrease in size or degree of pigment (usually associated with hormonal changes)
- Occasionally show hairs growing through surface

Assessment*

- Rule out other pigment spots
  1. Benign types
  2. Malignant types
- Determine type of nevus
- Examine old photographs if available

Plan

- On first presentation, document development of spot and any changes
- Photodocument if possible, or diagram and measure
- Reassure and advise on reporting any changes

Follow-up

- Monitor every 3 to 6 months if any suspicions
- Recheck annually if normal appearing without change
- Compare photographs, diagrams, and measurements each visit
- If significant changes occur (especially in higher risk types or suspicious lesions), refer for biopsy

J. PAPILLOMA (BENIGN EPITHELIAL TUMOR)

Subjective

- Greater in older patients
- No symptoms
- Rarely secondarily irritated by infection or inflammation
- Cosmetic concern

Objective

- Epithelial overgrowths (benign tumors)
- Size and shape vary considerably
- Pigmentation ranges from amelanotic to black
- May present singularly or in abundant multiples
- Can be located anywhere but frequently found at mucocutaneous border of the eyelid
- Mass is avascular
- Surface is usually roughened but not eroded
  1. Roughened "granulated" surface is reflection of redundant epithelial cell growth
  2. Quite different surface texture from normal, surrounding skin
- Little change in growth pattern once developed
- May outgrow underlying blood supply (with increased size, aging) and necrose (blacken and harden)

Assessment*

- Rule out
  1. Nevus (usually congenital)

---

*See also Appendix 3.

  2. Senile keratoses (usually "floating" plaque effect)
  3. Subcutaneous sebaceous cyst (normal overlying skin texture)
  4. Verrucae (umbilicated surface)
  5. Neoplasia
- Consider any history of changes in mass

Plan

- Reassurance and patient education
- Treat any secondary infection or inflammation with standard topical anti-infective or combination drugs
- If patient desires removal for cosmetic reasons:
  1. Grasp with toothed forcep and extend outward
  2. If width of base less than 1 to 2 mm, snip off with sharp (iris-type) scissor
  3. Small bleed controlled by direct pressure
  4. If base greater than 2 mm, refer for excision
- If lesion appears highly suspicious, refer to dermatologist for excision and biopsy

Follow-up

- If lesion is new or recently reported, photodocument and recheck in 3 to 6 months
- For longstanding lesions, recheck annually
- Any significant changes in mass (any mass) should be referred for excision and biopsy

K. SEBACEOUS CYST (FATTY FIBROUS CYST OF SEBACEOUS GLAND) (Color Plates 20 and 21)

Subjective

- No symptoms
- History may include recent onset or longstanding
- Two types
  1. Superficial type: very common
  2. Subcutaneous (deep) type: common
- Cosmetic concern

Objective

For Superficial Type
- Range in size from 0.5 to 1 mm, up to 8 to 10 mm (normal range about 2 to 5 mm)
- Caseous ("cheesy"), yellowish material in recently developed cysts (less than 3 to 6 months)
  1. Covered by thin flattened epithelial cell layer
  2. Occasionally, pigmented particles or dirt may be trapped inside cyst (inclusion)
- In older cysts, material becomes fibrotic with a paler yellow-white coloration
- May appear as single cysts or in multiples
- Common around lids, especially at inner and outer canthal regions

For Subcutaneous (Deep) Type
- Location could be anywhere on body, especially the axillary regions (e.g., armpits, groin)

- Slightly movable lump of variable size with normal skin (texture) overlying (skin slides minimally over lump with palpation and "pinching" procedure)
- Extensive range of sizes from 1 to 20 mm or greater
- Sometimes overlying skin may show prominent blood vessels, telangectasia or venous congestion (blue-red or purplish hue)

Assessment*

For Superficial Type
- Rule out sudoriferous cyst (clear versus caseous filled)
- Rule out pustules or infectious vesicles (e.g., herpetic, bacterial)
  1. Usually associated erythema and symptoms
  2. Sebaceous cysts are rarely symptomatic or "hot"

For Subcutaneous (Deep) Type
- Rule out papilloma (granulated surface)
- Rule out dermoid (congenital)
- Neoplasia

Plan

For Superficial Type
- Reassurance and patient education
- If detected as part of routine examination (common) and patient not concerned, do nothing
- If patient desires removal (for cosmetic purposes):
  1. Consider duration of cyst (from history)
     a. Less than 3 to 6 months, cysts usually soft and easy to drain
     b. Older cysts more fibrous and require considerable forceps manipulation
     c. Do the easier ones initially
  2. Clean surface (e.g., alcohol, Zephiran) and apply topical anesthetic (on cotton tip) for about 1 minute
  3. Incise epithelial surface (over cyst) with bevel of hypodermic needle or tip of jeweler's forceps
  4. Massage out contents of cyst by opposing two cotton-tip applicators or arms of forcep at base of gland until tinge of blood appears
  5. In older cyst, grasp and pull out fibrotic strands with jeweler's forceps
  6. Prophylax surface of drained cyst with topical antibiotic ointment (e.g., Polysporin) 1×
- Instruct patient on immediate and long-term hygiene

For Subcutaneous (Deep) Type
- Reassurance and patient education
- If patient desires cosmetic removal, refer for surgical excision
- If patient reports abundant axillary sebaceous cysts developing in conjunction with lid cyst(s),

consider medical evaluation for possible systemic cause

Follow-up
- For drained superficial type, recheck 1 week or PRN
- If cyst reoccurs (rarely), redrain and observe
- Advise patient to report any changes in status or characteristics of cyst(s)

L. SUDORIFEROUS CYST (SEROUS OR FLUID CYST OF GLAND OF MOLL) (Color Plate 22)

Subjective
- No symptoms
- Usually noted during routine external eye exam
- Occasionally cosmetic concern (if cyst observable)

Objective
- Single or multiple cyst(s) on superior or inferior lid margin
- May be fluid or sebum filled (clear or cloudy)
- Usually small (2 to 4 mm) and round

Assessment*
- Rule out amelanotic papilloma (solid versus cystic)
- Rule out milia of meibomianitis (inflamed lid)

Plan†
- Reassurance and patient education
- If patient desires removal:
  1. Lance with 18- to 25-gauge hypodermic needle
  2. Always direct lancing away from globe
  3. Prophylactic antibiotic (1 ×) optional
- Advise patient on lid hygiene

Follow-up
- Resolution usually immediate
- PRN

M. VERRUCAE (VIRAL WART) (Color Plate 23)

Subjective
- History of slow insidious development
- Reported as contagious lesion with autoinoculation tendency
  1. Attributable to viral origin
  2. Believed to be transmitted by hands and fingers
- Cosmetic concern

---

*See also Appendix 3.

†See also Appendix 4.

Objective

- Single or multiple, nonsecreting papillomatous wart
- Gray-brown to yellowish colorations
- Various shaped (types) presentations
  1. Verruca planar: relatively flat and round
  2. Verruca vulgaris: raised, irregular mass on a broad base (sessile)
  3. Verruca digitata: multiple cauliflower-like dentate projections on narrow stalk (pedunculated type)
- Smooth surfaces with petal-like or cauliflower-like redundant tissue waves
- Infrequently, lesions at lid margin may cause mild secondary viral keratoconjunctivitis

Assessment*

- Rule out (nonviral) papilloma (roughened surface)
- Rule out molluscum contagiosum (rounded wart with depressed productive central core)
- Rule out neoplasia

Plan

- Reassurance and patient education
- Advise on contagious nature of warts on touching
- If causing no distress (cosmetically or ocularly), do nothing
- If problematic or requested for cosmetic relief, consider removal
  1. First choice should be referral for excision
  2. Occasionally primary practitioners use chemical removal methods (e.g., bichloroacetic acid)
     a. Lengthy process (weeks) versus excision
     b. Produces undue patient discomfort

Follow-up

- Recheck annually or PRN
- If removed, advise patient on possible recurrences

N. XANTHALASMA (Color Plate 24)

Subjective

- Usually older patients (greater in females)
- Occasionally positive contributory history[22]

  1. Atherosclerosis
  2. Hyperlipidemias (e.g., hypercholesteremia)
  3. High-risk cardiovascular history (e.g., family, obesity, hypertension)
- Family history of xanthalasma most contributory factor
- Cosmetic concern

Objective

- Usually flat triangular masses (base nasalward) at inferior or superior inner canthal lid sulcus
- Light brown to yellowish coloration
- Usually bilateral symmetrical presentation
- May be small patches or moderate to large plaques
- Occasionally can produce a horseshoe-like appearance at the inner canthi within the orbital rims

Assessment*

- Consider family, systemic, and dietary factors
  1. Family history most common cause
  2. Positive family or patient cardiovascular history with lesions demand careful counseling regarding risk factor control
- Rule out syringomas in younger females (small yellow spots at inner canthi)
- Rule out large superficial sebaceous cysts (usually unilateral and asymmetrical)

Plan

- Reassurance and patient education
- If high-risk systemic history and not under medical management, refer for workup
- Counsel patient on potential cardiovascular risk factors
- Advise on familial tendency
- Photodocument if possible or diagram and measure
- Cosmetic removal should be discouraged because of likely recurrences

Follow-up

- Recheck annually and remeasure or redraw
- Check on risk factors (e.g., blood pressure)

IV. Lacrimal Drainage (Excretory) Problems†

A. DACRYOCYSTITIS (CONGENITAL AND ACQUIRED)

Background Information

1. Infection or inflammation of lacrimal sac
2. Usually secondary to obstruction in the system

---

*See also Appendix 3.
†In alphabetical order.

3. Most common infectors in decreasing order
   a. *Streptococcus*
   b. *Staphylococcus*
   c. Gram-negative bacteria
   d. Streptothrix and fungi (canaliculitis)

Subjective

Congenital (or Infantile) Form
- Frequent complication of congenital dacryostenosis
- Subacute (mild to moderate tenderness on palpation) or chronic (painless) presentation for weeks to months
- Occasionally a family history of condition
- May be unilateral or bilateral

Acquired (Adult) Form
- Most frequently a unilateral presentation
- Usually acute onset with moderate to severe pain
  1. Dramatic tenderness at inferior inner canthus
  2. Pain generally diffuse around eye and orbit
  3. Often patient reports associated headache
- May present as chronic low-grade insidious infection with pain only on firm palpation of inner canthus

Objective

Congenital and Acquired Form
- Almost always epiphora (wet eye presentation)
- Acute presentations
  1. Usually moderate swelling of sac
  2. Mild to moderate localized edema and erythema throughout inferior nasal region
  3. Occasionally a hardened distention of the sac (mucocele) will produce a focal enlargement in the swollen area
  4. Purulent discharge is usually present in varying degree (depending on nasal congestion)
  5. Frequently a secondary conjunctivitis
  6. In severe cases a secondary preseptal cellulitis
- Chronic presentation
  1. Similar to acute presentations but less severe
  2. More common congenital presentation
     i. Common pediatric referral
  3. Purulent discharge often exaggerated by massage of the lacrimal sac area (toward puncta)
  4. Condition can persist for up to 9 to 12 months in congenital form with spontaneous remission (opening of the valve of Hasner)

Assessment*

Congenital and Adult Forms
- Attempt to determine cause of obstruction
  1. In congenital form, usually valve of Hasner
  2. In adult forms, rule out tumor (bloody tears)
- Determine presence or absence of mucocele

- Rule out preseptal cellulitis
- Rule out streptothrix (solid regurgitate on massage)
- In severe or nonresponsive cases, culture discharge

Plan†

Congenital and Acquired Forms
- Reassure and educate parents or patient
- Acute presentations
  1. Hot pack (rapped around finger) qid
  2. Topical antibiotic drops (e.g., sulfacetamide) qid
  3. In moderate to severe cases or in patients with preseptal cellulitis, use broad-spectrum oral antibiotic (co-manage children on oral agents with pediatrician)
  4. Never dilate and irrigate (D&I) an acute case
  5. Upon resolution of symptoms (reduced tenderness), D&I (adults) and introduce gentle massage over sac (children and adults) qid
  6. Mucoceles must be surgically incised and drained
- Chronic presentations
  1. Introduce more vigorous (firm) massage on first presentation qid
  2. D&I adult patients
  3. Hot packs can be combined with massage by using rapped finger technique for both
  4. Medication is optional in chronic cases, if no infection (discharge) is noted
- Advise patients or parents on chronicity and need for ongoing care and compliance

Follow-up

Congenital Form
- Recheck acute presentations in 3 to 5 days
  1. If stable or improving, continue treatment for 10 to 14 days and taper over following week to hot packs and massage bid to tid for 3 months
  2. If condition worsening
     a. Culture (and sensitivities)
     b. Adjust medications on the basis of laboratory work
  3. If condition not resolving within 3 to 4 weeks, refer to pediatric ophthalmologist for D&I or nasolacrimal duct probing (Bowman's)
- Recheck chronic forms every 6 to 12 weeks until resolution or until child reaches 1 year of age
  1. Reassure parents continually and stress need for compliance in spite of apparent lack of progress
  2. Explain nature of problem (valve-opening delay) and likelihood of spontaneous opening by 12 months
  3. Treat secondary complications appropriately
  4. If no resolution by 9 to 12 months (or total

---

*See also Appendix 3.

†See also Appendix 4.

noncompliance or resistance of parents or child), refer for nasolacrimal probing

Acquired Form

- Manage acute presentations as for congenital form
- D&I procedure will frequently be unsuccessful in older patients with primary unresolved obstructions (e.g., dacryostenosis, strictures)
- Nonresponsive chronic conditions may require ongoing therapy or referral for reconstructive surgery of the lacrimal system (recommend oculoplastics specialist due to complexity of procedures and high failure rate)

B. LACERATION

Subjective

- Most common injury to lacrimal system
- Caused by penetrating or ripping wounds to eyelids
- Does not need emergency repair

Objective

- Usually extensive swelling and bleeding
- Puncta or canaliculi may be torn or cut

Assessment

- Differentiate lid laceration from canaliculi involvement
- If possible, differentiate puncta from canaliculi involvement
- Rule out presence of foreign matter in the wound

Plan

- Better to wait for 24 to 48 hours to permit swelling and bleeding to subside
- Frequent cold packs and mild pressure
- Refer to oculoplastics for surgical repair and possible conjunctivodacryocystorhinostomy (that's the biggest word in the book!)

Follow-up

- Lacrimal surgical procedures often take 2 months or more to heal and thus require diligent compliance
- Prognosis usually guarded regarding complete repair (i.e., often resolves with chronic residual tearing)

C. OBSTRUCTIONS (INCLUDING DACARYOSTENOSIS)

Subjective

- Most common congenital abnormality of the system

1. Up to 30 percent of newborns (delayed opening of valve of Hasner)
2. Most open spontaneously within weeks to months
- Not uncommon in adults, especially elderly
  1. Usually idiopathic (no established cause)
  2. Narrowing of canaliculi (dacryostenosis)
     a. Sometimes caused by eyedrops
        i. Phospholine iodide
        ii. Antiviral agents, especially idoxuridine (IDU)
        iii. Epinephrines
     b. Sometimes disease (e.g., ocular pemphigoid)
     c. Sometimes trauma (e.g., repeated probing)
  3. Occasionally obstruction is mechanical
     a. Trauma and resulting cicatrix (scarring)
     b. Tumors (benign or malignant)
     c. Localized strictures in system
     d. Occult matter (e.g., makeup, dirt particles)
     e. Dacryoliths (calcium deposits in tubules)
- Common complication of inflammation or infection
  1. Congenital or acquired dacryocystitis
  2. Mucous plugs
  3. Secondary strictures
- Infrequently, nasal or sinus disease or surgery may cause secondary obstruction

Objective

- Epiphora, usually from inner canthal region
- Punctal integrity, position usually normal
- Drainage tests (e.g., Jones, Saccharin) positive
- Dilation and irrigation difficult or impossible
- Dacryocystorhinogram (x-ray) (done only in serious or suspicious cases, usually definitive)

Assessment

- Congenital versus acquired
- Rule out inflammation or infection (pain, discharge)
- Rule out signs of tumor
- Rule out punctal anomalies
- Rule out nasal or sinus disease
- Do diagnostic tests if clinical picture confusing
  1. Drainage tests (e.g., dyes)
  2. D&I
  3. X-Ray studies if indicated

Plan

- Manage congenital and acquired dacryostenosis same as chronic dacryocystitis
- Treat primary cause of obstruction appropriately
- Often frequent heat and firm massage (hot cloth wrapped around massaging finger) with or without other therapies may have positive effect
- Dilation and irrigation procedure[23]

1. Usually effective for following causes
   a. Discrete obstructions (e.g., mechanical)
   b. Subacute inflammation or infection
2. Usually ineffective for following causes
   a. Dacryostenosis (primary or secondary), especially in elderly patients
   b. Strictures
   c. Disease causes (e.g., tumors, nasal or sinus)
- Probing (Bowman's) often required in resistant cases with limited success and risk of aggravation
- Referral for surgical repair should be limited to absolute necessity and serious requests only
   1. Reason is difficulty and guarded prognosis of lacrimal repair procedures (dacryocystorhinostomy)
   2. Refer to oculoplastics specialist
- Carefully advise and educate patients on condition, chronicity (if applicable), compliance to therapies, and prognosis of treatment, management, and surgical repair

Follow-up

- Follow-up on treatment of primary conditions as indicated
- Monitor untreated conditions at 3- to 6-month intervals
   1. For spontaneous resolution
   2. For deterioration
   3. For complications
- Recheck D&I procedures in 1 week (for resolution or retreatment)
   1. Occasionally sequential or periodic D&Is prove successful versus single procedure
   2. Noninvasive approach versus repeated probing
   3. Usually no hope after three to five unsuccessful attempts
- Stress compliance with any treatment regimen

D. PUNCTAL ANOMALIES

Subjective

- May be congenital or acquired
- Lower punctual problems usually most clinically significant
- Most often associated with signs and symptoms of associated (usually primary) disorder

Objective

- Epiphora, usually at inner canthus
- Examination of lower puncta area demonstrates
   1. Absence (imperforate) puncta (usually congenital)
   2. Atresia, stenosis, or closure (usually in elderly)
   3. Duplication or double puncta
   4. Punctal ectropion (puncta turning outward and not communicating with lacrimal lake)
      a. Rarely congenital (e.g., blepharophimosis)
      b. Commonly acquired (e.g., eyelid laxity in elderly)
      c. May also follow injury or burns (scarring)
- Simple blockage by foreign matter, lashes
- Tumors of the inner canthus (benign or malignant)
- Secondary to advanced ocular surface diseases, such as keratitis sicca-type syndromes, inflammation

Assessment

- Congenital versus acquired
- Determine primary cause
- Rule out canalicular involvement (by D&I)
- Rule out other causes of wet eye presentations

Plan

- Treat the primary cause as indicated
- Attempt gentle opening of closed puncta with sharp punctal dilator (e.g., Reudamann) or needle
- Dilate puncta with progressive-diameter dilators
- Hot pack surrounding tissue tid to qid for 1 week
- Refer serious cases or requests for surgical repair

Follow-up

- Outcome of any nonsurgical approaches usually unrewarding
- Surgical approaches such as silastic or glass tubing and bypass procedures like conjunctivodacryocystorhinostomy have guarded prognosis

E. TUMORS

Subjective

- May be benign or malignant
- Fortunately very uncommon
- Can mimic chronic dacryocystitis or stenosis and thus can go undiagnosed for extended period
- Can appear as painless swelling (or mucocele)
- Frequently associated nasal or sinus symptoms

Objective

- May be external or internal (usually lacrimal sac)
- Mimic common signs of obstructed system
   1. Epiphora
   2. Same response to dilation and irrigation
- Frequently produces "bloody tears"
- Usually some degree of palpable or observable mass in region of drainage system

Assessment

- Rule out dacryocystitis and dacryostenosis by lack of response to standard therapies
- Rule out other causes of obstruction
- If suspicious, refer for dacryocystography (x-rays)
- Refer suspicious masses in region for biopsy

Plan

- Refer for surgical excision (dacryocystectomy)
- Patient refusal for immediate care should be carefully documented in records
- Postoperative radiation therapy frequently applied

Follow-up

- Recheck after referral to confirm care
- Due to wide range of tumor types in the area (and attendant risks), prompt care and careful followup monitoring is essential

---

V. Other Associated Disorders*

A. LACRIMAL GLAND

1. Dacryoadenitis

Subjective

- Relatively rare condition
- More common in third- to fourth-decade women
- Sometimes referred to as Mikulicz's syndrome or lymphoepithelial lesion
- Acute or chronic onset
- Usually tenderness on superior temporal palpation
  1. Anatomical site of gland
  2. Tenderness usually spreads beyond gland alone
- Frequent history of mononucleosis

Objective

- Unilateral or bilateral
- Eyelid shows variable degree of edema and erythema
- Produces "S"-shaped lid (Fig. 2–3)
- Discharge may be associated
- Nonocular-related signs:
  1. Salivary gland involvement

---

*In alphabetical order

2. Preauricular lymphadenopathy
3. Mononucleosis-related symptoms

Assessment

- Rule out lacrimal gland tumor
- Rule out bacterial etiology (mucopurulence)
- Up to 30 percent caused by mononucleosis
- May be associated with collagen vascular disease
  1. Take careful medical history
  2. Sjögren's syndrome frequently associated

Plan

- Refer to internist for medical evaluation
- Treatment usually includes systemic antibiotics
- Treatment for underlying systemic causes, if any

Follow-up

- Syndrome often includes degeneration of gland
- May produce long-term dry eye problems[24]

2. Tumors of the Lacrimal Gland

Subjective

- Considered rare
- May be benign or malignant
- Granulomas are most common form

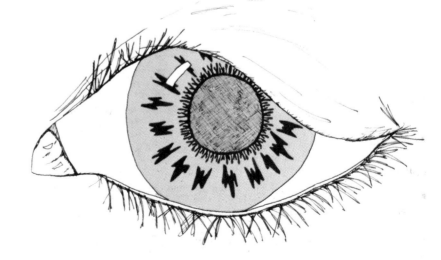

Figure 2–3.
S-shaped lid

- Onset may be insidious (slow) or fast
- Pain on palpation possible
- Patient may report diplopia

Objective

- Lid swelling may be moderate to severe
- Pseudoptosis common
- Variable degrees of proptosis (exophthalmos)
- Displacement of eyeball (down and in), causing diplopia

Assessment

- Rule out dacryoadenitis
- Slow progression usually implies benign nature
- Fast progression implies malignant mass

Plan

- Refer for surgical excision (possible exenturation)
- Usually extensive radiation therapy also required

Follow-up

- Malignant forms require close follow-up monitoring for metastasis or recurrence

B. ORBIT

1. Congenital Abnormalities

Subjective

- Very uncommon
- Most are cosmetically very obvious

Objective

- Anophthalmos: globe absent and orbit reduced
- Craniostenosis: prominent orbits and globes
- Hypertelorism: laterally displaced orbits
- Microphthalmos: small orbit(s) and globe(s)

Assessment

- Rule out developmental syndromes (e.g., Crouzon's)
- Rule out intracranial abnormalities

Plan

- Refer for pediatric (FLK) syndrome workup
- Assess potential visual function

Follow-up

- If pediatric diagnosis established, monitor eyes and associated structures for changes every 6 months
- Advice and counsel parents on visual prognosis

2. Exophthalmos

Subjective

- May be congenital or acquired
  1. Congenital forms usually associated with syndromes
  2. Acquired forms usually associated with potentially serious progressive disease
- Most common presentation of orbital disorders

Objective

- May be unilateral or bilateral
- Exophthalmometry (Hertel-type) readings
  1. Greater than 21 mm in either eye (bilaterally)
  2. Greater than 3 mm difference between eyes in unilateral conditions
- Resistance on repositing (pushing in) globe
- May show increased IOP[25]

Assessment*

- Most common cause in adults (unilateral or bilateral) is Graves' disease (hyperthyroidism)[26]
  1. Ballet's sign: EOM palsies (especially superior rectus)
  2. Cowen's sign: jerky consensual pupil reflex
  3. Dalrymple's sign: lid retraction
  4. Grove's sign: lid resistence on downward gaze
  5. Jellinek's sign: increased lid pigmentation
  6. Joffroy's sign: weak forehead wrinkling on upward gaze
  7. Knie's sign: unequal pupil dilation
  8. Moebius' sign: poor convergence
  9. Riesman's sign: bruit over closed eye
  10. Rosenback's sign: tremor of closed lids
  11. Stellwag's sign: infrequent blink rate
  12. Suker's sign: weak lateral-gaze fixation
  13. von Graefe's sign: lid lag on downward gaze
- Rule out other causes
  1. Space-occupying lesions
  2. Orbital cellulitis (most common cause of unilateral exophthalmos in children)
  3. Leukemia
  4. Pseudotumor
  5. Glaucoma
  6. High myopia (unilateral or bilateral)
- Rule out contralateral size reduction disorders

Plan

- Do exophthalmometry (unilateral and bilateral comparisons) with Hertel type or Luedde type (unilateral readings only)
- Refer Graves' disease suspects for thyroid screen
- If space-occupying lesion suspected
  1. B-scan ultrasonography
  2. Orbital x-rays (e.g., Caldwell, Waters)

*See also Appendix 3.

3. Computed tomography (CT) scan
4. Magnetic resonance imaging (MRI) studies
- Congenital forms should be monitored (by exophthalmometry) annually or upon apparent cosmetic change in appearance
- Treat secondary complications appropriately (e.g., corneal exposure from Graves' disease)

Follow-up

- Instruct patients on monitoring appearance
- Confirm diagnostic studies and care of referred patients

3. Orbital Cellulitis (Color Plate 8)

Subjective

- Acute or subacute presentation
- Diplopia
- Pain ranges from moderate to severe
- Occasionally patient suffering general malaise (i.e., fever, chills, vomiting)
- Most common in children (secondary to sinusitis)[27]

Objective

- Most commonly unilateral (in children)
- Progressive lid edema and erythema
  1. Usually deep, dark purple-red coloration
  2. Tender and warm on palpation
- Proptosis
- Conjunctival hyperemia and moderate to severe chemosis
- Restriction of ocular motility (painful)
- Vision often not significantly reduced

Assessment*

- Differentiate possible causes[28]
  1. Sinusitis (especially in children)
  2. Infection
    a. *Staphylococcus*
    b. *Streptococcus*
    c. *Hemophilus influenzae*
    d. Fungal
  3. Cavernous sinus thrombosis (especially bilateral)
  4. Trauma
  5. Neoplasia (primary or metastatic)
- Differentiate preseptal cellulitis
  1. Similar infectious causes
  2. Similar lid signs and symptoms
  3. Following signs essential to preseptal cellulitis diagnosis
    a. No diplopia
    b. No restrictions in ocular motility

*See also Appendix 3.

c. No proptosis
d. No conjunctival chemosis

Plan

- Refer emergently to medical practitioner[29]
  1. Pediatrician
  2. Pediatric ophthalmologist
  3. Primary care physician
  4. Internist
- Usually requires hospitalization, parenteral therapies and drainage (for abscesses)
- Condition is life-threatening, so act quickly

Follow-up

- Same-day verification of referral and care
- Verify resolution of cause before administering routine follow-up management or vision care

4. Trauma

Subjective

- Contusion injuries most frequent
- Can also be caused by head and facial injury
- Consider foreign body history as well
- Eyeball usually damaged from injury
- Pain on palpation, especially at fracture sites

Objective

- Surrounding soft tissue usually swollen and traumatized
- Rim may be spared or involved in any type of injury
- Orbit may fracture at numerous sites
  1. Roof
  2. Medial wall
  3. Apex (optic canal)
  4. Floor (blowout fracture: may be complicated by entrapment of inferior rectus muscle and resultant restriction of upward eye movement)

Assessment

- Measure visual acuity to determine damage to either the eye or optic nerve, or both
- Assess damage to eyeball (anterior and posterior)
- Rule out blowout fracture (restricted movement)
- Rule out foreign body (by history and x-ray)

Plan

- Treat damage to eye and other soft tissue
- Consider x-ray studies in seriously injured orbits
- Refer blowout fractures to oculoplastic surgeon if resultant diplopia on upward gaze problematic

Follow-up

- Monitor nonsurgical blowout fractures for 3 to 6 weeks for possible spontaneous release

- Occasionally untreated (nonsurgically repaired) blowouts result in "sinking" of the orbital fat into antrum, with resulting orbital asymetry and diplopia

5. Tumors

Subjective

- May be congenital or developmental
- Benign and malignant types

Objective

- Usually manifest as proptosis or exophthalmos
- May present as inflammatory conditions
- Usually unilateral

Assessment

- Common orbital tumors in children
  1. Capillary hemangioma
  2. Dermoid (e.g., epidermoids, choristomas)
  3. Lymphangioma
  4. Metastatic neuroblastoma
  5. Neurofibroma
  6. Optic nerve glioma
  7. Pseudotumor

  8. Rhabdomyosarcoma
- Common orbital tumors in adults
  1. Cavernous hemangioma
  2. Lymphangioma
  3. Lymphoma
  4. Meningioma
  5. Metastatic neoplasia
  6. Primary neoplasia
  7. Pseudotumor

Plan

- Refer all acquired space-occupying lesions
  1. B-scan ultrasonography
  2. X-ray evaluation
  3. CT scan
  4. MRI studies
- Monitor congenital, benign tumors every 6 months

Follow-up

- Discuss cosmetic removal of benign tumors if indicated
- Co-manage (e.g., alternate visits) metastatic and sight or life-threatening tumors with specialists

VI. Self-assessment Questions

1. The most common site for a benign epithelial tumor (papilloma) on the eyelid is:
   a. The inner canthus
   b. The outer canthus
   c. The mucocutaneous border
   d. The brow region
2. Subjective symptoms associated with a sudoriferous cyst (cyst of Gland of Moll) include each of the following *except:*
   a. Cosmesis
   b. Corneal irritation
   c. Concern
   d. No awareness
3. The leading cause of bacterial marginal forms of blepharitis is:
   a. *Pseudomonas*
   b. *Streptococcus*
   c. Herpes simplex
   d. *Staphylococcus*
4. The small single superficial subaceous cyst is best treated by:
   a. Expressing cyst contents
   b. Topical steroids

   c. Cauterization
   d. Oral antibiotics
5. Streptococcal invasion of lid tissue is frequently associated with:
   a. Rapid invasion after lid trauma
   b. Telangectasia (vascular zones on lid margins)
   c. Lash destruction (madarosis)
   d. Secondary hordeolii and chalazia
6. Primary care for chronic staphylococcal marginal blepharitis includes all of the following *except:*
   a. General hygiene
   b. Lid scrubs
   c. Oral steroids
   d. Topical antibiotics
7. The subjective hallmark of herpes zoster dermatoblepharitis is:
   a. Itching
   b. Severe pain
   c. Secondary venous congestion
   d. History of fever blisters
8. Demodex folliculorum infestation of the lids is best differentiated from chronic

staphylococcal marginal blepharitis by each of the following *except:*
   a. Collarettes
   b. Madarosis (loss of lashes)
   c. Pyramidal-shaped hair follicles
   d. Patient older than 50 years

9. Herpes simplex lesions on the lid will present with which of the following characteristics?
   a. Following dermatomes (nerve fiber course)
   b. Respect for facial midline
   c. Ulcerations resulting in scarring
   d. Pustules resolving without scarring

10. Colobomas of the lid margin are seen most frequently:
   a. Superior medially
   b. Inferior medially
   c. Superior laterally
   d. Inferior laterally

11. Recommended hot or cold compress therapy for ecchymosis (black eye) is:
   a. Hot packs for 1 week
   b. Cold packs for 1 week
   c. Hot for 24 hours, then cold for 1 week
   d. Cold for 24 hours, then hot for 1 week

12. Subjective and objective corneal signs may be noted with any of the following lid abnormalities *except:*
   a. Entropion
   b. Trichiasis
   c. Ptosis
   d. Viral warts

13. The most critical consideration in the evaluation of ptosis is:
   a. Unilateral versus bilateral
   b. Congenital versus acquired
   c. Partial versus complete
   d. Equal versus unequal

14. All of the following are therapies for chalazia *except:*
   a. Steroidal injections
   b. Oral steroids
   c. Hot packs
   d. Surgical excision

15. Which of the following is *not* a predisposing condition for basal cell carcinoma?
   a. Excessive UV skin exposure
   b. Previous history of basal cell lesions
   c. Fair complexion
   d. Previous history of metastatic carcinomas

16. Which of the following lid lesions *does not* have a viral etiology?
   a. Keratoacanthoma
   b. Molluscum contagiosum
   c. Xanthalasma
   d. Verrucae

17. The most significant diagnostic sign for internal hordeolum is:
   a. Focal palpable tenderness
   b. Diffuse lid edema
   c. Copious discharge
   d. Painless palpable mass

18. Which of the following is *not* a type of nevus?
   a. Dermal
   b. Junctional
   c. Transitional
   d. Melanoma

19. The most appropriate care for an atypical lid lesion of suspicious origin is:
   a. Ongoing watchful management
   b. Cultures and sensitivities
   c. Referral for systemic evaluation
   d. Biopsy

20. Common problems of the lacrimal drainage system include each of the following *except:*
   a. Dacryoadenitis
   b. Dacryocystitis
   c. Dacryostenosis
   d. Obstructions

For answers, refer to Appendix 6

REFERENCES

1. Malinovsky V: Benign essential blepharospasm. J Am Optom Assoc 58:646, 1987
2. Ruusuvaara P, Setala K: Use of botulinum toxin in blepharospasm and other facial spasms. Acta Ophthalmol (Copenh) 65:313, 1987
3. Canavan YM, Archer DB: Anterior segment consequences of blunt ocular trauma. Br J Ophthalmol 66:549, 1982
4. Wagoner MD, Albert DM, Lerner AB, et al: New observations on vitiligo and ocular disease. Am J Ophthalmol 96:16, 1983
5. McCulley JP, Dougherty JM: Bacterial aspects of chronic blepharitis. Trans Ophthalmol Soc UK 105:314, 1986
6. Dougherty JM, McCulley JP: Comparative bacteriology of chronic blepharitis. Br J Ophthalmol 68:524, 1984
7. Seal DV, McGill JI, Jacobs P, et al: Microbial and immunological investigations of chronic nonulcerative blepharitis and meibomianitis. Br J Ophthalmol 69:604, 1985

8. Catania, LJ: Staphylococcal risk reduction program. International Contact Lens Clinics 14:6, 1987

9. Norn M: Expressibility of meibomian secretion. Acta Ophthalmol (Copenh) 65:137, 1987

10. Oh JO (ed): Herpesvirus infections. Surv Ophthalmol 28:293, 1984

11. Cooper M: Epidemiology of herpes zoster. Eye 1:413, 1987

12. Womack, LW, Liesegange TG: Complications of herpes zoster ophthalmicus. Arch Ophthalmol 101:42, 1983

13. Heacock CE: Clinical manifestations of demodicosis. J Am Optom Assoc 57:914, 1986

14. English FP, Nutling WB: Demodicosis of ophthalmic concern. Am J Ophthalmol 91:364, 1981

15. Tesluk GC: Eyelid lesions: Incidence and comparison of benign and malignant lesions. Ann Ophthalmol 17:704, 1985

16. Wesley RE, Collin JW: Basal cell carcinoma of the eyelid as an indicator of multifocal malignancy. Am J Ophthalmol 94:164, 1982

17. Tierney DW: Basal cell epithelioma. J Am Optom Assoc 58:307, 1987

18. Pizzarello LD, Jakobiec FA, Mofeldt AJ, et al: Intralesional corticosteroid therapy of chalazia. Am J Ophthalmol 85:818, 1978

19. Doxanas MT, Iliff WJ, Iliff NT, et al: Squamous cell carcinoma of the eyelids. Ophthalmology 94:538, 1987

20. Lyndon WM, et al: Metastatic disease first presenting as eyelid tumors: A report of two cases and review of the literature. Am J Ophthalmol 19:13, 1987

21. Sturgis MD, Ashinskie LJ: Optometric management of eyelid malignancies. J Am Optom Assoc 58:307, 1987

22. Douste-Blazy P, Marcel YL, Cohen L, et al: Increased frequency of Apo E-ND phenotype and hyperpobeta-lipoproteinemeia in normolipidemic subjects with xanthalasmas of the eyelids. Am Intern Med 96:164, 1982

23. Semes L, Melore GG: Dilation and diagnostic irrigation of the lacrimal drainage system. J Am Optom Assoc 57:518, 1986

24. Rosen J, Atasia OG, Jakobiec FA: Aging changes in the human lacrimal gland: Role of the ducts. Contact Lens Association of Ophthalmologists Journal 11:237, 1985

25. Gamblin GT, et al: Prevalence of increased intraocular pressure in Graves' disease: Evidence of frequent subclinical ophthalmopathy. N Engl J Med 308:453, 1983

26. Gorum C: Ophthalmopathy of Graves' disease. N Engl J Med 308:453, 1983

27. Noel LP, Clarke WN, Addison D: Periorbital and orbital cellulitis in childhood. Am J Ophthalmol 16:178, 1981

28. Bergin DJ, Wright JE: Orbital cellulitis, Br J Ophthalmol 70:174, 1986

29. Mauriello JA, Flanagan JC: Management of orbital inflammatory disease. A protocol. Surv Ophthalmol 29:104, 1984

ANNOTATED REFERENCES

Anderson RL, Blodi FC, Boniuk M, et al: Symposium on diseases and surgery of the lids, lacrimal apparatus and orbit. Transactions of the New Orleans Academy of Ophthalmology, St. Louis, CV Mosby, 1982
Transcripts of presentation by leading authorities on general care and new concepts regarding common diseases of the lids, lacrimal, and orbit. Includes panel discussions on controversial issues regarding topics.

Duane DD, Jaeger EA (ed): Clinical Ophthalmology. Vol 2: Orbit, Philadelphia, Harper & Row, 1987
Chapters on standard approaches and new methods of care regarding orbital disease, injury, tumors, and so forth.

Duke-Elder WS, The Ocular Adnexa; Systems of Ophthalmology. Vol XIII. St. Louis, CV Mosby, 1976
Most comprehensive work on all congenital, developmental, anomalous, and disease entities of the lids, lacrimal, and orbit.

Eagling EM, Roper-Hall MJ: Eye Injuries: An illustrated guide. Philadelphia, JB Lippincott, 1986
Excellent color plates and illustrations of various eye injuries. Short descriptions of involvement and repair with each case.

Older JJ: Eyelid Tumors: Clinical Diagnosis and Surgical Treatment. New York, Raven Press, 1987
Two parts, one on diagnosis and one on surgical treatment. Diagnosis section uses excellent photographs with short descriptions to assist in differential diagnosis of benign and neoplastic tumors.

3

Diagnoses (by SOAP) of the Conjunctiva, Sclera, and Episclera

Chapter Outline

I. Bacterial Conjunctivitis (Color Plates 25 and 26)

A. ACUTE FORM[1]

Subjective

- Found in all age ranges

- Unilateral initially with frequent contralateral autoinoculation reported
- No frank pain (but may report nonspecific irritation)

- History of 2 to 3 days with increasing intensity of objective signs
- No associated reduction in vision
- There may be a positive medical history
  1. Especially in children
  2. Examples: upper respiratory infection (URI), otitis media (ear infection) in children
- Frequent reports of "lashes matting" or "eyes stuck shut" upon waking
- Frequently associated history of chronic blepharitis
- Patient usually concerned over increasing intensity of redness (main reason for visit)

Objective

- Grossly hyperemic, meaty red bulbar conjunctiva
  1. Hyperemia greater toward fornices
  2. Circumcorneal area relatively clear
  3. Injected vessels easily movable with cotton tip
  4. Injected vessels blanch with mild vasoconstrictors
  5. Vessels show irregular (nonradiating) pattern
  6. Combination of smaller- and larger-diameter vessels
- Cornea clear (always check with slit lamp)
- Palpebral conjunctival papillae usually present
  1. Papillae present as reddish vascular tufts, varying in diameter from small (velvety appearance when abundant) to large mounds
  2. Often blanched and congested by secondary edema
- Yellowish-greenish mucopurulent discharge
  1. Accumulations usually greater in the morning
  2. Tends to accumulate inferiorly and at inner canthus
  3. Accumulations may also produce hard crustations on lid margins (e.g., staphylococcal rosettes)

Assessment*

- Rule out other causes of red eyes
- Rule out other causes of conjunctivitis (see table entry on p. 61)
- Differentiate staphylococcal conjunctivitis (most common form of acute bacterial conjunctivitis) from other organisms
  1. No need for immediate cultures in acute forms because *Staphylococcus* is usually the cause and, inasmuch as *Staphylococcus* is normal flora to the eyelid and common to the ocular surface (75 percent of the time), cultures will be inconclusive and not as useful as clinical signs
  2. *Streptococcus* and gram-negative bacteria usually produce hyperacute bacterial conjunctivitis
  3. *Hemophilus influenzae (H. flu)* usually associated with a purplish (preseptal) flush or cellulitis on lids
     i. Frequently a URI or otitis media associated
  4. *Gonococcus* always hyperacute, plus venereal signs
  5. *Chlamydia* (Trachomatous–Inclusion conjunctivitis [TRIC]) usually more insidious
     a. 2- to 4-week history
     b. Mixed bacterial, viral and immune signs
     c. Positive genitourinary (venereal) history
     d. Nonresponsive or only temporary (returns after discontinuation) with topicals alone
  6. *Pseudomonas* is a hyperacute, rapidly advancing, secondary (usually history of injury) infection
- Rule out other secondary causes
  1. Blepharitis (usually staphylococcal)
  2. Systemic causes (e.g., acne rosacea)

Plan†

- Prescriptive considerations
  1. Topical anti-infective agents (ointments or drops)
     a. Broad-spectrum drugs (Table 3–1)
     b. Specific agents (Tables 3–1 and 3–2)
     c. General dosages (vary with degree of objective presentation)
        i. qid for 5 to 7 days (minimum)
        ii. Duration can be extended safely up to 10 to 14 days if necessary
     d. For resistant organisms:
        i. Change anti-infective agent
        ii. Extend course up to 21 days (maximum)
        iii. Consider culture and sensitivity tests
        iv. Oral antibiotics may be indicated
  2. Topical steroid combination drops or ointments (Table 3–2)
     a. Avoid use in mild to moderate cases
     b. With severe inflammatory responses or subjective discomfort, use cautiously (in lieu of any contraindications)
     c. Dosage: q4h for 3 to 5 days, then taper
        i. Maximum duration: 7 to 10 days
        ii. Check IOP for steroid-linked glaucoma
- Nonprescription (OTC) considerations
  1. Topical OTC broad-spectrum anti-infective ointment preparations containing bacitracin and polymyxin B (Table 3–2)
     a. Readily available (1/2-, 1-, and 2-oz. tubes)
     b. Inexpensive for patient (thus increasing compliance)
     c. Consider neomycin hypersensitivity risks
     d. Bacitracin component specific for staph (most common cause of acute bacterial forms)
     e. Polymyxin B specific against *Pseudomonas*
     f. Ointment vehicle (in most cases) preferable[2]

---

*See also Appendix 3

†See also Appendix 4

TABLE 3–1. SUSCEPTIBILITY OF SOME OCULAR PATHOGENS TO COMMON ANTI-INFECTIVE AGENTS: "THE BUGS" VERSUS "THE DRUGS"

THE "Bugs" → THE "Drugs" ↓	Gram-Positive		Gram-Negative				Suggested Dosages	
	Staphylococcus	Streptococcus pneumoniae	Haemophilus influenzae	Moraxella	Neisseria gonorrhoea	Pseudomonas	Ointments	Oral or Drops
Bacitracin	+ + + +	+	+ +	—	+	—	qid 5–7 days +	N/A
Cephalosporins (orals only)	+ + + +	+ + +	+ + +	+ +	+ + +	?	N/A	Oral 250 mg qid 5–10 days
Erythromycin	+ +	+ + +	+ + +	—	+ +	—	tid or qid 5–7 days +	Oral 250 mg qid, 5–10 days +
Gentamicin (and tobramycin)	+ + + +	?	+	?	+ + +	+ + + +	qid 7–10 days +[a]	Drops q3, 4, 6h 7–10 days +[a]
Neomycin	+ +	?	+ +	+	+	—	tid or qid 5 to 7 days +[b]	qid drops 5–7 days +[b]
Penicillins (orals only)	?	+ + +	+ + +	+ + +	+ + + +	—	N/A	Oral 250 mg qid 7–10 days +
Polymyxin B	—	—	+	—	?	+ + + +	qid 5–7 days +[c]	qid drops 5–7 days +[c]
Sulfonamides (15%)	+ + +	+	+	—	+	?	qid 5–7 days +	qid drops 5–7 days +
Tetracycline	+ +	+	?	—	+ +	—	tid or qid 5–7 days +	Oral 250 mg qid 7–10 days +

[a]Use as backup drug.
[b]Beware of hypersensitivities.
[c]Use in combination

Key: +, questionable efficacy; + +, effective; + + +, highly effective; + + + +, specific; ?, unknown; —, unapplicable.

TABLE 3–2. EXAMPLES OF RX AND OTC MEDICATIONS FOR CONJUNCTIVITIS (NOT INCLUSIVE)

Category	Generic Name	Trade Name	Route	Rx/OTC	Pharmaceuticals Firm
Antihistamines	Brompheniramine	Dimetane	Oral	OTC	Robbins
	Chlorpheniramine	Chlor-Trimeton	Oral	OTC	Schering
	Rose Pedal Infusion	Estivin	Topical	OTC	Alcon/bp
	Terfenadine	Seldane	Oral	Rx	Merrell Dow
Combinations	Chlorpheniramine and Pseudoephedrine	Chlor-Trimeton Plus	Oral	OTC	Schering
Anti-infectives	Bacitracin	Baciquent	Topical	OTC	Upjohn
		Bacitracin	Topical	OTC	Lilly
	Chloramphenicol	Chloromycetin	Topical	Rx	Parke-Davis
		Chloroptic	Topical	Rx	Allergan
		Econochlor	Topical	Rx	Alcon/bp
	Erythromycin	Illotycin	Topical	Rx	Dista
	Gentamicin	Garamycin	Topical	Rx	Schering
	Sulfonamides	Bleph 10/30	Topical	Rx	Allergan
		Sulf 10/30	Topical	Rx	Cooper
		Isopto Cetamide (15%)	Topical	Rx	Alcon/bp
	Sulfisoxazole	Gantrisin	Topical	Rx	Roche
	Tetracycline	Achromycin	Topical	Rx	Lederle
	Tobramycin	Tobrex	Topical	Rx	Alcon/bp
Broad-spectrum combinations	Neomycin, polymyxin B, and bacitracin	Neosporin	Topical	OTC	Burroughs Wellcome
	Polymyxin B and Bacitracin	Polysporin	Topical	OTC	Burroughs Wellcome
	Polymyxin B and Bacitracin	Polyspectin	Topical	Rx	Allergan
Antivirals	IDU	Stoxil	Topical	Rx	Smith Kline
	Vidarabine	Vira A	Topical	Rx	Parke-Davis
	Viroptic	Trifluridine	Topical	Rx	Burroughs Wellcome
	Acyclovir	Zovirax	Topical	Rx	Burroughs Wellcome
Astringents	Zinc sulfate	Zincfrin	Topical	OTC	Alcon/bp
		Prefrin Z	Topical	OTC	Allergan
Corticosteroids	Dexamethasone	Decadron	Topical	Rx	MSD
	Fluorometholone	FML	Topical	Rx	Allergan
	Hydrocortisone	Cortaid	Topical	OTC	Upjohn
	Medrysone	HMS	Topical	Rx	Allergan
	Prednisolone	Pred Mild	Topical	Rx	Allergan
		Pred Forte	Topical	Rx	Allergan
		Econopred	Topical	Rx	Alcon/bp
	Triamcinolone	Kenalog	Topical	Rx	Squibb
Anti-infective–steroid combinations	Chloramphenicol and prednisolone	Chloroptic-P	Topical	Rx	Allergan
	Neosporin and dexamethasone	Maxitrol	Topical	Rx	Alcon/bp
	Sulfonamides and prednisolone	Blephamide	Topical	Rx	Allergan
	Neosporin and hydrocortisone	Cortisporin	Topical	Rx	Burroughs Wellcome
Decongestants	Dimenhydrinate	Dramamine	Oral	OTC	Searle
	Diphenhydramine	Benadryl	Oral	OTC	Parke-Davis
	Naphazoline	Degest-2	Topical	OTC	Barnes Hind
		Naphcon	Topical	OTC	Alcon/bp
	Phenylephrine	Prefrin Liquifilm	Topical	OTC	Allergan
		Soothe	Topical	OTC	Alcon/bp
	Pseudoephedrine	Sudafed	Oral	OTC	Burroughs Wellcome
Combinations	Naphazoline and pheniramine	Naphcon-A	Topical	Rx	Alcon/bp
	Naphazoline and antazoline	Vasocon-A	Topical	Rx	SMP
		Albalon-A	Topical	Rx	Allergan
	Phenylephrine and pyrilamine	Prefrin-A	Topical	Rx	Allergan
	Ephedrine and antipyrine	Collyrium	Topical	OTC	Wyeth
	Pseudoephedrine and chlorpheniramine	Sudafed-Plus	Oral	OTC	Burroughs Wellcome
Mast cell stabilizer	Sodium cromoglycate	Opticrom 4%	Topical	Rx	Fisons

continued

TABLE 3–2. (Cont.)

Category	Generic Name	Trade Name	Route	Rx/OTC	Pharmaceuticals Firm
Irrigating solutions	Balanced salt solution with BAK	Eye Stream	Topical	OTC	Alcon/bp
	Isotonic solution with phenylmercuric acetone	Blinx	Topical	OTC	Barnes Hind
	Buffered solution with BAK	Dacriose	Topical	OTC	Cooper
Lubricants	Mucomimetics	Hypotears	Topical	OTC	Cooper
		Absorbotears	Topical	OTC	Alcon/bp
	Ointments	Lacrilube	Topical	OTC	Allergan
		Durotears	Topical	OTC	Alcon/bp
		Duolube	Topical	OTC	Muro
	Vitamin A drops	Vit-A-drops	Topical	OTC	Spectra

i. Up to 6 hours therapeutic value versus less than 20 minutes with drops

ii. No risk of corneal entrapment[3]

iii. No risk of clinical toxicity or systemic absorption (most carried off by mucous threads on the ocular surface) versus drops draining into the lacrimal canals[4]

g. Ointment most effective when applied on the external lid margins[4,5]

i. Site of greatest staphylococcal concentration

ii. Called reservoir effect (or technique)[4,6] (Table 3–3)

h. Some common topical ophthalmic antibacterial ointments have similar components and characteristics as their OTC ointment[7,8] counterpart (e.g., Polysporin ointments); the following have identical chemistry and formulation:[9]

i. Polymyxin B sulfate, 10,000 units

ii. Bacitracin zinc, 500 units

iii. Special white petrolatum qs[10] (best ointment vehicle)

iv. Same concentrations

v. Same pH (7.4), although eyes can tolerate range of 3.5 to 10.5 pH[11] due to tear buffering

vi. Bioequivalent

vii. Equal bioavailability

viii. Identical bioactivity

i. Any prescription versus OTC differences are offset by the "reservoir technique"

i. Sterile ophthalmic (Rx) requirements negated by fingertip and external eyelid application technique

ii. Also, consider that components in ointment itself are antibacterials

• Studies have shown no growth of pathogens in antibacterial ointments[12]

• Only contaminants found in Polysporin components have been subclinical colonies of molds (e.g., *Aspergillus*)[13]

• Bacteria cannot grow well in a nonaqueous media (ointment)[14,15]

• Ocular surface itself is not sterile and does not demand sterility due to tear lysozymes, secretory immunoglobin A (sIg A), lactoferrin, β-lysin and leukocytes themselves (which increase dramatically with threat of infection)[16–18]

iii. "Milling" process and any additional filtration (e.g., to reduce ointment base coagulates and particles) of no consequence due to melting effect during reservoir effect[19,20]

iv. One eighth ounce "sterile" ophthalmic tubes, originally mandated by Food and

TABLE 3–3. RESERVOIR EFFECT: STEP-BY-STEP APPROACH AND RESULTS

1. Squeeze out a ¼-inch ribbon of ointment onto your fingertip and discard (reduces risk of contaminants from tip).

2. Squeeze out a ½-inch ribbon of ointment onto your fingertip.

3. Wipe ointment onto the closed external lid margins of the affected eye.
   a. Tell patient to keep eye closed with normal pressure during application.
   b. When treating lid involvements directly, rub ointment in firmly.

4. Apply some extra ointment (dab on) at the inner and outer canthal portions of lid margin (outer canthus more preferable).

5. Body temperature will melt ointment base (white petrolatum) rapidly (30 to 60 seconds), and drug will begin to transport itself actively onto ocular surface (conjunctiva and cornea) by migration of mucous threads as patient is instructed to open eyes and resume normal blinking.

6. Patient will experience minimal blurring effect (versus ointment applied directly into eye in traditional method at inferior cul-de-sac).

7. Any excess ointment base or oils remaining on lid margins may be wiped off (for cosmesis) after 3 to 5 minutes without reducing therapeutic effect due to drug retention behind lid margins and on mucous threads in the fornices (resulting in a continuous reservoir effect for up to 6 hours).

Drug Administration (FDA) for one-time use in sterile surgical suites, of no value (and cost-ineffective) once opened and reused in nonsterile environment[21]

    v. Tapered tip on 1/8-oz tubes for intrapalpebral administration unnecessary in fingertip to lid margin application

  j. Irreconcilable (nonclinical) differences that must be considered

    i. FDA recommendations on OTC packaging describe external use only and state "Do not use in the eye"[22]

      • Such recommendations may be reconsidered relative to current research and clinical literature[23]

      • Reservoir technique can be considered external application[24]

    ii. Patients tend to save and reuse larger supplies of medications (e.g., ointments)

      • Carefully instruct against misuse

      • Monitor conditions to resolution

2. Topical astringents and heavy metals, such as zinc and mercuric oxides

  a. Reduce discharge

  b. Some antibacterial qualities (especially zinc against *Moraxella* angular conjunctivitis and blepharoconjunctivitis)

  c. Silver nitrate is too toxic for general use

3. Antibacterial preservatives found in low, but effective, concentrations in irrigating solutions

  a. Benzalkonium chloride (BAK)

  b. Chlorobutanol

  c. Disodium edetate

  d. Thimerosol (beware of toxicity)

■ Nontherapeutic (drugless) considerations

1. Can be used independently or in conjunction with therapeutic approaches

2. Irrigation with ophthalmic solutions or warm water to clear discharges and dilute or remove bacterial toxins

3. Warm packs to enhance body's immune–defense system (vasodilation with increased leukocytic action)

4. Noninvasive, nontoxic nature of these steps permit ad lib dosages

5. Instruct with 25–50–100 rule

  a. No worse in 24 ("25") hours

  b. Better in 48 ("50") hours

  c. Gone in 100 hours (about 4 days)

Follow-up

■ Reschedule patient within 3 to 5 days

■ Carefully advise (25–50–100 rule) or PRN

■ Preventive considerations (for patient and doctor)

1. Treat both eyes to reduce risk of autoinoculation

2. Instruct on general lid and skin hygiene

3. Instruct patient never to touch eyes during acute disease process (infection and reinfection usually originate from bacteria on skin and hands)

4. Never reuse medications beyond 6 to 8 weeks

5. *Never* patch conjunctivitis

6. Monitor cornea closely during follow-up evaluation

7. Many acute cases "lost to follow-up" probably improve themselves, but call patient to verify resolution

B. HYPERACUTE FORM[25]

Subjective

■ Found more frequently in younger age groups (children and young adults) and in parents of young children

■ Usually bilateral by time of presentation

■ Rapidly advancing acute bacterial signs and symptoms

■ Patient (or parents) anxious over rapid development

Objective

■ Advanced acute bacterial presentation

■ Copious mucopurulent discharge accumulating in lower cul-de-sac and overflowing (usually at inner canthus)

■ Varying degrees of secondary surrounding tissue involvement

1. Lid edema and erythema

2. Dermatoblepharoconjunctivitis

3. Preseptal cellulitis

4. Conjunctival chemosis (infiltrative edema)

5. Toxic corneal epithelial staining (beware of early ulceration)

■ Occasional hemorrhagic changes on bulbar conjunctiva ranging from petechiae (small dots) to larger areas of gross subconjunctival blood

■ Formations of true or pseudomembranes may develop in fornices and on palpebral conjunctiva

■ Frequent follicles and preauricular lymphadenopathy or enlargement present (mimicking viral presentation)

■ Laboratory workup indicated (versus optional in acute)[26]

1. Cultures and sensitivities

2. Gram stains

3. Cytology (usually demonstrates polymorphonuclear leukocytes [PMNs])

Assessment*

■ Rule out other causes of red eyes

■ Rule out other causes of conjunctivitis (see table entry on p. 61)

■ Possible organisms to consider (after *Staphylococcus*)

1. *Streptococcus pneumoniae*

  a. Usually bilateral

---

*See also Appendix 3.

b. Associated preseptal cellulitis

c. Often hemorrhagic

2. *H. flu*

   a. Children

   b. Associated medical history (i.e., URI, otitis)

   c. Frequent purplish preseptal cellulitis

3. *Neisseria gonorrhoeae*

   a. Rapid proliferation

   b. Extremely copious discharge (ballooning lid)

   c. Positive venereal history (or suspect)

4. *Pseudomonas* (secondary injury, usually corneal)

   a. Most rapidly proliferating bacteria

   b. Occasionally organism is phosphorescent with black light

5. Other gram-negative bacteria

   a. Especially common gastrointestinal (GI) organisms (e.g., *serratia, Escherichia coli*)

   b. Beware of mothers of children in diapers!

■ Always consider (and protect against) the risk of corneal invasion of hyperacute bacteria (not including *Pseudomonas,* surprisingly) through an intact cornea

   1. *Streptococcus*

   2. *Gonococcus*

   3. *H. flu* (Kochs–Weeks bacteria)

   4. *Cornybacterium* (uncommon)

   5. *Pseudomonas* requires an epithelial defect to enter cornea

■ Differential consideration for acute and hyperacute bacterial conjunctivitis can be accomplished fairly accurately by age alone (rule of fives)

Age Range	Leading Cause
0 to 5 days	*Gonococcus*
5 days to 5 weeks	*Chlamydia*
5 weeks to 5 years	*Streptococcus*
	H. flu
5 years and older	*Staphylococcus*

Plan*

■ Topical therapies (Rx, OTC, and "drugless") same as for acute bacterial conjunctivitis at q2–3h dosages

■ Oral antibiotics usually required in hyperacute forms

   1. Penicillins (or penicillinase-resistant penicillin against *Staphylococcus*) in standard recommended dosages

   2. Cephalosporins (e.g., Keflex)

   3. Erythromycin

   4. Children's oral dosages should be determined on the basis of body weight in conjunction with pediatrician

■ Refer systemic-related conditions for specific medical care (e.g., URIs, otitis media, venereal disease)

Follow-up

■ Reschedule in 24 to 48 hours on the basis of severity

■ Adjust initial broad-spectrum therapy to specific drug, upon receipt of laboratory results (if indicated)

■ If condition stable or improving within 24 to 48 hours, continue therapy at moderating dosages for minimum of 10 to 14 days

■ If condition unstable or worsening within 24 to 48 hours, adjust medications (per laboratory results), increase dosage, add oral medication (if absent), and reconsider diagnosis

■ Monitor cornea closely for bacterial keratitis

■ Upon resolution, advise and educate patient on prevention (see Table 2–1)

---

*See also Appendix 4.

II. Viral (and Other Follicular) Conjunctivitis (Color Plates 27 and 28)

A. ADENOVIRAL TYPES

Background Information

1. Viruses are single-cell organisms smaller than bacteria

2. Made up of single nucleic acid (DNA or RNA) that cannot grow or multiply independently

   a. Require protein synthesis from another source

   b. Host (infected) cells or chemical substances in our body (or on a contact lens surface)

3. Our susceptibility to viruses varies depending on many factors

   a. Age

   b. Chromosomal factors (genetic)

   c. Physiological factors

4. Defense mechanisms against viral infection

   a. Primary infection produces bodily resistance through immune system response (antibodies)

      i. Interferon

      ii. Immunoglobins (IgG, IgM, IgA)

      iii. Lymphoid system

      iv. B and T lymphocytes

v. Polymorphonuclear (PMN) leukocytes
vi. Killer and natural killer (NK) cells
b. Circulating antibodies persist (lifelong) as protection against reinfection of same virus
c. Additional defense is physical barrier to viral spread and penetration
   i. Epithelial surface
   ii. Tear film on ocular surface
   iii. Mucin tear layer and mucopolysaccharides
   iv. Phagocytosis (e.g., macrophages)
d. Factors that reduce immune response and physical barriers enhance viral susceptibility, spread, penetration, and length of acute infection
   i. General health
   ii. Nutrition
   iii. Genetic factors
   iv. Physiological factors
   v. Ocular surface inflammation
   vi. Immunosuppressive drugs (steroids)
   vii. Acquired immune deficiency syndrome (AIDS)
5. For unknown reasons, viruses live in ganglion or host (infected) cells as dormant obligate parasites and are activated by aggravating factors
   a. Physical (e.g., injury, irritation, contact lenses)
   b. Mental (e.g., excitment, stress)
   c. Emotional (e.g., aggravation, fear)
   d. Environmental (e.g., wind, air pollution, UV light)
   e. Physiological (e.g., illness, poor diet, lowered resistance)
6. Philosophies of treating virus
   a. No cures available
   b. Prevention before infection
      i. Health maintenance
      ii. Sanitation (personal, environmental)
      iii. Physiological (nutrition, immune system enhancement)
   c. For inactive infection
      i. Reduce aggravating factors
      ii. Enhance immune system function
   d. For active infection
      i. Paliative measures (symptom relief)
      ii. Inhibit or interfere with virus or host cell RNA, DNA protein synthesis with antiviral or antimetabolite drug
      iii. Trick of antiviral or antimetabolites is to affect virus or host (infected) cells without interfering with normal cells
         • Acyclovir (and some experimental drugs) accomplish this goal
         • Viroptic interferes with DNA of all cells and thus is toxic to normal (noninfected) cells
7. Some viruses known to affect the eye

DNA Virus	RNA Virus
Adenovirus	Coxsackie
Cytomegalovirus	Enterovirus 70 (*Hemophilus conjunctivitis*)
Epstein–Barr (mononucleosis)	Influenza
Herpes simplex	Measles (rubeola)
Molluscum contagiosum	Mumps
Papilloma (verrucae)	Newcastle disease
Vaccinia	Poliovirus
Variola (smallpox)	Rabies
Varicella (herpes zoster)	Rhinovirus
HTLV-III (AIDS virus)	Rubella

Subjective

- Most common form of acute conjunctivitis in children and adults
- Patient often does not seek care because of frequent mild and short-lived acute phase
- May be unilateral or bilateral (autoinoculation)
- History of onset and development usually 3 to 7 days
- Occasionally a prodromal medical history
  1. Upper respiratory infection (URI) such as cold, flu, sore throat
  2. Low-grade fever
  3. Most common in pharyngoconjunctival fever (PCF)
- Occasionally a previous history of conjunctivitis
- Mild visual fluctuations (transient)
- Usually mild to moderate burning irritation

Objective

- Presents as a purplish-pinkish bulbar hyperemia
- Injection usually begins at inner canthal (caruncle–plica area) and slowly spreads lateralward to involve entire bulbar conjunctiva (slightly greater inferior)
- Vessels may blanch slightly with mild vasoconstrictor
- Usually a quick NaFl tear breakup time (BUT)
  1. Can produce secondary exposure SPK response with associated corneal irritation
  2. Exposure SPK may stain with rose bengal
- Serous (tearing, watery) discharge (hyperlacrimation)

- Follicular changes (follicles)
  1. Pale mounds of infiltrative cellular accumulation on the palpebral conjunctiva of varying diameter
  2. Variable degrees of overlying (low-grade) inflammatory hyperemia with most vessels surrounding base of elevated accumulated areas
  3. When abundant, follicles produce "rugae"-like folds in lower cul-de-sac
  4. Follicular changes (folliculosis) in lower cul-de-sac of children considered normal in quiet eyes
  5. Follicular changes on superior tarsal plate (in children or adults) usually not normal
- Occasional preauricular lymphadenopathy (tenderness on palpation) or lymph node enlargement (more common)
- Laboratory workup (usually not done) usually reveals lymphocytes

Assessment*

- Rule out other causes of red eyes
- Rule out other causes of conjunctivitis (see table entry on p. 61)
- Rule out pharyngoconjunctival fever (PCF)
  1. Sometimes referred to as Beal's follicular conjunctivitis, or swimming pool conjunctivitis
  2. Found in children (usually under ages 15 to 18)
  3. Pharyngitis with low-grade fever precedes eye involvement by 1 to 2 weeks
  4. Often history of recent swimming pool exposure or hot tubs (in some adult presentations or precocious kids!)
  5. Rarely, a transient fine SPK or subepithelial infiltrates (usually peripheral)
- Rule out epidemic keratoconjunctivitis (EKC) in its early stages
  1. Frequently a history of exposure to another case
  2. Unilateral to bilateral
  3. Usually more hyperacute than mild adenoviruses
  4. Highly contagious during incubation (milder) stages (first 7 to 10 days)
- Rule out herpes simplex virus (HSV)
  1. Almost always has keratitic component
     a. Coarse SPK
     b. Dendriform pattern (75 to 80 percent of cases)
  2. Always unilateral
  3. Frequently recurrent history
  4. Reduced corneal sensitivity
- Rule out herpes zoster ophthalmicus (mimicker)
  1. Dermatoblepharitic component
  2. Severe pain
- Rule out *Chlamydia*
- Rule out other less common follicular forms of conjunctivitis

Plan†

- Prescription (Rx) considerations
  1. No Rx cure for viruses of any kind
  2. Antiviral agents are not effective against adenoviruses
  3. Prophylactic antibacterial use questionable as to value and efficiency
     a. Potential for creating resistant strains of bacterial (not yet proved)
     b. Antibacterial agents of no therapeutic value against conjunctival viral infection, as opposed to corneal viruses (see Chapter 4)
  4. Steroids and steroid combination drugs should be limited (as in bacterial conjunctivitis) to the more severe presentations
- Nonprescription (OTC) drug considerations
  1. Topical astringents and heavy metals such as zinc and mercuric oxides may (or may not) be of value
     a. Reduce discharge
     b. Secondary antibacterial effect may help(?)
  2. Ocular lubricants (mucomimetics) to supplement and protect tear film from dessication
  3. Topical vasoconstrictors (used limitedly) will improve appearance and may reduce symptoms
- Nontherapeutic (drugless) considerations
  1. Irrigation with ophthalmic solutions or warm or cold (for symptom relief) water to dilute or remove viral toxins
  2. Warm packs will enhance body's immune (defense) mechanism to fight viral spread (by vasodilation and increased leukocytic action) but will also produce added congestion and discomfort
     a. Suggest course of hot and cold (5 minutes each)
     b. Patient can decide on continuation based on subjective response to either or both
  3. Noninvasive nontoxic nature of these steps permits ad lib dosages
  4. If pseudomembranous fibrin deposits begin to form in fornices (hyperacute forms), remove by means of lavage, wet swabbing or toothed or jeweler's forceps
     a. May cause discomfort (even with topical anesthetic) and small petechial hemorrhages on removal
     b. True membranes would bleed heavily
- Instruction and preventive measures
  1. Same considerations as described for acute bacterial conjunctivitis
  2. Advise patient, "This may get worse before it gets better"
     a. Explain to patient (at first visit) risk of early presentation of more virulent viral infections (e.g., EKC) versus 7- to 10-day normal course of nonspecific adenoviruses

---

*See also Appendix 3.

†See also Appendix 4

b. Explain that impossible to tell until recheck visit
3. State clearly to patient, "You have a virus in your eye and there is *no* cure for viruses"
   a. Explain any treatment as palliative
   b. Autoimmune system will "treat" and control viral infection over period of time relative to potency of virus and response of system
4. Carefully instruct on contagious nature of some viruses, especially during early mild stage
   a. Advise on avoiding contact with eye
   b. If hyperacute, eliminate contact with others until reversal of clinical course
   c. School or work may require temporary discontinuance or limited activities

Follow-up

- Recheck acute presentations approximately 5 to 8 days after reported first signs of infection (or PRN)
   1. If nonspecific adenovirus, will improve
   2. If virulent adenovirus (e.g., EKC), will worsen
   3. Cornea usually becomes involved
- Educate patient to dormant obligate nature of ocular viruses and potential for intermittent mild to moderate exacerbations with varying stress factors

B. MISCELLANEOUS TYPES*

1. Axenfeld's Chronic Follicular Conjunctivitis

Subjective

- Always a low-grade, insidious, and asymptomatic course
- Only in children (called "orphan's conjunctivitis")

Objective

- Firm palpebral follicles most abundant on tarsal conjunctiva with no corneal involvement
- May produce mild, chronic, serous discharge

Assessment

- Rule out acute or subacute viral forms
- Probably a mild form of trachoma

Plan and Follow-up

- Usually a self-limiting course of months to years
- Monitor every 3 months and stress hygiene

2. Beal's (Swimming Pool) Conjunctivitis
Same as adenoviral types

---

*In alphabetical order.

3. Chlamydial (Inclusion) Conjunctivitis
Same as chlamydial keratoconjunctivitis

4. Folliculosis

Subjective

- Found mostly in young, healthy children
- May be sparse to florid

Objective

- Palpebral conjunctival follicles with no signs of inflammation
- Usually greatest in inferior cul-de-sac

Assessment

- Rule out causes of inflammatory follicle formation

Plan and Follow-up

- No treatment indicated
- Monitor routinely or PRN

5. Hemorrhagic (Acute) Conjunctivitis

Subjective

- Specific cause is Enterovirus 70
- Hyperacute clinical presentation with hemorrhages can be caused by EKC-type adenoviruses or any virulent microorganism (e.g., viral, chlamydial, bacterial)

Objective

- Rapid unilateral to bilateral presentation
- Dot to diffuse, spreading conjunctival hemorrhage

Assessment

- Rule out EKC syndrome
- Rule out other infectious syndromes

Plan and Follow-up

- Treat primary infectious cause
- Instruct on viral syndromes

6. Molluscum Contagiosum
Same as adenoviral types

7. Newcastle's Disease

Subjective

- Virus transmitted by infected bird (especially chicken droppings)
- Likely candidates are poultry workers

Objective

- Same as adenoviral types

Assessment

- Determine contact with viral carrier

Plan and Follow-up

- Remove infectious source and instruct
- Condition will self-limit on removal of source

8. Parinaud's Oculoglandular Fever

Subjective

- Ocular analogue of "cat-scratch fever"
- Frequent history of direct exposure to cat(s)
- Occasionally associated with systemic malaise, fever, and headache

Objective

- Always an acute unilateral presentation
- Large follicles with yellowish core associated with diffuse palpebral conjunctival granulomas
- Dramatic ipsilateral preauricular lymphadenopathy (tenderness) and enlargement (greater than 1 cm)

Assessment

- Determine association with cat(s)
- Consider systemic (cat-scratch fever) involvement

Plan and Follow-up

- Cat-scratch fever requires systemic treatment usually with antibiotics (of questionable value) and nonsteroidal anti-inflammatories (aspirin)
- If ocular involvement only, treat with a broad-spectrum antibiotic (e.g., gentamicin) q3–4h until remission of acute ocular symptoms
- Preauricular lymphadenopathy can persist for weeks to months

9. Toxic (Secondary) Conjunctivitis
Same as toxic or irritative conjunctivitis

10. Trachoma

Background Information
a. Caused by TRIC organisms (chlamydial trachomatis species)
b. Part of series of oculogenital diseases
   i. Trachoma
   ii. Inclusion blenorrhea (neonatal chlamydial disease)
   iii. Adult inclusion conjunctivitis
c. Tends to be endemic in underdeveloped countries and among certain ethnic groups
   i. Asia
   ii. Africa
   iii. South America
   iv. American Indians
d. Spread by direct contact (hands, sexual, cervical)
e. Associated genitourinary involvement often mild
f. Laboratory workup usually less reliable than clinical diagnosis
g. Severe (corneal scarring) forms far more sight threatening than milder conjunctival forms

Subjective

- Chronic insidious onset
- Measure epidemiological risk factors in patient
- Symptoms are usually absent in noncorneal forms
- Most cases seen in industrialized urban and suburban populations are usually old (and usually scarred)

Objective

- Moderate to severe upper tarsal follicles
- Papillary hypertrophy and moderate to severe inflammation and infiltration of superior palpebral conjunctiva
- Standard classification (MacCallan) based on conjunctival (not corneal) changes
   1. Follicles without scarring or papillae
   2. **A:** Follicles with papillary hypertrophy;
      B: Papillary hypertrophy obscures follicles
   3. Scarring develops with follicles
   4. Cicatricial scarring replaces follicles
- Superior half of cornea and upper lid secondarily involved and scarred (cicatrix) in numerous ways
   1. Trichiasis and entropion
   2. Superficial epithelial keratitis
   3. Superior panus (frequently very dense)
   4. Ulceration
   5. Limbal follicles, swelling, and subsequent depressed scarring (Herbert's pits)
   6. Linear scarring (fine in milder forms and broad lines in advanced cases) on tarsus (called Arlt's lines)

Assessment*

- Consider patient's ethnic background and country of origin (especially in old, scarred cases)
- Rule out active venereal (chlamydial) disease

---

*See also Appendix 3.

- Eliminate commonly associated secondary bacterial infections as cause by treating with topicals

Plan

- Treat all cases, mild to severe, with oral tetracycline (or erythromycin) 250 mg for 3 to 6 weeks
- Topical tetracycline ointment (Achromycin) bid for 2 to 3 months
- Treat family members, intimate associates with topical tetracycline ointment bid for 1 to 2 months
- Refer any suggestive venereal signs or symptoms for medical evaluation
- Active corneal involvement may require topical steroids (with guarded prognosis for response)

Follow-up

- Most cases usually result in some degree of conjunctival and corneal scarring (cicatrix) with or without treatment
- Active disease usually takes about 3 to 6 months to run its course (with or without treatment)
- Careful instructions to patients under care and to patients at high risk (exposed, endemic, or ethnic populations) should include hygiene and monitoring for early signs

11. Verrucae
Same as adenoviral types

III. Allergic Conjunctivitis

A. ATOPIC REACTIONS

Subjective

- Immediate (type I) reaction, within minutes, or delayed (type IV) reaction, within hours to days[27]
- Frequent patient or family history of allergies or asthma (especially type I)
- Often a seasonally related condition (e.g., hay fever)
- May or may not report specific allergen (substance)
- Predominant irritation is unrelenting itching

Objective

- May be unilateral (usually contact response) or bilateral (often from endogenous cause)
- Vision may fluctuate or remain unaffected
- Pink to red bulbar hyperemic injection
- "Glassy" appearing luster to mucous membranes
- Chemosis (subconjunctival infiltration and edema)
    1. Produces mild to dramatic swelling of bulbar conjunctiva
        a. Conjunctival tissue elevates and "rolls over" limbus (obvious with slit beam)
        b. "Watchglass" effect when complete peripheral cornea covered by conjunctiva
    2. More common and predominant on temporal conjunctiva due to eye-rubbing pattern at outer canthus (usually same side as dominant hand)
- Mucoid (stringy) whitish discharge
    1. Strands often spread across cornea
    2. Accumulates in fornices and at inner canthi
- Associated mild to severe lid edema and erythema
- Small "velvety" to "giant" papillary changes on upper and lower palpebral conjunctiva
    1. Frequently, follicular changes also present
    2. Associated edema often "buries" papillae (and follicles)
- Laboratory workup (if done) usually shows eosinophilia (type I) or basophils (type IV)

Assessment*

- Rule out other causes of red eyes
- Rule out other types of conjunctivitis (Table 3–4)
- Differentiate (if possible) by history or laboratory workup (optional), immediate versus delayed reaction
- If possible, determine specific causative agent (but don't drive yourself and your patient crazy!)
- Rule out vernal conjunctivitis

Plan†

- Prescriptive (Rx) considerations
    1. Limit Rx use to moderate to severe presentations
    2. Topical decongestant drops q3–4h for 24 to 28 hours
        a. Rarely effective alone (if at all!)
        b. Phenylephrine or naphozoline HCl (Table 3–2)
    3. Topical antihistamine drops q3–4h for 24 to 48 hours
        a. Rarely effective alone (if at all)
        b. Antazoline or pyrilamine (Table 3–2)
    4. Decongestant and antihistamine combination drops are slightly more effective because of synergism
    5. Delayed (type IV) reactions usually require ste-

---

*See also Appendix 3.
†See also Appendix 4.

TABLE 3–4. CONJUNCTIVITIS: CLINICAL PRESENTATIONS[a]

	Bacterial	Viral	Allergic	Chronic
Subjective	All age groups	Unilateral or bilateral	Onset in hours or days	Chronic
	Unilateral or bilateral	± systemic Hx	Unilateral or bilateral	Bilateral
	± irritation	3-7 day Hx	± allergic Hx	Cosmesis
	2–3 day Hx	Previous conjunctivitis	Seasonal	± Irritation
	No reduced VA	frequently reported	Itching	Sometimes
	May have URI Hx	Burning sensation	Hx of allergen	seasonal
	AM lashing matting	± VA	No reduced VA	No reduced VA
			(fluctuations)	Easily aggravated
Objective	Meaty red	Pink/purple	Pink/purple	Angular injection
	>toward fornices	>toward plica	Chemosis	Inferior hyperemia
	Movable vessels	Quick BUT (tear break up)	Mycoid	No discharge
	Blanch with mild vasoconstrictors	Tearing	± Lid edema	Papillae
	Cornea clear	Follicles	Papillae	Variable BUT
	Papillae	Enlarged preauricular node or	Occasional follicles	Occasional xerosis
	Mucopurulent	lymphadenopathy		
Assessment (Differential Diagnosis)	R/O	Secondary causes	Early bacterial	Staphylococcal
	Viral	Common (nonspecific)	Early viral	toxins
	Allergic	PCF	Seasonal reaction	UV radiation
	Secondary causes	EKC	Contact allergen	Tear disfunction
	Staph. aureus	Herpes simplex and zoster	Endogenous allergen	*Moraxella*
	Streptococcus pneumoniae	Adult inclusion/*Chlamydia*	Vernal	Allergens
	Hemophilus influenza	Lab: monocytes, inclusion	GPC associated with CLs	(seasonal)
	Chlamydia	bodies, giant cells	Lab: basophils, eosinophils	Lab: variable
	Gonococcus			
	Lab: PMNs			
Plan	Hygiene	Hygiene/contact	Remove allergen	Lid procedures
	Irrigation	Lubrication	Air conditioning (optional)	UV tints
	Warm compresses	Warm/cold compresses	Cold compresses	Lubricants
	Antibiotics (optional)	OTC ocular decongestant	OTC topical decongestant–	Zinc preparations
	Combo steroids (for severe	Educate and counsel	antihistamine (astringents)	Aminoglycosides
	cases)	Follow-up	Oral OTC or Rx	Oral antihistamine—
	Instructions and follow-up		decongestant–	decongestants
	Self-limiting		antihistamines	
			Opticrom 4%	

[a]by SOAP.

roids (not very responsive to decongestant–antihistamine drops)

  a. Topical drops or ointments

  b. Refer to Table 3–2 for selections

  c. Avoid fluorinated steroids (too strong)

  d. Limit use (if possible) to qid q48–72h

  e. Taper dosage (as always) with steroids

6. Mast cell stabilizers (cromolyn sodium, Opticrom 4%) useful in subacute cases

  a. Drug must be administered before acute phase (i.e., before significant symptoms appear)

  b. Dosage should be qid for 3 to 4 weeks

  c. Drug is more efficacious in seasonal condition as prophylactic over 6- to 8-week risk period

  d. Reduces subjective symptoms but not physical (objective) signs

  e. Effective as maintenance drug for symptom control upon tapering steroids after acute phase of chronic or recurring reactions

7. Oral (Rx) medications rarely required for ocular allergic reactions

  a. Oral steroids should be withheld as backup therapy in nonresponsive conditions

  b. Oral antihistamine–decongestant drugs can be administered freely (in lieu of contraindications), especially preparations of known effectivity for patient with allergic history (i.e., previously prescribed agents)

  c. Most oral antihistamine–decongestants available OTC

■ Nonprescriptive (OTC) drug considerations

1. Topical decongestant drops every 3, 4, or 6 hours ad lib

  a. Virtually equal response to Rx counterparts

b. Less irritating, hence greater compliance
c. Reduced concentrations (usually ½ Rx) reduce risk of vasodilatory rebound effect
2. Topical astringents in combo with decongestants
    a. Ephedrine (e.g., Collyrium)
    b. Synergistic with topical decongestants
3. Rose petal infusion
    a. Beats me how it works!
    b. But lots of people swear by it for relief
4. Oral antihistamines or decongestants
    a. Most now OTC
    b. Initial dose can effectively begin to reverse histamine release
    c. Diphenhydramine (Benadryl) effective
       i. Advise on drowsiness
       ii. Dosage per insert directions
    d. Many other excellent products (Table 3–2)
    e. Always rule out (by history) patients with potential idiosyncratic responses or contraindications to any drugs (Rx or OTC)
- Nontherapeutic (drugless) considerations
    1. Remove allergen (offending substance), if known
       a. Only complete cure for allergic reactions
       b. Allergen may be determined from careful history
       c. Contactants (e.g., external substances, eyedrops, cosmetics, soaps)
       d. Ingested (e.g., food, medicines)
       e. Injected (e.g., insect bite or sting)
       f. Airborne (e.g., pollen, spores, house dust)
       g. Pollutants (anything!)
    2. Frequent cold compresses (for vasoconstriction)
       a. One of the most valuable therapies for subjective and objective relief
       b. Always include with any combined treatment plan
    3. Air-conditioning for seasonal problems may be helpful
- Preventive measures
    1. Reasonable attempts to determine the allergen should be conducted so as to advise patient
    2. If appropriate (no contraindications or history of significant previous reactions), a "scratch test" may reveal offending substance
       a. Scratch clear skin (e.g., medial forearm) surface gently with needle to create slightly reddened area (approx. 5-mm diameter)
       b. Rub suspect substance (allergen) on area
       c. Wait 24 to 48 hours for mild localized edema or increased diameter (Arthus response)
       d. Positive reaction identifies allergen
    3. Counsel patient on risks of re-exposure
    4. Advise on chronicity and seasonal recurrences
    5. If reactions are severe or frequently recurrent, refer to allergist for complete workup and possible desensitization program

Follow-up

- In moderate to severe reactions, schedule patient for 24- to 48-hour checkup
- Reschedule beyond second visit only for slowly responding conditions or during steroid management
- Instruct on preventive measures

B. GIANT PAPILLARY CONJUNCTIVITIS (Color Plate 30)

Background Information

1. Probably a combined reaction: type I (mast cells and eosinophilia) and type IV (basophils)
2. Seen almost universally to some degree in soft lens wearers
3. Ten times more common in soft lens wear than hard[28]
4. Immune reaction probably incited by "microtrauma"
5. Reported causes in order of clinical frequency
    a. Soft contact lens wear
    b. Hard contact lens wear
    c. Protruding sutures postoperatively
    d. Prosthetic (artificial) eyes

Subjective

- Onset varies according to cause
    1. Soft lens wearers usually about 6 to 12 months
    2. Hard lens wearers usually greater than 3 to 5 years
    3. Protruding sutures within weeks to months
    4. Prosthetic eyes within months to years
- May show no symptoms with distinct physical findings or distinct symptoms with no findings
- Generally mild to moderate nonspecific irritation and itching
    1. Present both with and without lens wear
    2. May increase temporarily upon removal of lens
- Frequent reports of increased lens awareness and eventual loss of wearing time or inability to continue wear
- Lens movement on blinking becomes excessive
    1. Results in fluctuating vision or constant blur
    2. Frequent decentration of lens
    3. Ultimately dislodging and folding of lens(es)

Objective

- Almost always bilateral
- Mild to moderate conjunctival hyperemia (greater in superior bulbar regions)

- Small to giant diffuse papillae on tarsus
  1. Vary in areas of concentration
     a. Upper tarsus (near fold), sometimes called "zone 3", more common with soft lenses
     b. Close to lid margin (zone 1) with hard lenses
     c. Diffuse in more severe reactions
  2. Often associated with overlying infiltration and edema (which may even obscure papillae)
  3. Size range from less than 0.5 mm up to 2 to 3 mm
  4. Often tops of large papillae stain with NaFl
  5. Larger papillae may show whitish–yellowish central cores
- Lens surfaces usually show light to dense protein buildup on surfaces
- Varying degrees of mucoid discharge from absent to dense, stringy accumulations
- Occasionally, superior cornea may be involved
  1. SPK (greatest at limbus)
  2. Superior mucoid debri or filaments
  3. Limbal infiltrate(s)

Assessment*

- Rule out other causes of red eye
- Rule out other forms of conjunctivitis
- Rule out vernal conjunctivitis
  1. Usually more dramatic symptoms and signs
  2. Usually flat giant papillae
  3. Frequent corneal component
  4. Seasonal versus specific causative agent (i.e., contact lens)
- Rule out SLK
  1. Minimal tarsal reaction
  2. Pronounced corneal involvement
- Determine causative agent (usually obvious)
- Consider immune versus microtrauma versus combined etiology (Table 3–5)
  1. Increased hyperemia, infiltrates, heavy protein, corneal involvement, or positive response to steroids may suggest primary immune component
  2. Increased papillae (at zone 1 or 3), excessive lens movement (without heavy protein), hard lens materials, sutures, prosthetics or quick (less than 2 weeks) positive response to temporarily discontinued wear (without therapy) may suggest primary microtrauma component

Plan†

- Adjunctive therapies for mild presentations (i.e., minimal symptoms with or without physical signs)
  1. Reclean lens surfaces thoroughly
  2. Replace old lenses (older than 6 to 12 months) or those with poor surface quality

  3. Increase enzyme cleaning to twice a week
  4. Lubricant drops bid to tid
- Adjunctive therapies for moderate presentations, that is, symptoms with distinct physical findings
  1. All therapies for mild presentations, plus
  2. Enzyme cleaning every night at bedtime
  3. Lubricant drops qid to q4h
  4. Oral OTC antihistamines–decongestants
  5. Opticrom (with or without lenses)[29]
     a. qid for 3 to 4 weeks
     b. tid for 1 to 2 weeks
     c. bid for 1 to 2 weeks
     d. Recurrences may require retreatment
  6. Oral nonsteroidal anti-inflammatory agents (OTCs)[30]
     a. Prostaglandin inhibition may have effect
     b. Aspirin, 3 g/day (two 5-gr tabs q4h) for 1 week (in lieu of contraindications), or
     c. Ibuprofen (800 to 1200 mg/day) for 1 week
- Adjunctive therapies for severe presentations, that is, distressing symptoms and advanced physical signs
  1. All therapies for moderate presentations, plus
  2. Give 1 to 2 acetylcysteine (Mucomyst) drops qid for 2 weeks
  3. Topical steroid drops (e.g., 1 percent prednisolone)
     a. Most effective in primary immune reactions
     b. Dosage qid for 5 to 7 days, then begin to taper
     c. Introduce Opticrom during steroid taper
- Manage contact lens wear carefully in conjunction with adjunctive therapies (Table 3–5)

Follow-up

- Advise and educate patient on immune, mechanical nature of disorder and risk of recurrence(s)
- Reschedule patients based on degree of presentation and adjunctive therapies selected
- Sequential order of contact lens adaptations for giant papillary conjunctivitis (GPC) recurrences (with or without adjunctive therapy) (Table 3–5)
  1. Consider rewear of original lens
  2. Supply new lens of same material and design
  3. Refit new lens of different hydrophilic material (prime consideration in immune reactions)
  4. Refit new hydrophilic lens, same material as original with new design (e.g., diameter) (prime consideration in mechanical reactions)
  5. Refit new lens of different hydrophilic material and design
  6. Refit rigid gas-permeable lens
- Recheck patient with GPC history every 3 months on any lens

C. VERNAL CONJUNCTIVITIS

Refer to Vernal Keratoconjunctivitis in Chapter 4.

---

*See also Appendix 3.

†See also Appendix 4.

TABLE 3-5. CONTACT LENS MANAGEMENT IN GIANT PAPILLARY CONJUNCTIVITIS (GPC)

Management Considerations	Degree of GPC Clinical Presentation		
	Mild	**Moderate**	**Severe**
Lens wear	Continue wearing original lens	Temporarily discontinue wear	Temporarily discontinue wear
Positive Subjective and Objective response in less than 1–2 weeks			
s̄ Adjunctive therapies	Continue wearing original lens	Rewear original lens	Rewear new lens (original material and design)
c̄ Adjunctive therapies	Continue wearing original lens	Rewear original lens	Rewear new lens (new material or design)
Positive Subjective and Objective response in greater than 2 weeks			
s̄ Adjunctive therapies	Continue wearing original lens	Rewear new lens (original material and design)	Rewear new lens (new material or design)
c̄ Adjunctive therapies	Continue wear c̄ new lens (original material)	Rewear new lens (new material or design)	Rewear new lens (new material or design)
Suspected etiologies			
Immune	Opticrom and original lens	Opticrom and new material	Steroid→Opticrom and new material
Mechanical			
Hydrophilic lens	Lubrication and original lens	New lens design and lubrication	New lens design and Adjunctive therapies →lubrication
Hard lens	Lubrication and original lens	New lens design and lubrication	Discontinue lens wear
Protruding sutures	Remove sutures	Remove sutures and Adjunctive therapies	Remove sutures and Adjunctive therapies
Prosthetic eyes	Lubrication	Repolish prosthetic eye	Repolish or replace prosthetic eye

IV. Toxic and Irritative (Chronic) Conjunctivitis (Color Plate 31)

Subjective

- Common "red-eye" presentation easy to diagnose but difficult to establish primary cause as well as effective treatment
- Onset and history are always chronic and insidious
- Frequently "keeps company" with other anterior segment diseases
- Symptoms may be absent or mild to moderate nonspecific superficial irritation
- Patient usually most concerned with cosmesis
- Frequently associated with a history of a chronic irritating cause or toxic substance
  1. Some possible irritating causes
     a. Dry, arid conditions
     b. Airborne irritants (e.g., pollutants, pollen, dust)
     c. Allergens (i.e., any substance with the potential to cause a hypersensitive or immune-type reaction)
     d. Radiation (e.g., sun, reflectants, UV)
  2. Some possible toxic substances
     a. Chemicals (direct contact or fumes)
     b. Exogenous factors
        i. Bacterial toxins (especially staphylococcal exotoxins)
        ii. Viral toxins (e.g., molluscum, verrucae)
        iii. Topical medication (eyedrops or ointments), called medicamentosa
        iv. Cosmetics, soaps, perfumes
     c. Endogenous factors
        i. Internal medications
        ii. Systemic medications
        iii. Autoimmune responses

d. Morax Axenfeld *(Moraxella)* often reported as persistent (subclinical) cause
  i. Gram-negative bacteria
  ii. Produces scant, transient discharge and angular (palpebral fissure) hyperemia

- Condition reported as easily aggravated by external factors
  1. Wind
  2. Rubbing
  3. Contact lens wear

Objective

- Unilateral or bilateral, depending on primary cause
- Mild to moderate bulbar hyperemia often greater inferior
- Mixed papillary or follicular palpebral conjunctival response usually only mild to moderate in degree
  1. Predominance of one or the other based on primary cause
    a. Bacterial: greater papillary
    b. Viral: follicular
    c. Noninfectious irritants: usually papillary
    d. Noninfectious toxins: usually follicular
  2. Ultimately, combined effects over time produce mixed reactions
  3. Superior tarsus often presents greater involvement
- Never a pronounced discharge or exudates
- Frequently an angular, nasal and temporal hyperemic pattern, most prominent in the exposed palpebral fissure spaces
- Occasionally may demonstrate "phlyctenule" formation(s)
  1. Sometimes called "phlyctenular conjunctivitis"
  2. Pinkish-white epithelial nodule formed as focal reaction to localized toxin
  3. Greater in young children
  4. Sometimes subjectively uncomfortable (if densely infiltrated and secondarily inflamed)
  5. May show mild to moderate surrounding edema
  6. Usually singular lesions close to limbus
    a. May be multiple and located anywhere on bulbar conjunctiva
    b. If translimbal (onto cornea), symptoms increase and termed "phlyctenular keratoconjunctivitis"
- Infrequently, bulbar conjunctiva may keratinize (harden) producing yellow patches (xerosis or Bitot's spots)

Assessment*

- Rule out other causes of red eyes
- Rule out other forms of conjunctivitis (Table 3–4)
- Try to establish primary cause (e.g., irritant, toxin) through history and physical findings
- If no obvious primary cause from history or physical, consider nonspecific treatment plan(s) according to the following order of classic "nonspecific" diagnoses
  1. Staphylococcal toxins (look for other classic staphylococcal signs, e.g., lid problems, inferior patterns)
  2. Nonspecific allergic response
  3. Dry eye effects (with quick BUT, positive rose bengal stain: frequent corneal component)
  4. UV sensitivity (outdoor: sunlight irritant; exposure: palpebral aperture hyperemic pattern)
  5. Moraxella "angular conjunctivitis" (sometimes an associated angular blepharitis and scant discharge)

Plan†

- Treat primary cause if established
  1. Treatment plans should be appropriate for cause and should be modified based on chronicity of response
  2. Adjunctive topical steroids (in combination with primary therapeutic agents) often helpful in reducing secondary toxic, inflammatory response
  3. Avoid aggravating chronic condition or precipitating an acute response through introduction of additional toxic medications, eyedrops
- If primary cause is not established, introduce step-by-step treatment plan according to "classic causes"
  1. Explain to patient nature of "nonspecific" plan and establish understanding of "no guarantees!"
  2. Step-by-step plan
    a. Antistaphylococcal procedures (see Table 2–1) for 2 weeks
      i. Use all procedures (i.e., hygiene, hot packs, massage, scrubs, and bacitracin ointment) with or without clinical staphylococcal signs
      ii. Dosage: bid (minimum)
    b. Oral (not topical) antihistamine–decongestant for 2 weeks
    c. Lubricants 6 to 10 times daily for 2 weeks
      i. Mucomimetic agents useful
      ii. Most effective seems to be vitamin A drops
    d. Constant UV protection for 2 weeks
      i. Sunglasses outdoors (with or without bright sunlight)
      ii. UV tints or nonprescription UV protection for constant wear
    e. Ophthalmic zinc preparation for 2 weeks
      i. OTC agents effective against *Moraxella*
      ii. Dosage: qid with ointment at bedtime
    f. Tobramycin (Tobrex) or gentamicin for 2 weeks[31]
      i. Rx agents most effective against *Moraxella*

---

*See also Appendix 3.

†See also Appendix 4.

    ii. Sulfonamides also (but less) effective
    iii. Dosage: qid
  3. Steps may be combined, but positive results would not provide definitive diagnosis of primary cause

- Treatment plans on contact lens patients may be conducted with or without continued wear, depending on type of care

Follow-up

- Follow-up considerations should be based on nature of treatment plan for diagnosed primary causes
- In nonspecific step-by-step approach, recheck at 2-week intervals and add next step, when and if indicated
- Overall advice and education to patients
  1. Explain primary cause if established
  2. Counsel on measures to reduce associated aggravants
  3. Advise on potential chronicity, especially in cases of unknown cause(s)
- Suggest methods of effective self-care and maintenance
- Recommend brief periodic rechecks (should be advised for *all* chronic conditions) of ocular surface tissues at least once a year or PRN (Table 3–4)

V. Episcleritis (Color Plates 32 and 33)

A. SIMPLE FORM

Background Information

1. Episclera is connective tissue sheath between sclera and conjunctiva
2. Vascular (venules) plexus has regular, radiating pattern versus irregular, finer, movable overlying bulbar conjunctival vessels
3. May be associated with systemic disease etiologies
  a. Collagen vascular diseases (e.g., rheumatoid)
  b. Generally, causes remain unknown or idiopathic
  c. Sometimes mild trauma suggested due to common occurrence in exposed palpebral aperture(s)
4. Eighty percent of episcleritis: simple form (20 percent nodular)

Subjective

- Acute onset of signs and symptoms (sometimes as fast as minutes to hours)
- Greater in women (usually age 20 to 50) than men (age 30 to 60)
- Patient reports mild to moderate symptoms
  1. Nonspecific irritation (e.g., hot, uncomfortable)
  2. Tenderness on direct palpation to irritated site
- Frequent recurrent history of similar problem
- Vision never affected significantly
- Photophobia may be mild to moderate

Objective

- Wedge (sector) of deep injection and inflammation
  1. Usually apex of wedge toward limbus, base away
  2. Usually in interpalpebral areas (greater temporal)
  3. Deeper vessels show radiating pattern with net of irregular, overlying, finer conjunctival vessels
  4. Deeper injected vessels will not blanch with pressure (on palpation) or with mild vasoconstrictors
  5. Deeper (episcleral vessels) are immovable, while overlying conjunctival vessels move freely
- Usually unilateral but occasionally will present with bilateral inflammatory wedges
- Possible hyperlacrimation but never frank discharge
- Inflamed wedge may demonstrate diffuse infiltration or edema causing mild elevation of conjunctiva
- Deeper injection usually pinkish-purple coloration
- Anterior chamber reaction absent
- Palpebral conjunctiva and cornea remain clear

Assessment*

- Rule out other causes of "red eyes"
- Rule out common forms of conjunctivitis (Table 3–6)
- Also rule out inflamed pingueculas (painless) and phlyctenules associated with toxic conjunctivites
- Rule out scleritis
  1. Entirely separate disease category more severe and far less frequent than episcleritis
  2. Usually associated with systemic diseases
  3. Requires immediate referral for medical or ophthalmologic management (Table 3–7)

---

*See also Appendix 3.

TABLE 3-6. DIFFERENTIAL DIAGNOSIS OF EPISCLERITIS FROM CONJUNCTIVITIS

	Subjective Symptom	Injection	Discharge	Papillae or Bulbar Conjunctiva	Other Identifying Features
Episcleritis	Hot, gritty	Salmon pink	Waters occasionally	Bulbar focal hyperemia and infiltration	Wedge-shaped sectoral injection
Conjunctivitis					
Viral	Burn	Pink/purple toward plica	Tearing	Follicles	Perauricular lymph node
Allergic	Itch	Pink/purple	White stringy mucoid	Chemosis	Allergicv Hx, seasonal
Bacterial	Irritation, FB sensation	Bright red	Purulent mucopurulent	Papillae	Lids and lashes matted in AM
Phlyctenular keratoconjunc-tivitis	Corneal irritation	Localized pannus	Waters occasionally	Leash of vessels at phlycten	Phlycten invades cornea
Acne rosacea	Chronic recurring corneal irritation	Diffuse bulbar and circum-corneal	Occasional tearing or purulence	Chronic blepharocon-junctivitis	Skin lesions

(From Corcoran T, Catania L, 1986, p 544, with permission.[32])

- Rule out (by history) reported systemic disease causes reported in literature but rarely established in case presentations
  1. Rheumatoid arthritis
  2. Systemic lupus erythematosus (SLE)
  3. Giant cell arteritis
  4. Polyarteritis nodosa
  5. Sarcoidosis
  6. Herpes zoster
  7. Tuberculosis
  8. Syphilis
  9. Gout
  10. Thyrotoxicosis
- Rule out (from history) direct or indirect trauma
  1. Mechanical injury to ocular surface
  2. Chemical injury
  3. Radiation exposure
- Generally no cause will be established[32]

Plan*

- For mild cases, any treatment is optional
  1. Frequent hot packs (q3-4h for 3 to 5 days)
  2. Patient may prefer symptomatic and cosmetic relief
     a. Cold packs (for vasoconstriction)
     b. Topical vasoconstrictor (decongestant) drops
     c. Mild (1/8 percent) topical steroid (HMS, Pred Mild) (probably overkill!)
  3. Oral nonsteroidal anti-inflammatory agents (aspirin, ibuprofen) for analgesia and therapeusis (?)
- For moderate to severe (rare) simple episcleritis
  1. Same steps as for mild (above)

*See also Appendix 4.

TABLE 3-7. COMPARISON OF EPISCLERITIS AND SCLERITIS

	Subjective Symptom	Injection	Hyperemic Pattern	Cornea	Anterior Chamber	Associated with Systemic Condition
Episcleritis	Irritation, mild pain	Salmon pink	Sectoral wedge-shaped	No corneal involvement	No reaction	Low correlation with systemic tissue disease
Scleritis	Severe pain	Blue or purple	Diffuse involvement	Decreased corneal sensitivity, sclerosing stromal keratitis	Probable uveitic response with cells or flare	High correlation with systemic connective tissue disease (≈50%)

(From Corcoran T, Catania L, 1986, p 544, with permission.[32])

2. If indicated, use 1 percent prednisolone as steroid
3. Topical dosages from qid to q4h based on degree
4. Oral aspirin (3 g/day or two 5-gr tabs q4h) or ibuprofen (800 to 1600 mg/day)

- Episcleritis is one disease that occasionally will not respond to topical steroids as quickly as most
  1. Masking (eye whitening) effect may even be absent
  2. Always monitor such idiosyncratic cases closely

Follow-up

- Normal course (with or without treatment) is usually about 10 to 21 days (acute to subacute to resolution)
- Recheck patient on a weekly basis until resolved
- Advise patient at first visit of potential protracted (i.e., 10- to 21-day) course
- Advise on possible recurrences from 3-month to 3-year period
- Reschedule for annual recheck or PRN
- If more than three recurrences, recommend systemic medical workup

B. NODULAR FORM

Subjective

- Far less common than simple form
- Symptoms all similar to simple form, except more severe
- Pain present without palpation and tenderness on palpation (at site) usually greater than simple form
- Recurrent history not as frequent with nodular form
- Vision remains normal in spite of increased intensity of clinical presentation
- Photophobic response may be moderate to severe
- Systemic associations continue to be rare (as with simple form)

Objective

- All physical signs same as simple form except for increased intensity and development of a nodule

1. Nodule is an organized area of cellular infiltrate at the center of the sectorial inflamed wedge
2. Usually a single site but may be multiple
3. Frequently associated with increased edema in the immediate area and increased diffuse edema and infiltration throughout the inflamed sector

- Because of increased degree of inflammation, anterior chamber may begin to show mild secondary reaction in the form of trace cells and flare
- Cornea usually remains completely uninvolved
- Rarely, hyperemic sector may expand to involve up to 180° area and resist standard treatment for additional weeks or months
  1. Called episcleritis periodosis fugax
  2. Tends to reoccur more frequently than simple or standard nodular forms

Assessment*

- Differentiate nodular episcleritis from simple form
  1. Increased subjective and objective intensity
  2. Presence of nodule
- Remaining differential considerations same as for simple episcleritis

Plan†

- Same as for moderate to severe simple episcleritis
- Topical steroid dosages should be increased to range of q2–4h based on degree of presentation
- Rarely, in severe presentations, prolonged nonresponsive cases or periodosis fugax cases, a short course of oral steroids (prednisone) may be helpful
  1. Co-manage with internist
  2. Sometimes even with oral agents, response is slow

Follow-up

- Same as for moderate to severe simple episcleritis
- Course of nodule regression (melting) and sometimes associated signs and symptoms as well may extend into months (usually no more than 2 to 3 months) with or without continued treatment

---

*See also Appendix 3.
†See also Appendix 4.

VI. Noncorneal Ocular Surface Lesions (by Color)*

A. RED(DISH) TO DARK

1. Granuloma[33] (Color Plates 34 and 35)

---

*In alphabetical order.

Subjective

- Painless mass
- Usually insidious development
- Patient may be unaware or mildly concerned
- May have granulomas elsewhere on their body

Objective

- Variable position, size, shape, and redish color
- Most common presentation on palpebral conjunctiva
- Spongy vascularized tissue mass
- Occasional secondary surface inflammation or infection or ulceration with loose blood elements
- May be pedunculated (stalklike projection)

Assessment*

- Rule out systemic history of inflammatory or granulomatous disease (e.g., sarcoidosis)
- Frequently cause goes undiagnosed
  1. Ruptured chalazion
  2. Allergic reaction
  3. Infection (subclinical)
- Rule out mechanical causes of granuloma formation
  1. Foreign body
  2. Chronic irritant

Plan

- Usually self-limiting, self-resolving mass
- Refer for cause (e.g., systemic)
- Treat secondary superficial involvement (e.g., infection, inflammation)
- Heat therapy (compresses) useful for granuloma
- Photodocument if possible for follow-up purposes
- Consider surgical excision for cause or cosmesis

Follow-up

- Without referral and excision, recheck first presentations in 3 to 6 months
- Chronic masses should be rechecked every 6 months
- With significant changes, refer for excision

2. Hemangioma

Subjective

- Usually present congenitally or in early years
- May enlarge with age
- Cosmetically apparent and often disconcerting

Objective

- Raised broad-based bulbar conjunctival vascular tumor masses (benign)
- More frequently toward inner canthus or deep in fornices
- Reddish to darker purplish tortuous vessel masses

Assessment

- Differentiate lymphangioma (lighter color) or lymphoma (with history of lymphosarcoma)
- Rule out other red(dish) ocular surface masses

Plan

- Reassure and educate patient
- If requested (for cosmetic concern), refer to ophthalmology
  1. Excision
  2. Cautery
  3. Laser

Follow-up

- If no referral, check annually
- Advise on any changes PRN

3. Neoplasia[34]

Subjective

- Refer to "Neoplastic Considerations": Chapter 2, section III, part H

Objective

- Refer to "Neoplastic Considerations": Chapter 2, section III, part H

Assessment

- More common reddish conjunctival neoplasia
  1. Carcinomas
  2. Sarcomas
- Kaposi's sarcoma frequently associated with AIDS
  1. Hemorrhagic sarcoma
  2. Red papules and nodules on palpebral (less frequently bulbar) conjunctiva

Plan

- Suspect lesion should be referred for excision and biopsy
- Follow-up on referral to confirm care
- Refusal to accept referral advise should be carefully documented in records

Follow-up

- Excised patients with positive biopsy should be carefully instructed on possible recurrent signs
- Recheck every 6 months for 1 to 2 years (with surgeon), then annually or PRN

4. Papilloma

Subjective

- Occur most frequently in adults
- Asymptomatic

---

*See also Appendix 3.

- Development and growth can be rapid (weeks)
- Occasionally develop in multiple sites
- Usually fear or cosmetic concern

Objective

- Elevated, variable size and shape, benign epithelial tumor
- Most common at limbal juncture (transitional tissue site)
- Deeper vasculature may apear through surface
- Variable pigmentation
  1. Amelanotic (pinkish)
  2. Translucent (with vessels showing through)
  3. Moderate to heavily pigmented
- Frequently lobulated or pedunculated
- When at limbus, may give appearance of corneal involvement

Assessment*

- Rule out neoplasia
- Papilloma versus nevus or melanosis
- Rule out infectious or inflammatory associations

Plan

- Reassure and educate patient
- If suspicious or cosmetically requested, refer for excision and biopsy

Follow-up

- Without surgical referral, monitor qualitative and quantitative changes
  1. Papillomatous changes in size and shape are considered within normal limits
  2. Watch for neoplastic changes
- With surgery, continue to monitor patient every 3 to 6 months for recurrences (rather common)

5. Subconjunctival Hemorrhage† (Color Plate 36)

Subjective

- One of the most common ocular surface presentations
- Usually seen as an acute or subacute (STAT or ASAP) presentation
- Ominous, rapid-onset appearance of "blood" on the eye leads to dramatic patient concern
- Patient may or may not be able to elicit a positive history
  1. Trauma (e.g., ocular, head)
  2. Valsalva-like maneuvers
     a. Coughing
     b. Sneezing
     c. Vomiting
     d. Strangulation
     e. Constipation
     f. Seizure
  3. Systemic causes (e.g., vascular disease)
- Painless presentation

Objective

- Loose blood in the bulbar subconjunctival spaces
- Usually unilateral but could present bilaterally
- Flat sheaths of uniform red blood without vessel patterns (may show streaks as blood spreads)
- Blood accumulates more toward the limbus, where a clear space (line or ring) is usually visible as a border between the blood and cornea
- Spread of blood may occur in any direction, to any degree during the first few hours or days
- Over an average of 7 to 21 days, red color turns to orange to pink and back to clear white
- Rarely does permanent blood staining persist

Assessment*

- Rule out history of trauma
  1. Ocular
  2. Head
  3. Remote (to eyes or head)
- Rule out local inflammatory disease
  1. Hyperacute (hemorrhagic) conjunctivitis
  2. Usually produce small multiple hemorrhages
- Rule out associated systemic diseases
  1. Cardiovascular or blood dyscrasias
  2. Febrile diseases
  3. Leukemia[35]
- Other common causes
  1. Menstruation
  2. Telangiectasia (shows focal elevation within hemorrhagic area)
  3. Valsalva-like maneuvers (common)
- Idiopathic (probably most common)

Plan

- Attempt to determine cause
  1. Careful history
  2. Blood pressure
  3. Ocular examination (external and internal)
- Refer appropriately for cause, if indicated
- Reassure patient
- Advise on no need for (or effective) treatment
  1. May suggest alternate hot or cold packs to aid in reabsorption of loose blood
  2. Probably more a placebo than therapy
- Explain slow resolution (by color) over 7 to 21 days
  1. Dense blood (thick black sheaths) may take longer (3 to 6 weeks)
  2. Management remains the same

Follow-up

- Recheck at 1 week if patient (or physician) concerned

---

*See also Appendix 3.
†See also Appendix 2.

- If recurrent presentation, recheck at 3 to 6 months
- More than two recurrences within 1 year, obtain full medical workup by physician

6. Telangiectasia (Color Plate 36)

Subjective

- Asymptomatic patient (often general-examination patient)
- Patient may be concerned or completely unaware of finding
- Occurs in any age group

Objective

- Isolated, superficial, localized dilated, or convoluted blood vessel (arteriole) on bulbar conjunctival surface
- May appear as saccular-like aneurysms, berry shaped, or simple convolution
- Usually single finding but may be multiple
- More often unilateral (but could be bilateral)
- Rarely, increased prominence (and elevation) could produce secondary superficial irritation

Assessment

- Rule out any chronic superficial irritant
- Possible systemic causes
  1. Vascular disease
  2. Diabetes
  3. Collagen vascular diseases
  4. Acne rosacea
  5. Neoplasias (especially with elongated dilated vessel eminating from posterior eye)
- Idiopathic: most common

Plan

- No treatment indicated
- Reassure patient
- Document in patient's record (draw or photograph)

Follow-up

- Monitor routinely or PRN
- Patient at slightly higher risk for subconjunctival hemorrhage
  1. Produces ominous-appearing focal elevation within hemorrhagic area
  2. Previous documentation will rule out other remote causes for elevation (e.g., foreign body)

B. WHITE(ISH) TO YELLOW[36]

1. Calcium Concretions (Lithiasis)

Subjective

- Asymptomatic finding (usually during general examination)

- Occasional reports of very large concretions producing corneal irritation (rare)
- Common finding in elderly patients

Objective

- Small, white to yellowish hard spots on palpebral conjunctiva
  1. Usually about 1 to 3 mm in size
  2. Rarely larger than 5 mm
- May be single or multiple
- Common to both inferior and superior conjunctiva
- Usually flat, but may be slightly raised if large

Assessment*

- Differentiate from inclusion (lymphatic) cysts
  1. Cysts are clear or translucent to light or slit-lamp examination
  2. Solid masses are opaque to light examination
- Rule out other ocular surface lesions
- Rule out infectious or inflammatory causes (rare)

Plan

- If asymptomatic, no treatment indicated (usually)
- If irritating or disconcerting to patient, remove
  1. "Tease" out with jeweler's forceps or other instrument sharp enough to pry and lift
  2. Probable small conjunctival bleed will respond to direct pressure and self-resolve

Follow-up

- With no treatment PRN
- With removal, 5 to 7 days or PRN

2. Dermolipoma

Subjective

- Asymptomatic presentation
- Present congenitally, but may be too small for cosmetic awareness
  1. Tend to increase in size slowly
  2. First awareness or cosmetic distress may not occur until second or third decade of life
- Occasionally, infant's parent, caretaker, or pediatrician may note it initially in early childhood and report it as acquired lesion (with concern)

Objective

- Firm, elevated, distinctly yellow mass present at outer canthal (lateral) angle
  1. May be obscured (buried behind lid) in primary gaze position
  2. When eye turns inward, mass becomes visible
- Exposed surface may be perfectly smooth and clear or may contain surface appendages, including fatty tissue, glands, and hair follicles

---

*See also Appendix 2.

- Mass is slightly movable, hard to palpation, and painless
- If displaced superiorly, may be mistaken for lacrimal gland (superior temporal position); lacrimal gland usually larger and softer

Assessment

- Rule out other ocular surface lesions
- Rule out neoplasia
- Rule out cyst (versus mass)

Plan

- Reassure patient and explain nature and course
- If patient desires cosmetic removal, refer to experienced ophthalmic surgeon

Follow-up

- Without treatment, recheck annually or PRN
- With removal, routine follow-up evaluation

3. Icteric Sclera (Jaundice)

Subjective

- No associated ocular history
- Careful medical history (for liver disease)
- Cosmesis may dominate patient's concern

Objective

- Yellowing (rarely, greenish) diffuse discoloration to bilateral sclera (white of the eyes)
- Noninflammatory presentation with no associated ocular findings

Assessment

- Acute or chronic liver disease
- If undiagnosed, take careful medical history

Plan

- Recommend immediate medical examination and care if patient not actively under such care
- No treatment indicated for ocular finding

Follow-up

- Confirm medical care through phone contact with patient or physician
- Monitor (reversible) ocular finding in concert with medical care

4. Inclusion (Lymphatic) Cyst

Subjective

- Asymptomatic presentation
- Depending on position and size, may produce patient distress or cosmetic concern

Objective

- Small to moderate size (2 to 5 mm) cystic formations producing a clear to white to yellow color
- Locations are variable (in order of frequency)
  1. Deep fornices (inferior or superior)
  2. Inferior or superior palpebral conjunctiva
  3. Inner canthal caruncle and plica area
  4. Bulbar conjunctiva (greater nasalward)
- May be fluid filled (clear) or casseous (yellow)
- Frequently multiple in one or both eyes

Assessment

- Rule out other cystic ocular surface lesions
- Rule out infection, inflammation or trauma

Plan

- Treatment neither essential nor indicated
- If patient requests removal (usually cosmetic), primary drainage procedure may be attempted
  1. If fluid filled, simply lance with needle
  2. With casseous cysts, lance and massage
  3. Prophylactic antibiotic (1 ×) optional
  4. Generally, lancing puncture will close and cyst will refill within days
- Permanent removal best achieved by referral for surgical excision of entire cyst at its base

Follow-up

- Cysts are frequently recurrent (even with surgical excision), so advise and monitor postoperative patients (with surgeon)
- Advise patients on possibility of recurrences lancing or excision
- Follow up patient based on degree of presentation or within 1 week of any procedural approach

5. Keratinization (Xerosis or Bitot's Spot)

Subjective

- Asymptomatic or (rarely) mild distress
- Frequently patient cosmetically concerned
- Occasionally a history of poor or malnutrition
- Often a history of excessive exposure to UV light and dry, arid climate

Objective

- Dry, hardened, rough patch(es) on exposed areas of bulbar conjunctiva
- Granular, keratinized epithelial surface
- Rarely, a wet, frothy appearance may develop over roughened area (called Bitot's spot)

Assessment

- Possible vitamin A deficiency (avitaminosis A)
- Most often secondary to drying effects

1. Environmental
2. Mechanical
3. Exposure
4. Radiation (especially UV sunlight)
5. Allergic reactions)
- Retinoid dermatologic agents (Acutane) have been cited as aggravants

Plan

- Heavy lubrication therapy (drops or ointments every hour for relief of symptoms and reduction in tissue keratinization
  1. Mucomimetic agents helpful
  2. Most valuable therapy is vitamin A eyedrops
- Attempt to remove any aggravants or allergens
- Consider oral vitamin A supplements
- Bitot's spot(s) can be swabbed to reduce frothing effect (but without therapy, will recur)

Follow-up

- During active treatment plan, recheck every 2 to 4 weeks
- If condition worsens (with or without therapy), pursue cause aggressively and treat specifically
- Upon resolution of acute (or subacute) phase, continue vitamin A drops tid indefinitely unless primary cause completely removed
  1. Not usual because of nature of causes (e.g., UV)
  2. Recheck regularly (every 3 months) for complication

6. Lymphangiectasia (Color Plate 37)

Subjective

- Common ocular surface involvement
- Asymptomatic or (rarely) mildly uncomfortable
- Usually noted during general examination
- Occasionally patient may express concern or cosmetic distress over "bubble on white of eye"

Objective

- Variable-size and -shaped clear fluid-filled cyst on bulbar conjunctiva (greater temporalward)
  1. Usual size range from 2 to 10 mm
  2. Round or linear
- Focal or segmental dilations of fine thin-walled conjunctival lymphatic vessel(s)
- May be single or multiple sites and dilations
- Single cyst may be multilobulated
- Always clear and transparent (with slit-lamp examination

Assessment*

- Rule out other cystic ocular surface lesions
- Differentiate from inclusion (lymphatic) cyst

---

*See also Appendix 3.

1. Inclusion cyst has thicker walls, hence appears translucent (or yellowish)
2. Positioning of inclusion cysts more common nasalward and on palpebral conjunctiva

Plan

- For small asymptomatic cysts, no treatment
- For larger cysts or to allay patient concern or request
  1. Drain cyst by simple 25-gauge needle puncture (angled away from ocular surface)
  2. Gentle massage through close lid to flatten
  3. No medication necessary (tears do the job)
- Occasionally cyst(s) may drain spontaneously

Follow-up

- Best to advise, explain, and reassure patients, even those unaware of presence (they will notice it eventually and wonder whether you missed it, or worse, did not want to tell them!)
- With no treatment, follow routinely or PRN
- If drained, follow-up optional (1 week) and again in 3 to 6 months for possible reoccurrence (rare)

7. Neoplasia

Subjective

- Refer to "Neoplastic Considerations": Chapter 2, section III, part H

Objective

- Refer to "Neoplastic Considerations": Chapter 2, section III, part H

Assessment

- Rule out cystic or other solid ocular surface lesions
- Consider lymphoma in white(ish)-yellow neoplasia

Plan

- Suspect lesion should be referred for excision and biopsy
- Follow-up on referral to confirm care
- Refusal to accept referral advice should be carefully documented in records

Follow-up

- Excised patients with positive biopsy should be carefully instructed on possible recurrent signs
- Recheck every 6 months for 1 to 2 years (with surgeon), then annually or PRN

8. Pinguecula

Objective

- Common
- Frequent history of outdoor and UV exposure

- Usually asymptomatic and stable history
- Occasionally, patient will report acute onset
  1. More likely a first awareness
  2. Secondary inflammation often creates first awareness and alarm
  3. Frequent cosmetic concern

Objective

- Yellowish, slightly elevated triangular mass(es) with base toward limbus, adjacent to, but not on, corneal surface
- Found at exposed lateral areas on bulbar conjunctiva (greater nasal, but may be temporal)
- Usually bilateral presentation
- Generally free of blood vessels, but occasionally become surrounded by hyperemic injected vessels

Assessment*

- Rule out other ocular surface lesions
- Differentiate from pterygium
- Differentiate inflamed presentations
  1. From angular conjunctivitis
  2. From episcleritis

Plan

- No treatment indicated for quiet lesions
- If hyperemic, can be decongested with mild vasoconstrictors or cold packs
- Lubricants may be comforting to symptomatic patients
- Rarely done but can be excised and radiated for cosmetic purposes

Follow-up

- Because of association with sunlight (UV aggravant), UV tints and regular outdoor sunglasses may help to reduce increasing size, thickness, and color
- Routine follow-up evaluation or PRN

9. Pterygium
Refer to "Degenerations": Chapter 4, section III, part M

C. BLUE(ISH) TO BLACK
1. Axenfeld's Loops

Subjective

- No symptoms or patient concerns
- Usually noted on general external examination
- More prominent in black persons

Objective

- Blue to black ciliary nerve loops on the scleral surface
- Usually within a few millimeters of the limbus
- Diffuse on scleral surface (greater nasalward)
- May have small vessel loops (red or blue) adjacent to nerve loop

Assessment

- Rule out other darker-pigmented ocular surface lesions

Plan and Follow-up

- No treatment or special follow-up considerations

2. Blue Sclera

Subjective

- Asymptomatic presentation, usually with no patient awareness of variant
- Take careful history for possible causes in adult or patients with acquired changes
- May be parent concern in obvious presentations in young children and newborns

Objective

- Variable density, intensity, and distribution of pale to dark blue coloration to white of the eyes
- Rather common and generally normal in infants
  1. Relatively large globe size at birth versus thin scleral tunic transmits blue vascular choroid distinctly
  2. Often persists into early childhood
- Unilateral or bilateral (highly diagnostic sign)

Assessment*

- In children (and elderly) with negative history, presentation usually within normal limits
- In adults and acquired presentations, take careful systemic and developmental history
- Some systemic and developmental causes to consider
  1. Osteogenesis imperfecta
  2. Ehlers–Danlos syndrome
  3. Marfan's syndrome
  4. Paget's disease (pseudoxanthoma elasticum)
- Enlargement of globe
  1. Buphthalmos (infantile glaucoma): check IOP
  2. Keratoconus or keratoglobus: check cornea
  3. High myopia (sometimes unilateral): refract
- Pigmentations
  1. Melanosis (usually unilateral)
  2. Nevus of Ota (always unilateral)
  3. Intraocular foreign body (almost always unilateral)
  4. Medicamentosa

---

*See also Appendix 3.

Plan

- Refer appropriately for cause
- Reassure and explain phenomenon to parents of children and elderly, with thinning sclera effect

Follow-up

- Routine for normal patients
- For children or suspicious presentations, consider general overall recheck within 6 to 12 months

3. Hyaline Plaques (Focal Scleral Translucent Spots)

Subjective

- Common in older patients
- No associated symptoms or positive history
- Occasionally may produce patient concern

Objective

- Small (approximately 2 to 4 mm) translucent, grayish, flat round spots on the anterior scleral surface
- Multiple, bilateral and diffusely arranged

Assessment

- Rule out any severe collagen vascular diseases
- Rule out other ocular surface lesions
- Consider scleromalacia perforans
  1. Rare scleral melting disease in elderly
  2. Associated with pain and rheumatoid disease

Plan

- Reassure patient
- No treatment indicated

Follow-up

- Recheck annually (as part of routine examination) or PRN

4. Melanosis (Congenital Form) (Color Plate 38)

a. Conjunctival

Subjective

- Present at birth or shortly thereafter
- Greater in dark or black races
- May increase with age

Objective

- Flat pigmented patches, usually at limbus
- Variable size and shape
- Grayish brown to black coloration

Assessment*

- Differentiate from deeper, blueish, diffuse congenital scleral melanosis
- Rule out choroidal involvement (internal)

Plan

- Reassure patient or parent
- No treatment indicated

Follow-up

- Recheck annually during childhood or PRN
- Advise patient on slight long-range risk of melanoma (instruct on reporting changes in any pigmented lesions on body)

b. Scleral (Congenital Melanosis Oculi)

Subjective

- Unilateral congenital presentation
- Possible autosomal-dominant trait (i.e., 50 percent or more of immediate family shows signs)

Objective

- Deep (scleral or episcleral) blueish coloration
- Associated dark brown iris (unilateral)
- Increased choroidal pigmentation producing darker appearance to ipsilateral fundus
- Periorbital skin on affected side usually darker than opposite side
- If pigment distribution over C-V (cranial nerve 5) areas (forehead through cheek region), condition is called Nevus of Ota or oculodermomelanocytosis (much greater in Oriental race)

Assessment*

- Differentiate from congenital conjunctival melanosis
- Rule out blue scleral causes

Plan

- No treatment indicated
- Careful counseling necessary (especially in Caucasian presentations) regarding risks
  1. For malignant melanoma (choroid or body)
  2. For secondary glaucoma

Follow-up

- Annually or PRN
- Always be conscious of associated risks

---

*See also Appendices 2 and 3.

5. Melanosis (Acquired Form)*

Subjective

- Appears between 30 to 40 years of age
- Asymptomatic presentation
- Greater in males than females
- Patient generally concerned and apprehensive

Objective

- Spontaneous development of irregular, diffuse, flat patches of grayish-black bulbar conjunctival pigmentation
- May extend in more advanced cases onto palpebral conjunctiva
- Intensity and geography of pigmentation increase and diminish over 1 to 3 years, occasionally with complete disappearance

Assessment

- Differentiate from cancerous melanoma
- Rule out history of melanoma (or suspicious pigmented lesions, i.e., nevi) elsewhere on body or choroid
- Appearance can be secondary to dermatologic medications (e.g., monobenzone for vitiligo)

Plan

- Advise patient and reassure and educate
- Manage closely during active changes in pigmentation: every 3 months or PRN
- If any suspicious changes occur (e.g., erosion, elevation) refer for biopsy

Follow-up

- Fifteen to 17 percent of benign or precancerous melanosis converts to cancer (melanoma) within 30 years
- Higher percentage converts to choroidal melanoma than to melanoma elsewhere on body
- Mortality of choroidal melanoma is much less than melanoma elsewhere, but is still a threat!

6. Neoplasia

Subjective

- Refer to "Neoplastic Considerations": Chapter 2, section III, part H

Objective

- Refer to "Neoplastic Considerations": Chapter 2, section III, part H

---

*Benign or precancerous melanosis.

Assessment

- Rule out nevus
- Melanoma is a rare but high morbity and mortality cancer

Plan

- Suspect lesion should be referred for excision and biopsy
- Follow-up on referral to confirm care
- Refusal to accept referral advice should be carefully documented in records

Follow-up

- Excised patients with positive biopsy should be carefully instructed on possible recurrent signs
- Recheck every 6 months for 1 to 2 years (with surgeon), then annually or PRN

7. Nevus

Subjective

- Usually congenital or develop early in life
- Fairly common pigmented lesion
- Always asymptomatic, except for cosmetic distress
- Greater frequency at inner canthus

Objective

- Smooth, flat surface lesion with well-demarcated pigmented edges
- May have variable degrees and intensity of pigment ranging from negligible (amelanotic) to deep and dark
- Pigmentation may increase significantly during puberty and other hormonal changes
- Usually superficial (junctional) type on bulbar or palpebral conjunctiva with or without slight elevation
- Occasionally may show cystic type changes

Assessment

- Rule out other pigmented ocular surface lesions
- Rule out neoplastic changes

Plan

- If suspicious enough, refer for excisional biopsy
- Reassure and advise patient
- If referral not indicated, photodocument if possible or diagram and measure carefully

Follow-up

- Recall schedule
  1. Three months for first presentations
  2. Every 6 to 12 months routinely
  3. PRN

- Compare for qualitative and quantitative change at each follow-up visit
- If suspicious changes, obtain oculodermatologic consultation

8. Pigmentations

Subjective

- Positive history of contributory cause
  1. Exogenous (e.g., metal particles, eyedrops)
  2. Endogenous (e.g., disease, genetics)
  3. Medicamentosa
  4. Makeup
- Quiet, non-inflamed, painless presentations

Objective

- Argyrosis (caused by silver), most common
  1. Greatest effect in fornices as black line(s) or generalized graying of tissues
  2. May show pigment spot(s) on bulbar conjunctiva (greater at inner canthus)
- Medicines (topical and systemic)
  1. Adrenalin: brownish conjunctival cysts
  2. Epinephrine (topical ophthalmic forms): blackish particles
  3. Mercury: blueish gray (lids and conjunctiva)
  4. Other offending metals: gold, iron
- Makeup, primarily mascara (carbon black)
- Ochronosis is an acquired pigmentation (blueish or black deposits and tissue discoloration) secondary to recessive traits associated with metabolic involvement (alkaptonuria)
  1. Greater at extraocular muscle (EOM) insertion areas
  2. Also diffuse changes
  3. Patient may be suffering advanced osteoarthritis
  4. Pigment changes also seen on skin, ears

Assessment*

- Attempt to determine cause by careful history
- Rule out other pigmented lesions

*See also Appendix 2.

Plan

- Remove cause, if established
- Reassure, educate, and advise patient

Follow-up

- If cause not determined, monitor for any changes
- Counsel patient on possible causes
- Routine follow-up or PRN

9. Staphyloma

Subjective

- Relatively uncommon
- Usually developing in older patients with other ocular or systemic problems

Objective

- Bulging of uveal tissue through thinning sclera
- Dark blue (uvea) appearance to raised ectatic area
- May be circumferential (around cornea) or patchy
- Frequently associated with high myopia and posterior staphyloma

Assessment

- Rule out elevated pigmented (blue) lesions
- Carefully assess ocular, visual and systemic conditions and etiologies

Plan

- Refer appropriately for cause
- Attempt to ameliorate any associated visual or ocular conditions

Follow-up

- Monitor closely (every 3 months) for insidious advancement or complications
- Carefully instruct patient on preventive eye care and signs and symptoms of infections, inflammation, and so forth

VII. Injuries

A. BURNS

Chemical, thermal, radiation, and other burns to the ocular surface should always be treated as emergency keratoconjunctival conditions (i.e., assume corneal involvement) and are covered in detail in Chapter 4

B. FOREIGN BODIES

Subjective

- History of foreign material in eye
- Mild to moderate irritation (especially if cornea is secondarily involved)

Objective

- Palpebral conjunctival foreign bodies on tarsus
- Bulbar conjunctival foreign bodies imbed in the superficial conjunctival tissue (usually in areas of palpebral fissures)
- Immediate surrounding and diffuse hyperemia develops rapidly
- Occasionally as associated subconjunctival hemorrhage will appear
- If foreign body present for a prolonged period, a spongy vascularized mass (foreign body granuloma) may develop

Assessment

- Rule out corneal involvement
- Rule out penetrating or perforating intraocular involvement
    1. Nature of entry (i.e., high velocity projectile)
    2. Perform careful external and internal ocular examination
- Consider soft tissue (globe) x-ray or ultrasound evaluation

Plan

- Topical anesthesia for examination
- Remove foreign material from conjunctival tissue
    1. Lavage vigorously
    2. Swab with cotton-tip applicator
    3. Remove embedded particles with sharp instrument (e.g., needle, jeweler's forceps, spud)
- Irrigate copiously after removal
- Prophylax with broad-spectrum antibiotic 1 × optional or irrigation tid for 48 hours
- Reassure regarding secondary subconjunctival blood (iatrogenic if removed by sharp instrument)

Follow-up

- Recheck in 3 to 5 days or PRN
- If irritation persists, recheck for additional foreign material (frequent with granular or particular material or fiberglass)

C. LACERATION (Color Plate 39)

Subjective

- History of lacerating or abrading injury
- Usually mild irritation
- Patient gravely concerned by "bloody" appearance

Objective

- Relatively dramatic hemorrhagic response on bulbar conjunctival surface
- Conjunctiva becomes edematous and usually folds upon itself under traction exerted toward the outer canthus
- Full-thickness lacerations produce pure white (bare sclera) appearance at site of wound with excess surrounding tissue edema and blood
- Occasionally, associated laceration of episclera will produce a thickened white loose flap

Assessment

- Rule out corneal involvement
- Rule out penetration or perforation
- Check carefully for any foreign material

Plan*

- Topical anesthesia for examination
- Lavage tissue copiously
- Topical antibiotic (e.g., Polysporin) q4–6h for minimum 5 to 7 days or until significant healing begins
- Sutures not needed for conjunctival laceration alone[37]
- If episclera also involved (white flap), consider lid effect during blink
    1. If flap reduced and flattened during blink, no sutures indicated
    2. If flap elevated and rolled with each blink, may need suture repair
- Warm packs and continued irrigation (tid) will promote healing and insure asepsis

Follow-up

- Recheck in 48 to 72 hours to rule out complications and measure progress (probably minimal)
- Recheck in 5 to 7 days and subsequently every 5 to 7 days until completely healed (usually about 2 to 4 weeks)
- Monitor for any secondary infection or adverse ocular tissue effects: rare (e.g., fibrosis.)

---

*See also Appendix 4.

VIII. Self-assessment Questions

1. All of the following objective signs are directly associated with bacterial conjunctivitis, *except:*
    a. Mucopurulent discharge
    b. "Meaty red" bulbar hyperemia
    c. Slow, insidious course
    d. Papillary changes
2. Unilateral bacterial conjunctivitis in a 3-year-old child presenting with venous congestion (blueish preseptal cellulitis)

of the ipsilateral lid, suggests what organism?

  a. *Hemophilis influenzae*
  b. *Gonococcus*
  c. *Staphylococcus*
  d. *Streptococcus*

3. Chronic angular conjunctivitis caused by *Moraxella* is responsive to all of the following, *except:*

  a. Bacitracin
  b. Gentamicin
  c. Tobramycin
  d. Zinc sulfate

4. All of the following are typical objective diagnostic indicators for viral conjunctivitis, *except:*

  a. "Meaty red" bulbar hyperemia
  b. Follicular changes
  c. Tearing
  d. Preauricular lymphadenopathy

5. Which of the following pairings of associated conjunctival discharge and probable etiology are *incorrect?*

  a. Mucopurulence and bacterial
  b. Mucoid (white, stringy) and viral
  c. Tearing and viral
  d. No discharge and irritative or toxic

6. Among the following treatment modalities for allergic conjunctivitis, which represents a *cure?*

  a. Cold packs
  b. Antihistamines–decongestants
  c. Steroids
  d. Remove allergen

7. Appropriate therapy for acute bacterial conjunctivitis includes each of the following, *except:*

  a. Warm packs
  b. Irrigation
  c. Topical anti-infective agents
  d. Lubricants

8. Appropriate therapy for viral conjunctivitis includes each of the following, *except:*

  a. Lubricants
  b. Antiviral agents
  c. Irrigation
  d. Warm or cold packs

9. Appropriate therapy for allergic conjunctivitis includes each of the following steps, *except:*

  a. Cold packs
  b. Topical and oral antihistamines–decongestants
  c. Lubricants
  d. Steroids

10. The most significant consideration in treating toxic or irritative conjunctivitis is to:

  a. Determine primary cause
  b. Treat each sign separately
  c. Monitor recurrence rates
  d. Evaluate family history

11. Each of the following sign and symptoms are diagnostic for episcleritis, *except:*

  a. Deep episcleral injection
  b. Mild to moderate pain
  c. Sector injection
  d. Mucoid discharge

12. Unilateral facial pigmentation associated with ipsilateral blue sclera (Nevus of Ota) is most frequently found in:

  a. Caucasians
  b. Orientals
  c. Blacks
  d. Equal distribution

13. Acquired benign or precancerous ocular melanosis usually presents in what age range?

  a. 10 to 20 years old
  b. 30 to 40 years old
  c. 50 to 60 years old

14. Appropriate primary care for scleritis is:

  a. Immediate referral
  b. Treat as granulomatous uveits
  c. Monitor closely during self-resolution
  d. Initiate topical therapy

15. Treatment for subconjunctival hemorrhage includes any of the following, *except:*

  a. Hot packs
  b. Cold packs
  c. Topical steroids
  d. Self-resolution

16. A scleral condition requiring medical referral would be:

  a. Icteric sclera
  b. Blue sclera
  c. Hyaline plaques
  d. Staphyloma

17. The most common site for a conjunctival dermolipoma is:

  a. Inferior
  b. Superior
  c. Inner canthus
  d. Outer canthus

18. Hyaline plaques found on the sclera are caused by:

  a. Vessel loops
  b. Nerve loops
  c. Focal thinnings
  d. Pigmentation

19. Keratinization (xerosis or Bitot's spot) may be caused by any of the following, *except:*
   a. Vitamin A deficiency
   b. Vitamin B deficiency
   c. Drying
   d. Aging
20. Treatment for a conjunctival laceration is:
   a. Self-resolution
   b. Topical steroids
   c. Oral steroids
   d. Surgical repair

For answers, refer to Appendix 6

REFERENCES

1. McGill JI: Bacterial conjunctivitis. Trans Ophthalmol Soc UK 105:37, 1986
2. Fraunfelder, Hanna: Trends in topical ocular medication. Ann Ophthalmol 10:85, 1978
3. Fraunfelder, Hanna: Entrapment of ophthalmic ointment in the cornea. Am Ophthalmol 76:475, 1973
4. Norn MS: Role of the vehicle in local treatment of the eye, Acta Ophthalmol (Copenh) 42:727, 1964
5. Norn MS: Eyelid ointment penetrating into conjunctival sac. Acta Ophthalmol (Copenh) 50:206, 1972
6. Wallace, Hanna, Boozman F, et al: New application of ophthalmic ointments. JAMA 233:418, 1975
7. Jawetz E: Polymyxin, neomycin, bacitracin. Antibiot Monog 5. 1956
8. Physician's Desk Reference. Oradeli, N.J., Medical Economics, 1986
9. Personal communications with Burroughs Wellcome, Inc. 1984
10. Berkow R (ed): The Merck Manual, ed 14. Rahway, N.J., Merck Sharp & Dohme Research Laboratories, 1982
11. Moses RA (ed): Adler's Physiology of the Eye. Clinical Application, ed 7. St. Louis, Mo., C.V. Mosby, 1981
12. Bowman FW, et al: Survey of microbial contamination of ophthalmic ointments. Pharmaceut Sci 61:532, 1972
13. Vander Wyck RW, Granston CE: A bacteriological study of ophthalmic ointments. J Am Pharm Assoc 47:193, 1958
14. Klein M, Millwood E.G: On the sterility of eye ointments. Br J Ophthalmol 48:285, 1964
15. Schwartz TW: Sterile ointments and preservatives. Am Perfumer Cosmet J 86:39, 1971
16. Allansmith MR: Defense of the ocular surface. Int Ophthalmol Clin 19:2, 1979
17. Sen DK, Sain GS: Biological variations of lysozyme concentrations in the tear fluid of healthy persons. Br J Ophthalmol 70:246, 1986
18. Holly FJ, Lemp MA: Tear Physiology and dry eyes. Surv Ophthalmol 22(2):69, 1977
19. Mullen C, Shepherd W, Labovitz J: Ophthalmic preservatives and vehicles. Surv Ophthalmol 17:469, 1973
20. Osol A, Chase GD, Gennaro AR, et al: Remington's Pharmaceutical Sciences, ed 16. Easton, Penn., Mack Publishing Co., 1980
21. Robin JS, Ellis PP: Ophthalmic ointments. Surv Ophthalmol 22:335, 1978
22. Roth SH: Drug use, the package insert, and the practice of medicine. Arch Intern Med 142:871, 1982
23. Casser L, Catania L: An internal "reservoir" delivery method using non-ophthalmic, OTC, anti-infective ointments in the treatment of superficial eye disease. (abst) Am Acad Optom 60:10:46, 1983
24. Archer JD: The FDA does not approve uses of drugs. JAMA 252:1054, 1984
25. McGill JI: Bacterial conjunctivitis. Trans Ophthalmol Soc UK 105:37, 1986
26. Stenson S, Newman R, Fedukowicz H: Laboratory studies in acute conjunctivitis. Arch Ophthalmol 100:1275, 1982
27. Friedlander MH, Okumoto M, Kelley J: Diagnosis of allergic conjunctivitis. Arch Ophthalmol 102:1198, 1984
28. Allansmith MR, Korb DR, Greiner JV: Giant papillary conjunctivitis in contact lens wearers. Am J Ophthalmol 83:697, 1977
29. Adler RJ, Wenderoth FA: Sodium cromolyn eyedrops in allergic soft lens users. Contact Lens Forum 11:36, 1986
30. Abelson MB, Butrus SI, Weston JH: Aspirin therapy in vernal conjunctivitis. Am J Ophthalmol 95:502, 1983
31. Kowalski MS, Harwick MD: Incidence of moraxella conjunctival infection. Am J Ophthalmol 101:437, 1986
32. Corcoran TJ, Catania LJ: Management of episcleritis. J Am Optom Assoc 57:544 1986
33. Jennings BJ: Pyogenic granulomas. J Am Optom Assoc 58:664, 1987
34. Grossniklaus ME, Green WR, Luckenback M, et al: Conjunctival lesions in adults: A clinical and histopatholic review. Cornea 6:78, 1987
35. Kincaid MC, Green WL: Ocular and orbital movement in leukemia. Surv Ophthalmol 27:4:211, 1983
36. Panda A, et al: Cystic lesions of the conjunctiva. Am Ophthalmol 19:60, 1987
37. Casser-Locke L: Conjunctival abrasions and lacerations. J Am Optom Assoc 58:488, 1987

ANNOTATED REFERENCES

Catania LJ: "Primary care treatment procedures for the eyelids, in "Videocare" (Videocassette series-2A and 2B), Dresher, Primary Eyecare, Inc., 1986 Video presentations on procedures used for eyelid and ocular surface care. Comprehensive description and demonstration of "reservoir technique" for doctor and patient.

Donaldson DD: Atlas of External Diseases of the Eye, vol. I–V. St. Louis, CV Mosby, 1968
Comprehensive black-and-white atlas of major conditions of the anterior segment. Concentration on the ocular surface abnormalities, with brief descriptions and case reports.

Duane DD, Jaeger EA (ed): Clinical Ophthalmology, vol IV: External Disease. Philadelphia, Harper & Row, 1987
Chapters on standard approaches and new methods of care regarding conjunctival, and sclera and episcleral disorders.

Duke-Elder WS: Diseases of the Outer Eye; Systems of Ophthalmology, vol VIII, pt 1. St. Louis, CV Mosby, 1976
Most comprehensive work on all congenital, developmental, anomalous, and disease entities of the conjunctiva, sclera, and episclera.

Fedukowicz MB: "External infections of the eye, ed 3. E. Norwalk, CT, Appleton-Century-Crofts, 1985
Comprehensive descriptions of common infections and inflammations affecting the ocular surface. Good presentations on various forms of conjunctivitis.

4

Diagnoses of the Cornea

Chapter Outline

I. Congenital Abnormalities

A. MEGALOCORNEA

1. A visible horizontal iris diameter of 13 mm or greater
2. Ninety percent in males
3. Usually bilateral
4. Often high refractive errors, especially astigmia
   a. May cause reduced best correctable visions
5. Occasional iridodonesis (tremulous, unstable iris)
6. Most important management consideration is intraocular pressure (IOP) monitoring
   a. Increased risk of elevated IOP
   b. May occur congenitally or insidiously at any age
   c. Monitor IOP every 3 to 6 months under 5 to 6 years of age and annually thereafter (for lifetime)
   d. Increased IOPs (usually difficult to manage) should be referred to glaucoma specialist
7. All other findings can be managed routinely

B. MICROCORNEA

1. Visible horizontal iris diameter of 10 mm or less
2. Often associated with systemic or ocular syndrome(s)
   a. May be part of a microphthalmic syndrome
   b. Consider systemic relationship in "funny looking kids" (FLK) syndromes
   c. If in doubt, refer for pediatric evaluation
3. Associated findings and considerations
   a. High refractive errors
   b. About a 20 percent risk of increased IOP by adulthood (less than megalocornea risk)
   c. Anterior chamber syndromes

C. SCLEROCORNEA (Fig. 4–1)

1. A bilateral, superior prominence of scleral tissue into the corneal zone
   a. Occasionally, inferior involvement produces truncated corneal appearance
   b. Least likely is 360° involvement producing the appearance of microcornea
2. Sometimes considered mild stage of anterior chamber syndrome (Fig. 4–2)
3. Superficial scleral vessels create prominent limbal arcades mimicking neovascularization
   a. Arcades anastomose, hence not neovascular
   b. Also, blood cells usually traceable in and out of corneal zone

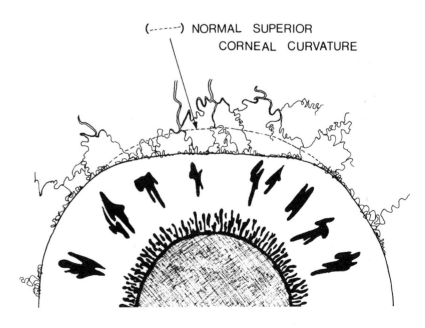

(-------) NORMAL SUPERIOR
CORNEAL CURVATURE

Figure 4–1.
Sclerocornea

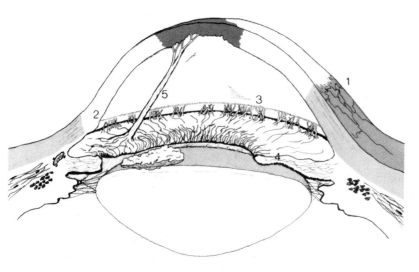

Figure 4–2.
Anterior chamber (cleavage) syndromes. **1.** Sclerocornea. **2.** Posterior embryotoxon. **3.** Axenfeld's anomaly. **4.** Rieger's anomaly. **5.** Peter's anomaly. *(Adapted from Reese, Ellsworth: The anterior chamber cleavage syndrome. Arch Opthalmol 75:307, 1966, with permission.)*

4. Other associated findings and considerations
   a. Flat corneas (cornea plana)
   b. High refractive errors
   c. Other anterior chamber syndrome signs: monitor IOP annually
   d. Consider systemic syndromes (e.g., FLK)
5. Always assess and photograph or diagram sclerocornea in general examinations and especially in prefit contact lens evaluations
   a. Do not consider it a contraindication for lens
   b. Try to avoid chronic edge insult to area by fitting small diameter rigid gas permeable (RGP) or large soft contact lens

D. ANTERIOR CHAMBER (CLEAVAGE) SYNDROMES (Fig. 4–2)

1. Synonyms
   a. Anterior angle syndromes
   b. Mesodermal dysgenesis syndromes
   c. Goniodysgenesis syndromes
   d. Iridocorneal (mesodermal) syndromes
   e. Axenfeld–Rieger (A–R) syndrome (newest title)[1]
2. New research suggests an arrest in neural crest cell development (rather than mesodermal dysgenesis) in the third trimester of pregnancy
   a. New theory accounts for the dental, facial, systemic manifestations and increased A–R syndrome glaucoma risks
   b. New theory creates differential between A–R (neural crest) syndromes and iridocorneal endothelial (ICE) syndromes (true mesodermal abnormalities) with decreased glaucoma risk
3. A–R syndrome clinical findings follow a graduating or "stepladder" diagnostic approach[2]
   a. Sclerocornea may or may not be an early or mild finding
   b. Posterior embryotoxon
      i. Exaggerated, thickened, prominent Schwalbe's line (or ring), usually an invisible demarcation line between trabeculum and posterior cornea
      ii. Partial or complete bilateral ring
      iii. Greater at 3 and 9 o'clock positions
      iv. Frequently visible on gross externals
      v. Slit-lamp examination reveals it to be on posterior cornea versus anterior Bowman's layer
      vi. Best evaluation is by gonioscopy
      vii. Risk of glaucoma is low, but monitor IOP biannually (even in children with signs)
   c. Axenfeld's anomaly or syndrome[3] (Color Plate 40)
      i. Posterior embryotoxon (plus)
      ii. Prominent iris processes attached to Schwalbe's line (usually abundant)

iii. Rarely, pupil abnormalities (e.g., corectopia, dyscoria)
iv. Prominent iris sphincter muscle (especially on dilation)
v. Bilateral gonioscopy and diagramming should be done biannually
vi. Glaucoma risk from 25 to 50 percent
vii. IOP can rise anytime during life
viii. Monitor IOP annually
ix. Normal IOP: Axenfeld's anomaly
x. Elevated IOP: Axenfeld's syndrome
xi. Associated glaucoma resistant to therapy, so try to refer to a glaucoma specialist

d. Rieger's anomaly or syndrome (Color Plate 41)
 i. Axenfeld's findings (plus)
 ii. Iris hypoplasia (i.e., shallow crypts, furrows, and thinned iris stroma)
 iii. Sphincter muscle prominent with multiple pupillary defects and distortions
 iv. Often other associated ocular problems (e.g., strabismus, corneal defects)

v. Glaucoma risk from 50 to 75 percent
vi. IOP can rise anytime during life
vii. Monitor IOP every 6 to 12 months
viii. Anomaly: eye findings only
ix. Syndrome: eye findings plus the following:
 • Lower facial abnormalities, including maxillary hypoplasia, flattened nose, and mouth and dental malformations (FLK)
 • Other systemic malformations and disorders involving hands, feet, spine, heart, hearing, and occasional mental retardation
e. Peter's anomaly (no longer considered A–R syndrome finding)

4. Differential diagnostic considerations (uncommon mesodermal and other abnormalities)* to rule out (Table 4–1)
 a. Peter's anomaly or syndrome
  i. Congenital iris hypoplasia
  ii. Iris strands to posterior cornea, causing posterior keratoconus and leucoma
  iii. Occasional anterior polar cataract

---

*See also Appendices 2 and 3.

TABLE 4–1. CONSIDERATIONS IN ANTERIOR CHAMBER ABNORMALITIES

Differential Considerations	A–R Syndromes		Mesodermal Dysgenesis Syndromes		
	Axenfeld's	Rieger's	Peter's	PPD[a]	ICE[b]
Age of onset	Congenital	Congenital	Congenital	Congenital or early years	Adolescence
Sex prediliction	Equal distribution	Equal distribution	Equal distribution	Equal distribution	Females
Inheritance pattern	Autosomal dominant	Autosomal dominant	Variable	Usually autosomal dominant	Variable
Laterality	Bilateral	Bilateral	80% Bilateral	Bilateral	Unilateral
Posterior embryotoxon	Present	Present	Absent	Absent	Absent
Iris strands (anterior synchiae)	Variable	Prominent	To central cornea	Occasional	Variable
Iris or pupil abnormalities	None	Prominent	Variable	Occasional	Prominent
Corneal involvement	None	None	Central Posterior Keratoconus	Posterior cornea	Edema occasional posterior
Systemic manifestations	Rare	Facial, dental, systemic	None	None	None
Glaucoma risk	25–50%	50–75%	50%	<25%	≈25%

[a]Posterior Polymorphous Dystrophy
[b]Iridocorneal Endothelial (Syndrome).

iv. Glaucoma risk about 50 percent (= syndrome)

v. Child requires early keratoplasty

vi. No systemic manifestations

b. Posterior polymorphous dystrophy (PPD)

i. Occasional iris involvements similar to A–R syndromes

ii. Glaucoma risk less than 25 percent

iii. No systemic manifestations

c. ICE syndromes

i. Chandler's syndrome (iris atrophy, pupil anomalies, corneal edema, and glaucoma)

ii. Progressive (essential) iris atrophy

iii. Cogan–Reese syndrome (Chandler's plus iris nevi and ectropion uveae)

iv. Posterior embryotoxin never present

v. Glaucoma risk about 25 percent

vi. No systemic manifestations

E. OTHERS (CONGENITAL ABNORMALITIES) (Color Plate 42)

1. Congenital glaucoma

a. Central corneal haze

b. Descemet's and endothelial folds and tears (Haab's striae)

c. Buphthalmos (enlarged globe)

d. If present at birth, medical–surgical prognosis poor

e. If acquired in early months or years (infantile glaucoma), better prognosis

2. Birth trauma

a. Epithelial edema

b. Vertically oriented ruptures in Descemet's

c. Findings usually greater in the left eye, owing to common left–occiput–anterior position

3. Numerous other corneal abnormalities related to congenital ocular and systemic syndromes (see Chapter 6)

II. Dystrophies

Background Information[4,5]

A. Most corneal dystrophies are relatively rare and seen infrequently in primary care practice

B. Generally diagnosed during routine (asymptomatic) slit-lamp examination (often first diagnosis in children)

C. Standard clinical characteristics of corneal dystrophy

1. Autosomal-dominant hereditary pattern

a. This means that 50 percent or more of family will show similar findings

b. Usually equal sex distribution

c. Variable penetration (frequency) and severity (expressivity)

d. Good clinical care dictates seeing other family members when evaluating dystrophies

2. No associated systemic disease history

a. Infectious or inflammatory conditions

b. Syndromes and congenital abnormalities

3. No primary ocular disease history

a. Acute or chronic ocular history must be ruled out before definitive diagnosis of dystrophy (e.g., herpetic, uveitis)

b. Rule out history of corneal scarring (from old trauma) mimicking dystrophic changes

4. Usual onset of findings by age 20

a. Dystrophy tends to present during the first or second decade of life

b. Mostly a first diagnosis in children

c. Major exception: Fuchs' endothelial dystrophy

5. Bilateral condition

a. No exceptions to this rule

b. Findings in second eye may be subtle

c. Second eye may advance slower or may arrest sooner than first

6. Slowly progressive changes

a. Dystrophy never presents suddenly or acutely

i. Complications may cause acute reactions

ii. Generally, dystrophic findings are slow and insidious in their progress

b. Changes usually start early, develop over years, and stabilize by 20 to 30 years of age

c. Changes after age 40 are usually degenerations (exception: Fuchs' endothelial dystrophy)

7. Generally centrally located findings
   a. Many exceptions to this rule (see specific dystrophies and Table 4–2)
   b. Some exceptions start centrally and then spread to periphery

8. Primary involvement of single corneal layer
   a. This is the most important clinical characteristic of dystrophy
      i. Used to classify the many types
      ii. Useful in simplifying diagnostic workup
   b. Break down cornea to major layers
      i. Epithelial
      ii. Bowman's
      iii. Stroma (90 percent thickness of cornea, thus, further subdivided)
         • Anterior
         • Full thickness
         • Deep (posterior)
      iv. Posterior (Descemet's and endothelium)
   c. Step-by-step diagnostic strategy
      i. Confirm other standard clinical characteristics of corneal dystrophy
      ii. Determine major layer of involvement
      iii. Consider the two to four dystrophies affecting that layer (Table 4–2)
      iv. Compare the lesions your finding to the description of the two to four types
      v. One dystrophy will fit the characteristics you are observing more than the others, usually rather obviously (each dystrophy having relatively distinct lesions and patterns)
      vi. Consider the course and prognosis of the dystrophy you choose and
         • Manage patient accordingly
         • Schedule other family members for slit-lamp examination
         • Advise and counsel the patient (family)
         • If prognosis is poor or clinical findings (expressivity) and vision loss are substantial, recommend genetic counseling

Clinical Conditions

A. EPITHELIAL LAYER DYSTROPHIES

1. Epithelial basement membrane dystrophy
   a. Also called map–dot–fingerprint dystrophy
   b. Separate description in Section V of this chapter, "Epithelial Basement Membrane Disorders"

2. Meesman's juvenile epithelial dystrophy
   a. Clinical features
      i. Epithelial, cyst-like vesicles
      ii. Seen best under indirect retroillumination
   b. Exceptions to standard rules for dystrophy: extends to limbus
   c. Potential complications
      i. Irregular astigmatisms
      ii. Mild epithelial erosions (after age 40)
      iii. Vision reduction
   d. Management
      i. Routine follow (every 1 to 2 years) or PRN
      ii. Treat symptoms
   e. Prognosis: excellent

B. BOWMAN'S LAYER DYSTROPHIES

1. Reis–Buckler's (ring-shaped) dystrophy
   a. Clinical features
      i. Irregular "fishnet" swirls
      ii. Superficial stromal haze
   b. Exceptions to standard rules for dystrophy: none
   c. Potential complications
      i. Painful, recurrent epithelial erosions usually decreasing by age 30
      ii. Anterior stromal opacification
   d. Management
      i. Erosion therapy
      ii. Keratoplasty
   e. Prognosis: guarded

2. Anterior mosaic dystrophy (anterior crocodile shagreen)
   a. Clinical features
      i. Central gray polygonal opacities with clear spaces
      ii. Resembles crocodile skin
      iii. Blanches with limbal pressure (returns on removal)
   b. Exceptions to standard rules for dystrophy
      i. None
      ii. Transient findings associated with ocular surface pressure (e.g., con-

TABLE 4–2. CLINICAL HIGHLIGHTS OF CORNEAL DYSTROPHIES

Primary Layer	Specific Dystrophy	Autosomal Dominant	No Systemic Disease	No Ocular Disease	Onset By Age 20	Bilateral	Slowly Progressive	Central	Single Layer	Visual	Epithelial	Stromal	Other[a]	Possible Keratoplasty	For Symptoms	For Edema	Genetic Counseling	Excellent	Good	Guarded	Poor
		Exceptions to Standard Clinical Characteristics of Dystrophy								*Secondary Complications*				*Management Considerations*				*General Prognosis*			
Epithelium	EBMD				✓	✓				✓					✓	✓			✓		
	Messman's														✓			✓			
Bowman's	Reis–Buck							✓		✓		✓		✓	✓		✓			✓	
	Anterior Mosaic					✓												✓			
Anterior Stromal	Granular (Groenouw's I)							✓		✓		✓		✓					✓		
	Lattice							✓		✓	✓			✓	✓		✓			✓	
	Central Crystalline		✓					✓		✓			1						✓		
Full Stromal	Macular (Groenouw's II)	✓						✓	✓	✓	✓			✓	✓	✓	✓			✓	
	Fleck												2								
Deep Stromal	Central Cloudy							✓	✓									✓			
	Posterior-Amorphous							✓		✓					✓			✓			
Posterior Cornea	Pre-Descemet	✓			✓			✓					3				✓	✓			
	Fuchs'	?			✓			✓		✓	✓	✓	4	✓	✓	✓	✓			✓	
	Posterior-Polymorphous						✓	✓		✓	✓	✓			✓	✓	✓		✓		
	Congenital Hereditary	✓					✓	✓		✓	✓	✓		✓	✓	✓	✓				✓

[a] 1, cardiovascular complications can result from uncontrolled hypercholesterolemia; 2, associated with congenital findings (e.g., lens opacities, dermoids); 3, may appear with other dystrophies; 4, increased risk of glaucoma (mesodermal dysgenesis?)

tact lens wear, eye rubbing) not dystrophy[6]

c. Potential complications: none

d. Management: none

e. Prognosis: excellent

C. ANTERIOR STROMAL DYSTROPHIES

1. Granular (Groenouw's I) dystrophy
   a. Clinical features
      i. First-decade presentation
      ii. Discrete focal white (translucent) spots
         • Hard white ("cornflake") spots
         • Powdery (small) dots
         • Ring-shaped opacities
      iii. Visual acuity (VA) reduces gradually (no worse than 20/200)
   b. Exceptions to standard rules for dystrophy: none
   c. Potential complications: reduced vision
   d. Management: keratoplasty
   e. Prognosis: good
2. Lattice dystrophy (of Biber)
   a. Clinical features
      i. Anterior stromal refractile lines
      ii. Central haze (after third to fourth decade of life)
      iii. Lines may thicken or bead
   b. Exceptions to standard rules for dystrophy: none
   c. Potential complications: epithelial erosions in advanced cases
   d. Management
      i. Treat erosions
      ii. Keratoplasty with severe VA reductions
   e. Prognosis: guarded
3. Central crystalline dystrophy (of Schnyder)
   a. Clinical features
      i. Central crystals form annulus during first to second decade of life
      ii. Dense arcus ring forms during third to fourth decade of life
   b. Exceptions to standard rules for dystrophy
      i. Associated with systemic hypercholesterolemia
      ii. Only dystrophy associated with systemic disease
   c. Potential complications
      i. Cardiovascular risks of hypercholesterol

ii. VA usually mildly effected

d. Management
   i. Refer to general medicine
   ii. Monitor ocular changes annually

e. Prognosis
   i. Good systemically with proper controls
   ii. Ocular signs not reversible, even with systemic control

D. FULL-THICKNESS STROMAL DYSTROPHIES

1. Macular (Groenouw's II) dystrophy
   a. Clinical features
      i. Diffuse ground-glass haze
      ii. Focal gray or white opacities
      iii. Increases to full thickness by teens
   b. Exceptions to standard rules for dystrophy
      i. Autosomal-recessive type (more severe)
      ii. Extends to periphery
   c. Complications
      i. VA reduces substantially by age 30
      ii. Corneal guttata with secondary erosions (a late occurrence in course)
   d. Management
      i. Treat erosions
      ii. Keratoplasty for VA
   e. Prognosis: guarded
2. Fleck dystrophy (François–Neetens)
   a. Clinical features
      i. Congenital or by 2 years of age
      ii. Asymmetry between eyes
      iii. Gray to white ring or comma-shaped spots
      iv. Lesions remain stable from early years
   b. Exceptions to standard rules for dystrophy: extends to periphery
   c. Complications
      i. Occasional congenital lens opacity
      ii. Occasional dermoids
   d. Management: none
   e. Prognosis: excellent

E. DEEP (POSTERIOR) STROMAL DYSTROPHIES

1. Central cloudy dystrophy (of François)
   a. Clinical features
      i. Fuzzy gray areas in deep central stroma
      ii. Slight polygonal pattern

b. Exceptions to standard rules for dystrophy: none

c. Complications: none

d. Management: none

e. Prognosis: excellent

2. Posterior amorphous dystrophy

   a. Clinical features

     i. Gray sheets develop across stroma

     ii. First decade

     iii. Occasional endothelial mosaic disruption

   b. Exceptions to standard rules for dystrophy: extends to periphery

   c. Complications: may reduce VA to about 20/40

   d. Management: none

   e. Prognosis: good

3. Pre-Descemet's dystrophy

   a. Clinical features

     i. Deep punctate or filamentous gray opacities

     ii. Indentations in Descemet's membrane

     iii. Fine "flour-like" dusting of gray specks of varying size and shapes
- Dendriform
- Boomerang
- Circular
- Comma
- Linear

     iv. All shapes may be in same cornea

     v. May be annular or diffuse pattern

   b. Exceptions to standard rules for dystrophy

     i. May present in older age initially (probably degeneration called corneal farinata)

     ii. May extend to periphery

     iii. Questionable hereditary pattern

     iv. Found with other dystrophies

   c. Complications: none

   d. Management

     i. Rule out degeneration versus dystrophy

     ii. Diagnosis other combined dystrophies

   e. Prognosis: excellent

F. POSTERIOR CORNEAL DYSTROPHIES

1. Fuchs' (late) endothelial dystrophy (Color Plate 43)

   a. Clinical features

     i. Three levels of guttata (depressions in endothelium, best seen by retroillumination)
- Few scattered guttata (ages 20 to 30)
- Early endothelial dystrophy: increasing guttata (ages 30 to 40)
- Late (Fuchs') endothelial dystrophy: guttata plus other signs (age greater than 40 years)

     ii. Pigment dusting on endothelium

     iii. Stromal edema and thickening (variable)

     iv. Epithelial edema (variable)
- Microcystic (diffuse)
- Wet, ground-glass effect (bedewing)
- Bullae (bullous keratopathy)

     v. Advanced edema produces subepithelial connective tissue opacities (permanent)

   b. Exceptions to standard rules for dystrophy

     i. Much higher prevalence in females (postmenopausal)

     ii. Late-age onset

     iii. Some forms extend to periphery with age

     iv. Appears as multilayer involvement

     v. May be far more common (in milder forms) than traditionally reported

   c. Complications

     i. Generally reduces VA in advancing stages

     ii. Increased stromal edema (thickening) in AM (secondary to closed lid edematous effect) produces VA fluctuation with transient increases in myopic errors

     iii. Advanced edema (and bullous keratopathy) produce AM erosions (morning syndrome). The four morning syndromes are
- Marginal keratitis (toxic staph)
- Epithelial basement membrane disorders (EBMD)
- Recurrent corneal erosion (RCE)
- Fuchs' endothelial dystrophy

     iv. Prolonged untreated edema produces connective tissue clouding of cornea

   d. Management (with symptoms or advancing signs)*

---

*See also Appendix 4.

i. Hot packs for edema
ii. Hypertonic saline (drops and hs ointment)
iii. Hot air (hair) blow dryer in AM
   • 5 to 10 minutes at arms length
   • Keep moving dryer back and forth
iv. Increased minus Rx for AM use if needed
v. Pupil dilation to increase light pathway around central clouding may help
   • Sometimes increased luminance is interpreted as increased VA
   • Use a sympathomimetic dilator (2.5 percent Neo-Synephrine) to avoid cycloplegia
   • Mydriacyl will require higher add due to cycloplegic effect
vi. High water, soft lenses
   • With chronic discomfort and erosions
   • Definitely with bullous keratopathy
vii. Keratoplasty
   • If VA in better eye nonfunctional
   • If dystrophic changes spreading to periphery with increased density
viii. Follow patient every 3 to 6 months
ix. Genetic counseling in severe cases
e. Prognosis
   i. Most cases remain stable and respond to simple antiedema therapies
   ii. Keratoplasty works well in central cases
   iii. Guarded prognosis in peripheral cases

2. Posterior polymorphous dystrophy (of Schlicting)
a. Clinical features
   i. Grouped vesicles of varying shape and distribution
      • Peripheral ring distribution
      • Focal wedge
      • Diffuse "Swiss cheese" pattern
   ii. Gray thickenings of Descemet's between vesicles
      • Often produce linear patterns
      • Lines tend to present as parrallel pairs (resembling railroad tracks)
   iii. Congenital or very early onset
   iv. Very slow changes, if any
b. Exceptions to standard rules for dystrophy

   i. Occasional ring pattern
   ii. Occasional congenital presentation
   iii. Suggested association with mesodermal dysgenesis syndromes[7]
c. Complications
   i. Mild stromal or epithelial edema
   ii. Rare reduction in VA to ≈ 20/30
   iii. Increased risk of glaucoma
d. Management
   i. Hypertonics for edema if indicated
   ii. Annual IOP checks throughout life
e. Prognosis: good

3. Congenital hereditary endothelial dystrophy
a. Clinical features
   i. Recessive form (congenital) with nystagmus
   ii. Dominant form (onset during first to second decade of life) with no nystagmus
   iii. Diffuse ground-glass edema (stromal and epithelial)
   iv. Increased corneal thickness (two to three times)
   v. "Peau d'orange" (orange peel) effect of Descemet's
b. Exceptions to standard rules for dystrophy
   i. Congenital recessive form
   ii. Extends to periphery
   iii. Appears as multilayer involvement
      • Occasionally mistaken for interstitial keratitis
      • Interstitial keratitis defined as
        Full thickness infiltration
        Stromal thinning
        Neovascularization
      • Dystrophy (all types) shows no true infiltrates, thinning or neovascularization
c. Complications
   i. Secondary epithelial reactions cause pain and photophobia
   ii. Frequently progressive to blindness by early age
d. Management
   i. Refer early for keratoplasty to reduce risk of amblyopia
   ii. Strongly recommend genetic counseling
e. Prognosis
   i. Poor for recessive forms
   ii. Guarded for the dominant forms (Table 4–2)

III. Degenerations* (Fig. 4–3A and 4–3B)

For a diagramatic summary of corneal degener- ations, refer to Figure 4–3A (peripherally ori- ented) and Figure 4–3B (variable positioning)

A. ARCUS SENILIS

Subjective

- Asymptomatic
- More common and pronounced among blacks
- Fifty percent by age 50 and up to 100 percent by age 80

Objective

- Usually bilateral
- Broad (1 to 2 mm) whitish mid-peripheral ring of lipids substances
- Found at level of Bowman's layer
- Gradual development
  1. Inferior first
  2. Superior second
  3. Ultimately a complete ring

Assessment[†]

- Most commonly a familial trait[8]
- Rule out risk factors for hyperlipidemias
  1. Usually not a factor after age 40
  2. Blood work not indicated without risk factors
- Considered cardiovascular risk factor under age 40 or combined with other classic risk factors
  1. Familial history of cardiovascular disease
  2. Hypertension
  3. Obesity
  4. Diets of polyunsaturated fats, high cholester- ols, increased salt
  5. Stress
  6. Smoking
  7. No exercise

Plan and Follow-up

- Advise patients under age 40 on increased risk and preventive measures
- Refer any patient under age 40 for medical workup if no medical care for more than 2 to 3 years
- Monitor eye changes routinely

B. BAND KERATOPATHY (Color Plate 95)

Subjective

- Usually asymptomatic in early development
- Late-stage painful epithelial erosions common

Objective

- Calcium accumulation in the palpebral fissure (band) region of cornea (usually bilateral)
- Whitish-yellow haze in epithelium and Bowman's
- Occasionally a Swiss cheese-like pattern
- Usually starts at nasal or temporal limbus and spreads centrally over months to years

Assessment[‡]

- Rule out Still's triad (juvenile rheumatoid arthritis) in early age presentations

Plan and Follow-up

- Refer for hyperparathyroid (hypercalcemic) workup in adult presentations
- Lubrication for mildly symptomatic presentations
- Chelation (usually with EDTA, a preservative) for severe symptoms
- Monitor suspicious development every 3 to 4 months

C. BULLOUS KERATOPATHY (Color Plate 44)

Subjective

- May present acutely, subacutely, or insidiously
- Often a contributory history of primary cause
- Extremely painful in moderate to severe cases

Objective

- Result of advanced, prolonged epithelial edema (from any primary cause)
- Formation of epithelial bullae (bubbling effect) which recurrently breakdown and reform
- Eventually, fibrosis occurs under bullae producing chronically painful and scarred epithelial layer

Assessment*

- Fundamental cause is reduced endothelial count producing poor corneal dehydration and resultant secondary epithelial edema
- Three most common primary causes (in rank or- der)
  1. Postoperative complication

---

*In alphabetical order.
†See also Appendix 3.

‡See also Appendix 2.
*See also Appendix 3.

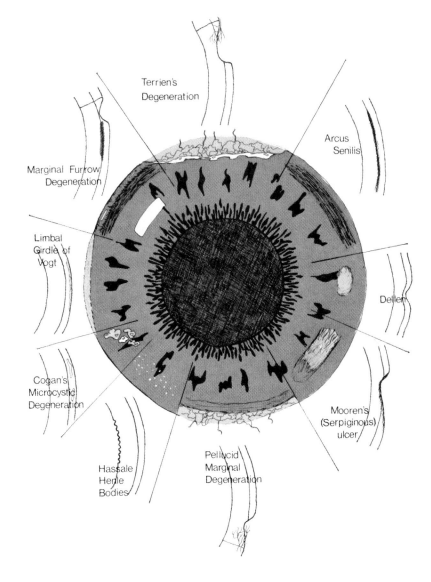

Figure 4–3A.
Diagramatic summary of peripherally oriented corneal degenerations

2. Fuchs' endothelial dystrophy
3. Degeneration (from cumulative loss of nonregenerative endothelial cells over lifetime)

Plan and Follow-up

- Consider qualitative and quantitative (cell count) endothelial integrity as indication (or contraindication) for elective intraocular surgery
- Treat advancing epithelial edema aggressively with all antiedema therapies before bullae form
- Treat bullae (early) with soft lens bandages and prophylactic antibiotics[9]
- With advanced (fibrosed) bullae, treat symptoms but poor prognosis for visual restoration

D. COGAN'S MICROCYSTIC DEGENERATION

Subjective

- Sometimes considered form of epithelial basement membrane (dot) dystrophy

- Generally found in older males
- Painful if spontaneous epithelial erosions occur

Objective

- Unilateral or bilateral presentations
- Usually peripheral single or groupings of large (1- to 2-mm) clear or gray intraepithelial microcysts

Assessment

- Differentiate from epithelial basement membrane (dot) dystrophy by following variations
  1. Unilateral presentations
  2. Older age presentation
  3. Male prevalence
  4. Larger cyst formations
  5. Peripheral versus central
- Rule out other causes of spontaneous erosions

Plan and Follow-up

- Monitor asymptomatic cases every 6 to 12 months or PRN
- Treat acute erosions same as EBMD

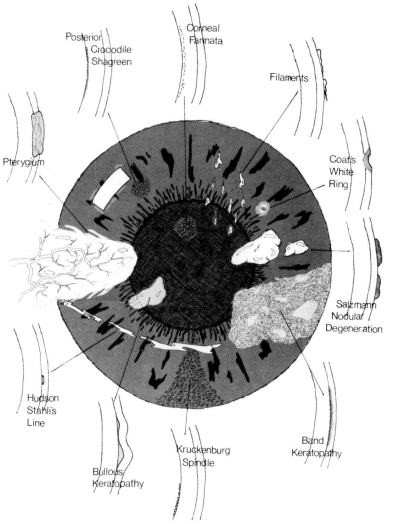

Figure 4–3B.
Diagramatic summary of variable-positioning corneal degenerations

(labels on figure:)
Posterior Crocodile Shagreen
Corneal Farinata
Filaments
Pterygium
Coats White Ring
Salzmann Nodular Degeneration
Hudson Stahli's Line
Kruckenburg Spindle
Band Keratopathy
Bullous Keratopathy

E. CORNEAL FARINATA

Refer to pre-Descemet's dystrophy.

F. DELLEN (GAULE SPOT) (Fig. 4–4)

Subjective

- Asymptomatic presentation (usually general exam)
- Any age range

Objective

- Focal, peripheral depressions (thinnings) adjacent to the limbus usually 0.5- to 1-mm diameter
- Borders may slope gently or frequently are sharp and well-defined producing appearance of a "hole"
  1. Hole may approximate one half of the corneal thickness
  2. Tissue remains clear or slight haze
- Eye is never inflamed or hyperemic
- Epithelium remains intact (no staining or symptoms)

- Elongation (along limbal border) may extend 2 to 3 mm
- Most frequent positioning at 3 and 9 o'clock
- Usually associated with an adjacent raised "mass"
  1. Conjunctival
     a. Pinguecula (most common)
     b. Chemosis
     c. Subconjunctival hemorrhage (thick)
     d. Other raised lesions
  2. Eyelid
     a. Internal chalazion
     b. Other causes of raised or irregular tarsus
     c. Also possible with lagophthalmos
  3. Thick edge of a firm contact lens

Assessment*

- Determine cause (raised mass)
- Reason for limited patient risk for dellen unclear
  1. Many people have thick pinguecula, but only small percentage develop dellen

*See also Appendix 2.

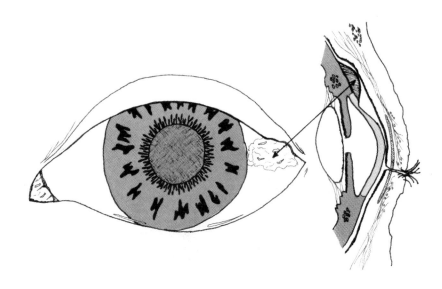

Fig. 4–4.
Dellen formation.

2. May be associated with a specific HLA factor
■ No risk of perforation (even though it looks it)

Plan and Follow-up*

■ Where possible, remove or reduce cause (mass)
   1. Adjust contact lens (edge)
   2. Remove chalazion
   3. Reduce or control pinguecula
■ Removal or protection achieved by lubrication
   1. Eyedrops or ointments q3–4h for 1 week
   2. Soft contact lens coverage
   3. Lid closure (patching) for 24 hours
■ If no treatment indicated, monitor yearly or PRN

G. DEPOSITS (ON OR IN CORNEA)

   1. Amyloid (systemic manifestation)
   2. Calcareous (degenerative)
   3. Coats' white ring (associated with foreign bodies)
   4. Filaments (epithelial or mucin debris)†
       (Color Plate 45)
   5. Hyalin (degenerative)
   6. Keloid (associated with scarring)
   7. Lipid (degenerative)

H. HASSALL–HENLE BODIES (DESCEMET'S WARTS)

Subjective

■ Asymptomatic presentation (usually general exam)

Objective

■ Small, round, peripheral endothelial indentations produced by thickening of Descemet's membrane
■ Appear as corneal guttata (but peripheral)
■ Usually associated peripheral edema (may be full thickness)

Assessment

■ Rule out Fuchs' endothelial dystrophy (central)
■ Peripheral edema sometimes produces appearance of an atypical arcus (diffuse versus defined ring)

Plan and Follow-up

■ No treatment indicated
■ Consider (endothelial) risk in elective surgery

Plan and Follow-up

■ No treatment indicated
■ Consider (endothelial) risk in elective surgery

I. MARGINAL FURROW DEGENERATION

Subjective

■ Asymptomatic presentation (usually general examination)

Objective

■ Bilateral thinning (furrowing) of peripheral cornea adjacent to limbus (usually 360°)
■ Generally presents with prominent arcus ring
   1. Furrowed trough (thinned cornea) diagnosed by depression of slit between arcus ring and limbal border

*See also Appendix 4.
†See also Appendix 2.

2. NaFl stain may pool in trough area but no positive staining because epithelium intact

Assessment*

- No risk of perforation
- Rule out other marginal (thinning) degenerations
  1. Pellucid marginal degeneration
  2. Terrien's marginal degeneration
- Rule out Mooren's ulcer (inflamed lesion)
- Rule out rheumatoid disease

Plan and Follow-up

- No treatment indicated
- Recheck annually or PRN

J. MOOREN'S ULCER

Subjective

- Acute or subacute painful presentation
- Two forms
  1. Older patients present with a unilateral, less severe inflammation
  2. Younger patients (rare) present a bilateral, severe type

Objective

- Inflammatory peripheral, serpiginous (creeping) type ulceration of unknown etiology (refer to section VII, part C, of this chapter, "Fungal Keratitis", under "Assessment" for serpiginous ulceration test)
- Usually a lateral to medial limbal presentation
- No discharge associated with stromal ulceration
- Often neovascularization develops early

Assessment*

- Major risk of scarring and possible perforation
- Rule out noninflammatory marginal degenerations
  1. Marginal furrow (painless)
  2. Pellucid (inferior)
  3. Terrien's (superior)
- Rule out marginal staphylococcal keratitis (no thinning)
- Rule out fungal keratitis (traumatic history)

Plan and Follow-up

- Responds poorly to therapies including steroids
- Frequently unrelenting course for 6 to 12 months
- Refer to corneal specialist

---

*See also Appendix 3.

K. PELLUCID MARGINAL DEGENERATION

Subjective

- Rare condition of unknown etiology
- Usually asymptomatic

Objective

- Inferior corneal thinning (noninflammatory)
- Occasionally found with keratoconus[10]

Assessment

- Rule out other marginal degenerations
- No risk of perforation or significant scarring

Plan and Follow-up

- No treatment indicated
- Monitor patient for keratoconic changes

L. POSTERIOR CROCODILE SHAGREEN

1. Diffuse, grayish polygonal degeneration of posterior corneal surface
2. No associated visual or ocular complications

M. PTERYGIUM (Color Plate 46)

Subjective

- Stable (occasionally advancing) lesion
- More common in outdoor people
  1. Stimulated by UV exposure and arid climate
  2. Probably a tissue response to irritants rather than a true degeneration
- Usually cosmetically unappealing
- May produce subacute symptoms
  1. Irritation and hyperemic appearance
  2. Foreign-body sensation
  3. Reduction of vision
     a. Secondary irregular astigmatisms
     b. Obstruction of the visual axis

Objective

- Thick, fleshy triangular mass of tissue (apex toward cornea) growing (stable or slow, insidious growth) onto nasal corneal surface
- Frequently a bilateral presentation with varying degree of advancement in each eye
- Usually yellowish coloration
- Relatively rich surface vascularization
- Occasionally a ferric line (orange-brown) seen at leading (corneal) edge called Stocker's line

Assessment*

- Differentiate from pinguecula
  1. Corneal involvement with pterygium
  2. Apex toward cornea with pterygium
  3. Rich vascular supply with pterygium
- Assess stable versus progressive nature
- Rule out other raised ocular surface lesions

Plan and Follow-up

- Measure and diagram (photodocument if possible)
  1. Recheck first observed lesions in 6 to 12 months
  2. Longstanding lesions usually stable
- If asymptomatic and stable, no treatment; monitor at 1- to 2-year intervals or PRN
- If symptomatic (but stable)
  1. Vasoconstrictors for hyperemia
  2. Lubrication for foreign body sensations
  3. Corrective lenses for induced visual astigma
     a. Add UV tints to reduce potential cause
     b. Lens also reduces exposure to irritants
- If progressive (towards pupil) or cosmetically unacceptable (patient requesting repair)
  1. Recommend surgical reduction before leading edge approximates border of dilated (dim illumination) pupil
  2. Postoperative focal radiation usually necessary
- Advise patients on guarded postoperative prognosis regarding redevelopment of growth pattern

N. SALZMAN'S NODULAR DEGENERATION

Subjective

- Usually asymptomatic presentation
- May present acutely with epithelial breakdown
- Uncommon presentation (more prevalent in females)

Objective

- Bilateral formations of elevated, grayish-blue nodules on corneal surface
- May be central or peripheral numbering (1 to 10)
- Vision effects depend on location of nodules

Assessment

- Rule out bullous keratopathy (more painful)

Plan and Follow-up

- If asymptomatic, no treatment but monitor closely (every 6 months or PRN)
- If epithelium chronically breaks down over nodules, use bandage soft lenses and prophylactic antibiotics qid
- Consider partial penetrating keratoplasty if patient desires (possible) permanent repair

O. TERRIEN'S MARGINAL DEGENERATION

Subjective

- Occurs in males, usually 20 to 50 years of age
- Generally a painful presentation

Objective

- Usually unilateral (rarely bilateral), superior nasal circumlimbal thinning with opacification
- Thinning is usually extensive, leading to corneal distortions and permanent visual loss (astigma)
- Acute presentations produce secondary inflammation and subsequent neovascularization of effected area

Assessment

- Rule out other marginal degenerations
- Rule out inflammatory causes
  1. Mooren's ulcer
  2. Fungal ulcer (history of trauma)
  3. Rheumatoid disease

Plan and Follow-up

- Heavy topical steroids may or may not help
- If thinning progresses to precarious stage, consider penetrating keratoplasty for protection
- Condition usually stabilizes (with permanent scarring) after initial attack

P. WHITE LIMBAL GIRDLE OF VOGT

1. Common presentation in women over age 50
2. Narrow band of fine crystal-like opacities lined up along nasal or temporal limbal border(s)
3. Usually bilateral and always asymptomatic
4. Old literature related it to band keratopathy and sunlight exposure due to palpebral fissure orientation (both theories unproven)

---

*See also Appendix 3.

IV. Other Funny-looking Corneal Conditions

A. KERATOCONUS

Subjective

- Sometimes referred to as corneal ectasia or ectatic cornea (connotes thinning and bulging)
- Patient begins to demonstrate slow, insidious, refractive changes and reduced best visual acuity (BVA) over months to years
  1. First signs usually about 15 to 25 years of age
  2. Progressive refractive changes for 5 to 6 years
  3. Changes usually stabilize but may recur 10 to 15 years later (uncommon)
- Frequent history of asthma, allergies, atopias, with reports of chronic eye rubbing
  1. Supports mechanical (environmental) etiology
  2. Hereditary etiology also possible
- Most cases remain painless unless secondarily complicated (e.g., epithelial breakdown, hydrops)
- Serious problems with glare and visual discomfort
- Mild to moderate phtophobia
- Occasionally diplopia (or polyopia) reported
- Not uncommon to find onset after hard lens wear
  1. Lens-induced theory unproven but reasonable
  2. May be latent trait manifested by hard lens
  3. May be coincidental based on age range and frequency of contact lens wear

Objective

- Early clinical signs (other than frequent, irregular refractive changes and reducing BVA) are usually subtle and difficult to discern
- Bilateral condition with one eye usually less involved or completely arrested (forme fruste)
- Earliest signs are refractive and visual
  1. Retinoscopy produces scissor type reflex
  2. Irregular, asymmetric astigmatic changes occur with each subsequent refraction
  3. Keratometry readings begin to steepen (most common course) and mires begin to distort
  4. Placebo disc (if used) will begin to show irregular ring patterns
  5. BVA will be reduced with spectacle correction and improved by pinhole, stenopaic slit, and contact lenses
- With advancing changes, the central to inferior (most frequent) cornea will begin to present a bulging, protruding profile (Munson's sign)
- Mild to moderate stromal thinning can be observed early at or proximal to the bulging "cone" area
- Eventually, a brownish-orangish ferrous ring will be observable at the base (or 360°) of the cone (Fleischer's ring)
- Fine, fibrillary lines will begin to be noticed at the subepithelial and anterior stromal levels

- The posterior cornea will reveal slightly thicker, vertically oriented stress lines or Vogt lines, usually centrally and frequently aligned with the minus axis of the refractive cylinder
- Stromal nerve fibers (in irregular orientation) will appear more prominent (central and peripheral)
- Scarred corneal lamellae may appear at Bowman's and anterior stromal levels
- Rarely, in advanced cases, corneal hydrops occurs
  1. Breaks in posterior cornea cause dense edema
  2. Onset can be acute and painful
  3. Full-thickness stromal edema can dramatically reduce vision
  4. Resolution occurs (with no specific therapy) over 2 to 3 months with guaranteed scarring
- Risk of perforation is almost nil

Assessment

- Rule out other thinning disorders[11]
  1. Marginal furrow (peripheral in older patient)
  2. Pellucid (inferior limbal)
  3. Terrien's (superior and usually acute onset)
- Rule out keratoglobus (thinning and bulging to periphery)
- Differentiate posterior keratoconus findings[12]
  1. Thinning occurs from posterior surface toward anterior with early disruption of endohelium and resultant stromal edema
  2. Probably a form of ICE syndrome (mesodermal)
- Rule out herpes simplex disciform keratitis by history and clinical findings
- Rule out associated systemic syndromes

Plan

- There is no known specific treatment, cure, or prevention for this unknown etiologic ectatic condition
- Visual treatment with spectacle lenses may offer assistance in early stages or mild cases
- Moderate to advanced changes require visual correction through contact lenses (discussed in detail in Chapter 7)
- Care for acute or painful hydrops is usually conservative with limited use of medication
  1. Extensive antiedema therapies
  2. Prophylactic antibiotics, if epithelial surface is severely compromised
  3. Rarely, a short-course topical steroid may be of value to reduce scarring
     a. However, risk of retarded healing with steroid may contraindicate its use
     b. Should be avoided
- Primary indication for penetrating keratoplasty

should be functional need or severe cosmetic distress

1. Indicated when better functioning eye is below acceptable (patient) standards with best visual correction system (contact lens)
2. Indicated when scarred cornea is emotionally, psychologically unacceptable to patient
3. Prognosis for corneal graft is generally good to excellent

Follow-up

- Monitor active refractive changes every 6 months
- Monitor contact lens patients closely
- Post keratoplasty patients usually require contact lens correction and close monitoring

B. PIGMENTATIONS*

1. Arlt's triangle (brownish coloration)
   a. Triangular-shaped pigment deposition at 6 o'clock position on posterior cornea
   b. Pathognomonic of old uveitis
2. Brawny edema (brownish coloration)
   a. Brownish edematous haze in epithelium
   b. Pathognomonic of epithelial basement membrane disorders or recurrent corneal erosions
3. Ferry's line (orangish-brown coloration)
   a. Ferric ions around a surgical filtering bleb
   b. No pathognomonic indications
4. Fleischer's ring (orangish-brown coloration)
   a. Ferric ions around or at base of cone in keratoconus
   b. No additional pathognomonic indications regarding keratoconus or other conditions
5. Goar's line
   a. Pigment granules forming horizontal line on inferior cornea
   b. Pathognomonic for pigmentary glaucoma
6. Hemosiderosis
   a. Intracorneal or posterior corneal surface blood straining
   b. Pathognomonic for
      i. Intracorneal bleed (neovascularization)
      ii. Hyphema (posterior surface staining)

7. Hudson–Stähli line (orangish-brown coloration) (Color Plate 47)
   a. Level of Bowman's layer in band region of cornea where margins of lids meet on blink may be produced by migration of ions over time into line from blinking action
   b. More frequent in males
   c. Frequency parallels age (e.g., 20 = 20 percent, 30 = 30 percent)
   d. Three typical presentations
      i. Faint segmented line
      ii. Continuous distinct line
      iii. Line with surrounding (whitish-yellow) opacities
   e. Frequent site of spontaneous or recurrent corneal epithelial erosions
8. Kaiser–Fleischer ring (orangish coloration) (Color Plate 48)
   a. Posterior corneal (and anterior angle) ring
      i. Best observed by gonioscopy
      ii. Advanced presentations may be grossly visible or observed by slit lamp alone
   b. Copper deposition specifically pathognomonic of Wilson's hepaticolenticular disease[13]
9. Keratitic (keratic) precipitates (white or pigmented)
   a. Endothelial surface pigment cells
   b. Almost universal with age
   c. May be pathognomonic (check history and associated findings) for
      i. Uveitis
      ii. Trauma
      iii. Aging
10. Keratomelanocystosis (striate melanokeratosis)
    a. Pigmented spokes radiating into cornea from limbal juncture
    b. Seen mostly in dark or black races
    c. Usually greater inferiorly, especially at 4 and 8 o'clock positions
    d. Pathognomonic for
       i. Trauma
       ii. Infection
       iii. Focal, toxic inflammation (e.g., *Staphylococcus* at 4 and 8 o'clock positions)
11. Kruckenburg's spindle (brownish coloration)
    a. A vertical spindle-shaped pigment deposition on inferior one third to one half posterior cornea

---

*In alphabetical order.

b. Pathognomonic for
  i. Old uveitis
  ii. Pigment dispersion syndrome
12. Salmon patch (orangish coloration)
  a. Discoloration of mid-stroma in interstitial keratitis (usually 3 to 6 weeks after onset)
  b. Pathognomonic of syphilitic keratitis
13. Sampaolesi's line
  a. Pigment granules are deposited at Schwalbe's line
  b. Pathognomonic for pigmentary glaucoma

14. Stocker's line (orangish-brown coloration)
  a. Ferric ions at leading edge of pterygium
  b. No pathognomonic indications to pterygium or other conditions
15. "Tattooing" (variable colorations)
  a. Staining of mucocutaneous membranes by heavy metallic substances or certain drugs
  b. Usually diagnosed through history

V. Epithelial Basement Membrane Disorders

Background Information

A. HISTORICAL BACKGROUND

1. Funny-looking changes in the epithelium (intraepithelial) were first noted by Vogt during the 1920s
2. Again reported by Guerry[14] during the 1950s as rare (1 in 4000) findings
3. Cogan et al[15] documented microcysts (dots) as part of an "epithelial dystrophy" during the 1960s
   a. Called it Cogan's microcystic dystrophy
   b. More generic term for findings became map–dot–fingerprint dystrophy
4. Finally, during the 1970s, many investigators began to describe these findings as epithelial basement membrane dystrophy (EBMD)[16–18]
   a. Autosomal-dominant pattern of inheritance
   b. Prevalence reported at approximately 2 to 6 percent[4]
5. Increased prevalence (from Guerry, in the 1930s, to Laibson, in the 1970s) probably a result of improved slit-lamp instrumentation and capabilities
6. Better understanding of etiology was a product of advanced electron microscopic techniques during the 1970s

B. ANATOMY OF THE EPITHELIAL BASEMENT MEMBRANE (Fig. 4–5)

1. Also called the basal lamina
2. Separates the epithelial cells from Bowman's layer
3. Thin mucoproteinous membrane secreted by basal epithelial cells
   a. Takes 6 to 8 weeks to form or resecrete membrane
   b. Thus, loss or damage to membrane requires extended period (much greater than expected hours for squamous epithelium and days for deeper epithelial cells to regenerate)
4. Function of basement membrane is to attach epithelial cells firmly to stroma (Bowman's layer)
   a. Does so on epithelial side by fibrils called hemidesmosomes, which extend into epithelium
   b. On stromal side, fine fibrils (anchoring fibrils) bind membrane and epithelium down to Bowman's layer
5. Thus, the contemporary concept of corneal anatomy differs slightly from traditional
   a. Epithelial layer
     i. Mucin layer of tears ("stolen" from the tear guys)
     ii. Squamous epithelial cells
     iii. Wing-shaped epithelial cells

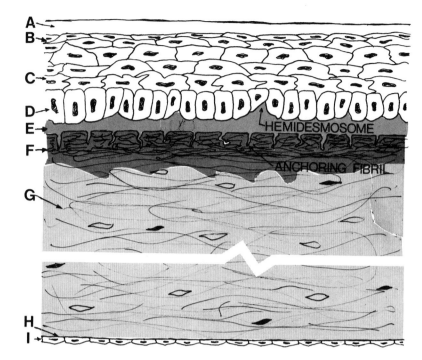

A →
B →
C →
D →
E →   HEMIDESMOSOME
F →   ANCHORING FIBRIL
G →
H →
I →

Figure 4–5.
Diagrammatic corneal anatomy. *Epithelial layer:* **A.** Mucin layer of tears; **B.** Squamous epithelial cells; **C.** Wing-shaped epithelial cells; **D.** Basal (columnar-shaped) epithelial cells; **E.** Epithelial basement membrane. *Stromal layer:* **F.** Bowman's layer (condensed collagen fibers); **G.** Stroma (loose collagen fibers). **H.** Descemet's membrane. **I.** Endothelium.

iv. Basal (columnar shaped) epithelial cells
v. Epithelial basement membrane
b. Stromal layer
i. Bowman's layer (condensed collagen fibers)
ii. Stroma (loose collagen fibers)
c. Descemet's membrane
d. Endothelium

C. HISTOPATHOLOGY OF EBMD

1. Basal epithelial cells produce abnormal fingerlike projections off basement membrane
   a. Generate off hemidesmosome thickenings
   b. Produce intraepithelial "map" configurations by slit-lamp examination (most common finding)
   c. Projections with fibrogranular ridges produce "fingerprint" patterns (least common finding)
2. Fingerlike projections bend intraepithelially and trap epithelial cells and debri to form microcysts (or pseudocysts)
   a. Microcysts appear clinically, under slit lamp as "dots" (common with maps)
   b. Migration of microcysts to surface produce subjective and objective corneal signs and symptoms (morning

syndrome #2) and epithelial erosions (Fig. 4–6)
3. All these intraepithelial changes create an irregular epithelial surface
   a. Clinical result is negative NaFl staining
   b. When extensive, results are irregular astigmia or reduced best correctable VA

Clinical Considerations in EBMD

Subjective

- Onset of symptoms may be insidious, subacute, or acute
- Often objective signs will be noted without symptoms (especially in general examination patients)
  1. More frequently, symptoms will be reported (in varying degree) with no objective signs
  2. Probably subclinical findings
- Appears to be slightly more common in females
- Wide range of symptoms depending on degree of condition (Table 4–3)
  1. Mild degree
     a. Usually asymptomatic
     b. Mild, short-lived corneal irritation on waking (morning syndrome)
  2. Moderate degree
     a. Morning syndrome or chronic corneal irritation
     b. May be awakened during sleep by reaction
     c. Transient or constant visual fluctuation
     d. Mild to moderate photophobia and glare

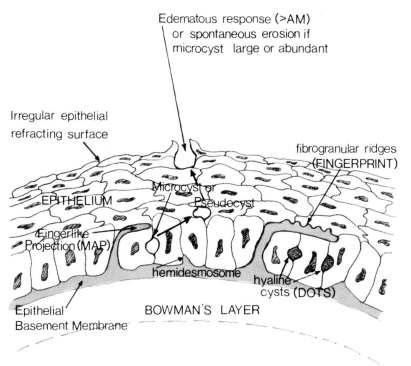

Edematous response (>AM) or spontaneous erosion if microcyst large or abundant

Irregular epithelial refracting surface

fibrogranular ridges (FINGERPRINT)

Microcyst or Pseudocyst

EPITHELIUM

Fingerlike Projection (MAP)

hemidesmosome

hyaline cysts (DOTS)

Epithelial Basement Membrane

BOWMAN'S LAYER

Figure 4–6.
Diagram of intra-epithelial histopathology of EBMD. (Adapted from Waring, et al, 1978, p. 71, with permission[4])

3. Severe degree
  a. Reduced best correctable visual acuity
  b. History of spontaneous (nontraumatic) painful epithelial erosions
  c. Slow epithelial healing time with re-erosions during treatment
  d. Recurrent corneal erosion syndrome (RCE) (morning syndrome #3)

Objective

- Usually bilateral presentation
  a. One eye may be more advanced than the other
  b. One eye may show no signs at all
- Findings seen best under high magnification, indirect, or retroillumination
  1. Even easier and more vivid with dilated pupil
  2. Observable without dilation, *but*
    a. Must have good slit-lamp illumination and optics in dark room
    b. Must know what to look for and be looking
- Occasionally signs are subtle, difficult to find
  1. If subjective symptoms present and you have ruled out other causes, follow cornea closely (especially after trauma), and they will probably show up in time
  2. Sometimes symptoms (e.g., morning syndrome) show up before physical signs
- Negative staining frequently presents early (alone or before other signs) (Color Plate 53)
  1. Instant tear breakup over same area(s) after each blink frequently in horizontal, linear cascades

  2. Different from BUT (tear-breakup time), which is not an instantaneous process
- Maps (usually central but could reach periphery) (Color Plate 49)
  1. Grayish patches or sheets of clear zones, geographic lines and amorphous patterns
  2. May be distinct lines or have fading edges
  3. Thicken and become more dense with aging or recurrent corneal erosions
  4. Size and shapes of patterns vary from short (<1 mm) to long (>3 mm), round, oval, sinuous, and irregular
  5. Frequently present with associated dots
- Dots (usually inferior central or just below pupil border) (Color Plates 50 and 51)
  1. Grayish (hyaline filled) microcysts or clear fluid-filled cysts
  2. Round ameboid, or comma shaped
  3. Often found in multiple clusters
  4. May be pinpoint but never much larger than 0.5 to 1 mm
  5. Sometimes form polygonal type rows, or "nets"
  6. Negative staining when intraepithelial
    a. Will stain positive if they erupt
    b. Will also be symptomatic at that point
  7. Seen frequently with maps
- Fingerprints (larger patterns and usually central) (Color Plate 52)
  1. Swirled refractile lines resembling a thumb print on corneal epithelium
  2. Look like "shift lines", "slipped rug", or "tramlines" seen in other corneal conditions (e.g., bullous keratopathy, ulcers)

TABLE 4–3. CLINICAL SUMMARY OF EPITHELIAL BASEMENT MEMBRANE DISORDERS

	Mild	Moderate	Severe
Subjective	AM Irritation	AM Irritation Chronic irritation Reduced (±) BVA Photophobia	AM Irritation Chronic irritation Reduced (±) BVA Photophobia Irregular astigmatism Spontaneous erosion RCE after injury Slow corneal healing

Objective	No observable signs
	Bilateral (occasionally
	   unilateral)
	   Maps or dots
	   Fingerprints (rare)
	   Negative staining
		Bilateral (occasionally
		   unilateral)
		   Maps or dots
		   Fingerprints (rare)
		Negative staining
		Tramlines
		"Mare's tail"
		Positive staining
		Diffuse epithelial edema
			Bilateral (occasionally
			   unilateral)
			   Maps or dots
			   Fingerprints (rare)
			Negative staining
			Tramlines
			"Mare's tail"
			Postive staining
			Diffuse epithelial edema
			Dendrites or filaments
			Spontaneous erosion
			Brawny edema

Assessment	Keratitis sicca
	Dry eye syndrome
	Fuchs' endothelial dystrophy
	Other epithelial or endothelial
	   dystrophy
		Keratitis sicca
		Dry eye syndrome
		Fuchs' endothelial dystrophy
		Other epithelial or endothelial
		   dystrophy
		Cogan's degeneration
		Traumatic aggravant
			Keratitis sicca
			Dry eye syndrome
			Fuchs' endothelial dystrophy
			Other epithelial or endothelial
			   dystrophy
			Cogan's degeneration
			Traumatic aggravant
			Infection or inflammation
			Other degenerations

Plan	Advise and educate patient
	Lubricant drops
		Advise and educate patient
		Lubricant drops
		Lubricant ointments
		Evaluate family
		Hypertonic drops and
		   ointments
		Soft lens wear
			Advise and educate patient
			Lubricant drops
			Lubricant ointments
			Evaluate family
			Hypertonic drops and
			   ointments
			Soft lens wear
			RCE therapy
			Bandage lens

Follow-up	PRN Annual Check	PRN Annual check Every 3 months with SL Every 6 months without SL	PRN Annual check Every 3 months with SL Every 6 months without SL Every 4 to 6 weeks with bandage

3. Clear to gray with indirect or retroillumination
4. Least common presenting sign in EBMD
5. May appear alone or with maps or dots
6. Occasionally lines come off central point (dot), giving appearance of a "mare's trail"

■ As condition advances, complications can occur on epithelial surface and anterior stroma
1. Positive NaFl staining
2. Edematous clouding and bullae
3. Dendriform (infiltrative) keratitis
4. Filamentary keratitis
5. "Brawny" (brownish) edema
   a. Especially after trauma and RCE
   b. Persists for months to years with RCE

6. Spontaneous (nontraumatic) epithelial erosions
   a. Usually "biggies" (25 to 50 percent corneal surface involvement)
   b. Usually followed by RCE
   c. Typically situated at inferior cornea
   d. May be loosely associated with Hudson–Stähli's line (e.g., frequency, risk?)[19]
7. Once epithelium compromised in advanced conditions, increased risk of infection
8. Advanced EBMD with RCE can also produce an anterior stromal haze and potential scarring[20]

■ RCE complications can be predicted quite well with relative accuracy by checking Bell's phenomenon[21]

1. Positive EBMD clinical findings with a negative Bell's (eyes do not roll upward on forced lid closure) indicates significant risk (>75 percent) for spontaneous corneal erosion
2. Simple test: Hold upper lids firmly with thumbs and ask patient to shut lids forcefully while you observe eye movements
3. Negative Bell's with EBMD findings indicates need for preventive therapy with or without symptoms

Assessment*

- Rule out dry eye–keratitis sicca-type syndromes
  1. Sicca symptoms usually increase in later day versus EBMD morning syndrome
  2. Sicca stains positively with NaFl and rose bengal versus negative staining and negative rose bengal in EBMD
  3. BUT less than 10 seconds (but greater than instantaneous) versus instantaneous breakup of tears (cascading) in EBMD
  4. Presence of band SPK, etc., versus map–dot–fingerprint changes in EBMD
- Rule out epithelial (and endothelial) dystrophies
- Rule out Cogan's microcystic degeneration
- Rule out corneal infection or inflammation
  1. Diagnose ''by the company they keep''
  2. Good history is critical
- Rule out corneal degenerations

Plan†

- In advanced presentations or positive findings in patients under age 20, consider dystrophy etiology
  1. Examine other family members
  2. Advise, educate, and counsel family
- In asymptomatic presentations (with positive clinical findings and normal Bell's)
  1. Advise and educate patient to findings
  2. Instruct on possible symptoms and care
- In asymptomatic presentations (with positive clinical findings and negative–absent Bell's)
  1. Advise and educate patient as to findings and as to increased risk of spontaneous erosion
  2. Instruct on possible symptoms and care
  3. Discuss prophylactic (mild) therapies as optional and available (patient's decision)
- Mild symptoms (morning syndrome) with or without objective signs
  1. Treatment optional
  2. Hypertonic ointment at bedtime
  3. Hot packs ad lid
  4. Lubricants ad lib
- Moderate symptoms with or without objective signs
  1. Hypertonic saline drops q3–4h daily
  2. Hypertonic saline ointments at bedtime

---

*See also Appendix 3.
†See also Appendix 4.

3. Antiedema therapies (heat) in AM
4. Consider contact lens wear, if best visual acuity (BVA) reduced[22]
- Severe symptoms or complications (e.g., RCE)
  1. Treat uncomplicated symptoms with same regime as moderate, at more frequent dose rates
  2. For spontaneous erosions and RCE
     a. Use standard abrasion protocol
     b. Avoid prolonged patching (more than 2 to 3 days); it causes edema complications
     c. Run minimum 1-week postabrasion course of hypertonic ointment q2–3h and hs
     d. Consider bandage soft lens for RCE (see Chapter 7)
  3. Use prophylactic gentamicin drops qid during any complication with epithelial compromise
  4. Treat any secondary infection or inflammation appropriately, avoiding steroids if possible

Follow-up

- Asymptomatic and mild cases followed routinely
- Moderate cases, PRN *or*
  1. Every 3 months with contact lens wear
  2. Every 6 months without contact lens wear
- Manage severe cases closely during acute complications or bandage lens therapies
- After complications phase, carefully advise and educate patient on early signs and symptoms and monitor corneal integrity every 3 months
- Remember to explain chronic nature of condition
  1. No cures
  2. Long-term prognosis guarded, but prognosis for individual episodes of complications and pain are generally favorable for complete resolution (average time approximately 6 to 12 weeks, but could take up to 1 year)
  3. Substantial risk of exacerbation

Concepts and Controversies in EBMD

A. In 1981 Werblin et al[23] documented significantly greater frequencies than in previously reported map–dot–fingerprint changes in corneas

1. Forty-three percent of the general population
2. Seventy-six percent (or greater) in patient's over age 50

B. In late 1983, Alvarado et al[24] were able to prove that the human epithelial basement membrane thickens substantially through membrane reduplication in focal areas from age 20 and older (almost 100 percent thickening from age 20 to 60)

1. The thickening occurs in all individuals
2. The process is aggravated or accelerated

by trauma or chronic irritation (cell injury and death)

    a. Abrasion

    b. Ulceration

    c. Infection or inflammation

    d. Contact lenses (as chronic irritant)

    e. Corneal surgery (e.g., radial keratotomy)[25]

3. Changes below age 20 (infrequent) are probably primary (dystrophic) changes, unless an aggravant is present

4. Membrane thickenings weaken attachments and even "buries anchoring fibrils" over time producing "significant disruption in terms of adhesion and stability of the corneal epithelium"[24]

5. Thus, EBM changes are age related, very prevalent, perhaps universal, and varying in degree of clinical appearance and significance (i.e., signs and symptoms)

C. Factors challenging "dystrophy" diagnosis

  1. Highly prevalent (versus uncommon)

  2. Age related (versus early childhood)

  3. Aggravating causes (versus dystrophic origin)

  4. Other exceptions to the "standard clinical characteristics of corneal dystrophy"

    a. Questionable hereditary pattern

    b. Ocular disease and trauma aggravants

    c. Onset after age 20

    d. Twenty-five percent of cases appear to be unilateral

    e. More prevalent in women

D. Reasonable clinical conclusions

  1. There probably is a true EBMD

    a. Probably infrequent (less than 2 to 5 percent)

    b. Seen initially in age ranges under 20

    c. Autosomal-dominant (check family)

    d. Free of traumatic or ocular disease history or causes

    e. Relatively prominent clinical features

  2. There are probably a fair number of nondystrophic map–dot–fingerprint changes found in patients secondary to EBM insult or injury (acute or chronic disease, trauma, or irritation)

    a. Frequency relative to nature of patients

      i. Frequency of disease

      ii. Risks and rate of ocular trauma (see "Examples of EBMD-like presentations")

    b. Population of hard lens patients (see "Examples of EBMD-like presentations")

    c. Possibly even the nature of air and climate in specific areas could effect frequency

      i. Sandy, gritty environments

      ii. Wind, dust, other

  3. There probably is a high frequency of EBM changes (probably called atypical or "garden-variety" dry eye–keratitis sicca) in older and aging patients (see EBM-like presentations)

    a. The frequency is probably highest because of the increasing age of the population

    b. Age is a relative term because the degree of EBM changes (while advancing with age beyond 20) can be clinically significant by 30 to 40, or subclinical at 60 to 80

  4. In any case, any one or all possibilities have significant practical clinical implications to primary eye care practitioners

    a. Regarding frequent symptomatic patients

    b. Regarding accurate objective examination and differential diagnosis of common corneal findings

  5. Almost all presentations, regardless of true etiology, can be successfully managed by very basic techniques and procedures

    a. Supportive therapies

    b. Hypertonics

    c. Standard abrasion care

    d. Bandage soft lens therapy

    e. Careful patient advise and counseling

E. Examples of some EBMD-like presentations (pseudodystrophy)

  1. Tangential corneal abrasive injury (e.g., fingernail injury, paper cut, branch, twig, and radial keratotomy) frequently precipitates chronic, sometimes permanent, EBMD-like signs in the corneal epithelium

    a. Map–dot–fingerprint changes

    b. Brawny edema

    c. Recurrent corneal erosion

    d. Nontangential corneal trauma does not affect the epithelial basement membrane, hence never causes EBMD-like signs

      i. Contact lenses

      ii. UV radiation

      iii. Corneal foreign bodies

      iv. Blunt injury

e. Thus, post-traumatic effects of tangential corneal injuries are probably often misdiagnosed as EBMD

2. The 10- to 15-year polymethylmethacrylate (PMMA) hard lens patient who can no longer wear lenses comfortably
   a. Patient usually about age 25 to 35
   b. Wearing time and comfort decreasing
   c. Fit and cornea appear perfect
   d. Discontinuation or refit with soft or (sometimes) rigid gas-permeable lens solves problem
   e. This may have been a weak (nondystrophic) EBM, mechanically or physiologically aggravated by PMMA material
      i. Soft lens creates bandage effect
      ii. RGP lens relieves hypoxic effect
3. Dry eye–keratitis sicca syndromes common in aging patients often demonstrate EBMD-like signs and symptoms; however, consider:
   a. Morning syndrome (AM irritation versus typical later-day symptoms in dry eye)

b. No rose bengal staining
c. Negative NaFl staining versus BUT
d. Possible map–dot–fingerprint changes present
e. No apparent tear-film abnormality
f. This is more likely a nondystrophic EBM aging (or degenerative) change than a true dry eye–keratitis sicca syndrome

F. Suggestion

1. Retain EBMD as the mnemonic device
2. But instead of *Epithelial Basement Membrane Dystrophy*, broaden the mnemonic to *Epithelial Basement Membrane Disorders*
   a. Dystrophic (< 2 to 6 percent from age 20 up)
   b. Acquired (variable frequency at all ages
   c. Degenerative (frequency as high as 50 percent from age 20 and older and greater than 50 percent from age 60 and up)

VI. Superficial Keratitis* (Color Plates 54 and 55)

Background Information

A. SUBJECTIVE CONSIDERATIONS

1. Presentation of corneal symptoms with no associated history of corneal injury, irritation, or foreign body
2. Corneal symptoms usually reported in one of three classic descriptions
   a. Report of a sandy, gritty feeling in eye(s)
   b. Description of a foreign-body sensation
   c. Report of "something under upper lid"
      i. Effect of upper lid pressure during blink
      ii. Worth everting upper lid to rule out any possibility of tarsal foreign body
3. Symptoms are generally acute or subacute
4. Always conduct careful, comprehensive history to help establish nontraumatic etiology
5. Associated symptoms may also help establish etiology
   a. Inflammatory pain and congested feeling
   b. Allergic (hypersensitivity) itching
   c. Viral burning sensation

B. OBJECTIVE CONSIDERATIONS

1. Designation superficial keratitis assumes primary disease process limited to the epithelial layer of cornea
   a. Secondary effects, such as edema and infiltration, should be limited to anterior stroma
   b. Full-thickness stromal involvement should be considered deep keratitis with different diagnostic, therapeutic, and prognostic implications
2. Classic physical finding is superficial punctate keratitis (SPK)
   a. Epithelial surface irregularities caused by multiple etiologic factors and mechanics

---

*In alphabetical order.

i. Superficial erosions (usually well defined)
ii. Microcystic edema (intercellular spaces)
iii. Punctate infiltrates (usually larger with ill-defined borders)
b. All types cause cell juncture breaks that stain with NaFl as small punctate dots (from pinpoint in size to 1 to 2 mm for some infiltrates)
c. Often small punctate dots can concentrate into a focal confluent patch of stain and appear as a single larger lesion

3. Infiltrates (white blood cells) can remain as superficial (punctate infiltrates) or may penetrate deeper
   a. Epithelial infiltrate (full epithelial thickness)
      i. Usually focal toxic or immune response
      ii. Such as staphylococcal marginal infiltrate
   b. Subepithelial infiltrate (between epithelium and anterior surface of Bowman's layer of anterior stroma)
      i. Usually associated with virus (lymphocytes)
      ii. Proximity to anterior stroma may result in mild stromal scar secondary to antigen–antibody reaction over prolonged exposure
         • Scar(s) often mistaken for infiltrates
         • Process can occur with any infiltrate

4. Chronic superficial toxic or hypersensitive irritation will tend to stimulate translimbal immunological vascular responses

a. Increased prominence of limbal arcades
b. Pannus (superficial neovascular process)
c. Neovascularization (deeper, fine, weak, terminal arborizing vessels)

C. ASSESSMENT (DIFFERENTIAL DIAGNOSTIC) CONSIDERATIONS

1. Diagnose superficial keratitis "by the company it keeps," both subjectively and objectively
   a. Bacterial
   b. Viral
   c. Toxic or hypersensitive (immunological)
   d. Mechanical
   e. Irritative
   f. Systemic manifestations
   g. Other associated clinical findings
2. Geographic (topographic) pattern of SPK usually of significant differential diagnostic value in superficial keratitis (localization of predominance of SPK)
   a. Diffuse SPK (in approximate order of frequency) (Fig. 4–7)
      i. Adenovirus
      ii. Toxic staphylococcal reaction
      iii. Medicamentosa (reaction to diagnostic or therapeutic eyedrops)
      iv. Herpes simplex
      v. Herpes zoster
      vi. SPK of Thygeson
      vii. Veruccae
      viii. Molluscum contagiosum
   b. Inferior SPK (in approximate order of frequency) (Fig. 4–8)
      i. Toxic staphylococcal reaction

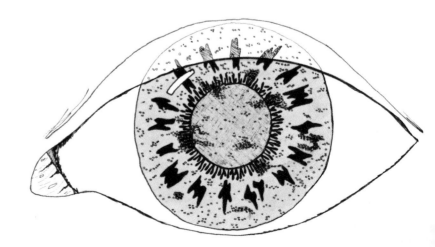

Figure 4–7.
Diffuse SPK pattern

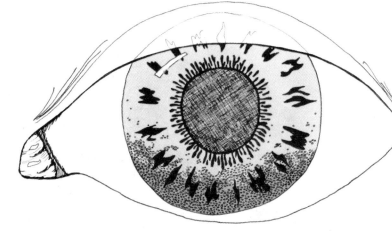

Figure 4–8.
Inferior SPK pattern

ii. Trichiasis (usually vertical or irregular foreign-body tracking)
iii. Medicamentosa (gravitational effect)
iv. Entropion (same pattern as trichiasis)
c. Band-region SPK (usually epithelial erosions) (Fig. 4–9)
   i. Dry-eye syndrome
   ii. Keratoconjunctivitis sicca
   iii. Exposure
      • Lagophthalmos
      • Radiation burns
      • Chemical burns
   iv. Neurotropic
d. Superior SPK (in approximate order of frequency) (Fig. 4–10)
   i. Atopic keratoconjunctivitis
   ii. Superior limbic keratoconjunctivitis (SLK)
   iii. Inclusion (chlamydial) keratoconjunctivitis
   iv. Vernal keratoconjunctivitis
   v. Trachoma (old scarring or active stage)

3. Most important differential consideration in assessing superficial keratitis is differentiating infiltration (process) from ulceration (process)
   a. Infiltrative keratitis usually superficial (epithelial) and noninfectious (sterile on culture)
   b. Ulcerative keratitis deeper (stromal) and usually infectious (e.g., bacterial, fungal)

D. PLAN AND FOLLOW-UP (TREATMENT AND MANAGEMENT)

1. Aminoglycoside(s) (e.g., gentamicin, tobramycin), as therapeutic or prophylactic agent
   a. Minimum standard for acute or subacute keratitis
   b. Minimum therapeutic dosage, qid for 5 to 7 days depending on diagnosis and degree of presentation
   c. Minimum prophylactic dosage, bid for 2 to 3 days

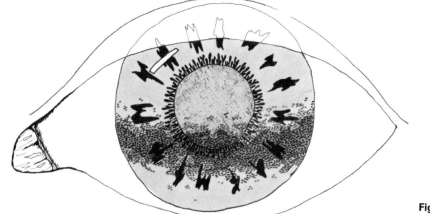

Figure 4–9.
Band region SPK pattern

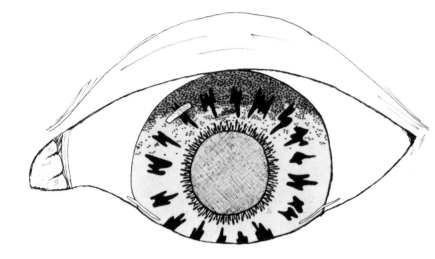

Figure 4– 10.
Superior SPK pattern

2. Topical steroids are indicated in superficial corneal involvements, including cellular or tissue damage, destruction, infiltration, or scarring being produced by noninfectious-induced immune response
   a. Contraindicated in infectious (ulcerative) keratitis or any superficial keratitis of suspicious origin
   b. With suspicion (of infection or ulceration) or risk factors for ulcer, do not introduce steroids for minimum of 24 to 48 hours or until clinical picture or cultures reveal noninfectious etiology
3. Lubricants are valuable adjunctive agents with or without other therapy
   a. Can be used to monitor a suspicious keratitis
   b. Tend to reduce subjective corneal symptoms
   c. Should not be used exclusively (e.g., without prophylactic antibiotic) in acute or subacute keratitis (SPK with inflammation)
4. Hypertonic saline (drops or ointments) can be used to reduce secondary epithelial edema
   a. Not effective in deeper stromal edemas
   b. Not effective in larger (than SPK) epithelial defects
5. Standard cycloplegic-dilation therapy may be indicated in moderate to severe SPKs to reduce risk of (or actual) secondary anterior uveitis
   a. Prostaglandins (inflammogenic agents) released in aqueous with any degree of corneal insult
   b. High probability of secondary anterior uveitis in moderate to severe superficial keratitis
   c. Minimum dosage, tid (e.g., 1 percent tropicamide, 2 or 5 percent homatropine) based on degree of corneal and anterior chamber sign and symptoms
6. Heat is useful adjunctive therapy to reduce ciliary muscle spasms and to promote epithelial healing
7. Oral medications are rarely indicated in superficial keratitis because of the avascular nature of the cornea and subclinical tear level concentrations
8. Complications from superficial keratitis are usually nonepithelial, but rather a product of compromised surface epithelial defense mechanisms, tissue damage from immune responses, and secondary anterior stromal infiltration and scarring
   a. Secondary infectious or ulcerative complications
   b. Risk of toxic or hypersensitive, antigen–antibody immune responses causing anterior stromal damage

Clinical Conditions

A. ATOPIC KERATOCONJUNCTIVITIS

Subjective

- Greater in men, age range approximately 20 to 50
- Frequently an active or inactive (history of) atopic dermatitis in patient and family

- Always report itching (moderate to severe) with "insatiable" need to rub the eyes vigorously
  1. Often results in excoriated tissue leading to further discomfort
  2. May also be associated with increased risk of keratoconus
- Symptoms persist year-round (as opposed to vernal or seasonal conditions)
- Additional burning sensation, corneal symptoms and nonspecific irritation is frequently reported

Objective

- Always a bilateral condition
- Discharge includes tearing and often thicker, white, stringy mucoid accumulations on ocular surface
- Lids are usually moderately edematous and mild to moderately erythematous
  1. Also secondary excoriation
  2. Occasionally, chronic edema produces hardening of soft tissues (induration) and leathery textures
- Inferior palpebral conjunctiva produces moderate to dramatic papillary changes
- Bulbar conjunctiva varies from no hyperemia to mild or moderate degrees, but no chemosis
- Corneal findings are concentrated superiorly
  1. Limbal infiltrates (usually circumlimbal)
  2. Trantas' dots
     a. Usually about 1 to 2 mm round, slightly raised whitish dots (eosinophilic accumulations)
     b. Rarely more than two to five present on limbus
  3. Moderate to severe SPK
  4. Chronic forms may show prominent limbal arcades, pannus, and neovascularization
- Long term complications generally produce an anterior stromal haze and scarring
  1. Superior arcus-like band may develop (called pseudogeronotoxon)
  2. Sterile ulceration can occur (usually shallow, oval, and horizontally oriented)
- Superior tarsus generally spared of advanced changes
- Reports of increased frequency of premature cataracts

Assessment

- Rule out vernal keratoconjunctivitis (seasonal)
- Rule out SLK (no dermatitis or atopic history)
- Rule out GPC (dramatic superior tarsal involvement)

Plan

- Cold packs as frequent as possible
- Oral antihistamines or decongestants (OTCs)
- Topical 1 percent prednisolone (dramatically effective)

  1. Dosage q2–4h for short course (maximum 7 to 10 days)
  2. Taper to cromolyn sodium regimen
- Lubricants may provide increased comfort initially

Follow-up

- Counsel and advise patient on chronic nature
- Condition does self-limit over time, but may take many years
- Minimize topical steroids by using only during acute phases and running short courses, replaced as soon as possible with cromolyn sodium (e.g., Opticrom 4%)
  1. Run minimum 6- to 8-week courses of cromolyn at qid
  2. Taper and monitor for exacerbations every 6 months
  3. Advise patient to reinstitute cromolyn therapy at first sign of symptoms or PRN appointments

B. BACTERIAL KERATITIS

1. Synonyms
   a. Bacterial ulcer
   b. Central corneal ulcer
   c. Corneal ulcer
   d. Infectious keratitis
   e. Microbial keratitis
2. See "Infectious keratitis"

C. FILAMENTARY KERATITIS (Color Plate 45)

Subjective

- A secondary nonspecific diagnosis resulting from a primary precipitating clinical condition which disrupts corneal epithelial integrity
- Onset may be acute, subacute, or insidious
- Symptoms range from annoying (in chronic, low-grade forms) to severe in acute presentations
- Corneal foreign-body sensation (as lid tugs on filaments with each successive blink)
- Symptoms of primary causative disease process may also be present

Objective

- Dead epithelial cells combine with mucin debri to form chains (helices) in the form of small round buds and elongated threads (or filaments) from 1 to 3 mm or greater
  1. One end of filament becomes adherent to dry spot on cornea
  2. Unattached portion of filament hangs loosely over corneal surface and moves slightly with the blink
- Filaments tend to accumulate on corneal region most aggravated by underlying, primary disease process (often superior, under upper lid)

- Filaments (or buds) stain with both NaFl and rose bengal
- Signs of primary disease usually associated with filamentary findings

Assessment*

- Determine primary, underlying, causative disease
- Most common possibilities†
  1. Atopic keratoconjunctivitis
  2. Burns to cornea (radiation, thermal, chemical)
  3. Dry eye–keratitis sicca syndromes
  4. Epidemic keratoconjunctivitis
  5. Herpes simplex keratitis
  6. Herpes zoster ophthalmicus
  7. Mechanical (chronic) corneal irritation (e.g., poor contact lens surfaces or edges, tarsal FB)
  8. Postoperative response
  9. Prolonged pressure patching
  10. Recurrent corneal erosion
  11. Superior limbic keratoconjunctivitis (SLK)
  12. Thygeson's superficial punctate keratitis (SPK)
  13. Vernal keratoconjunctivitis

Plan

- Treat primary, underlying disease
- Reduce or remove in situ filaments
  1. Heavy lubrication will reduce filaments over a 3- to 5-day period
  2. Short-term pressure patch (in nonprolonged patch cases) usually melt existing filaments
  3. Mechanically remove filaments
     a. Grasp at base with jeweler's forceps and lift off cornea with upward twist
     b. Gently swab or roll filament onto a wetted cotton tipped aplicator in upward sweep
  4. Acetylcysteine (Mucomyst) 1 × or qid for 24 hours
  5. Low to medium water bandage soft lens for 24 to 48 hours

Follow-up

- Manage primary condition appropriately
- Advise patient on risk of recurrence and PRN recheck

D. INFILTRATIVE KERATITIS

1. Synonyms
   a. Marginal infiltrative keratitis
   b. Marginal keratitis
   c. Marginal ulcer (misnomer)
   d. Staphylococcal infiltrative keratitis
   e. Sterile infiltrative keratitis
   f. Sterile keratitis
2. See Marginal keratitis

---

*See also Appendix 2.
†In alphabetical order.

E. KERATOCONJUNCTIVITIS SICCA SYNDROMES

Refer to section X, part D of this chapter, "Dry Eye–Keratitis Sicca-type Syndromes", for a complete discussion

F. MARGINAL KERATITIS (Color Plates 56 and 57)

Background Information[26]

1. Synonyms
   a. Marginal infiltrative keratitis
   b. Marginal staphylococcal keratitis
   c. Marginal ulcer (misnomer)
   d. Staphylococcal infiltrative keratitis
   e. Sterile infiltrative keratitis
2. Caused by infiltrative immune response to staphylococcal exotoxins (usually from inferior lid margin glands)[27]
   a. Most vulnerable sites at 4 and 8 o'clock positions of peripheral cornea (approximately), where the lid margin crosses corneolimbal juncture (4–8 syndrome)[28]
   b. Exotoxins are enzymes that produce superficial toxic (infiltrative/immune) responses
   c. Result in intraepithelial infiltrates on mid-peripheral cornea (usually inferior)
      i. Raised lesions due to accumulated excess of infiltrative cells and debri
      ii. Lesions are always "islands" on peripheral cornea with clear interval (called interval of Vogt) between limbus and distal border of lesion (antigen–antibody response)
3. Corneal lesion (infiltrate) is sterile response to bacterial (staphylococcal) toxins on corneal surface[29]
   a. Keratitis is sterile keratitis, as opposed to infectious keratitis, which has live bacteria on, or in, the cornea (producing ulceration)
   b. Cultures of sterile infiltrative keratitis will be negative, even though primary cause is *Staphylococcus*
   c. Clinical diagnosis (of symptoms, risk factors, and physical signs) usually more useful than laboratory work (versus necessity for cultures in ulcers)
4. Appropriate therapy for infiltrative or immune process is to reverse the infiltration and "melt" the excess accumulated infil-

trative cells and debris by immunosuppressing the tissue with corticosteroids

   a. Simultaneous antistaphylococcal therapy helps reduce primary cause of toxins with resultant immune response and its adverse corneal tissue effects and potential risk of scarring

   b. Ulcerative process requires deep stromal immune response to reduce penetration and thus contraindicates immunosuppressive corticosteroid use

Subjective

- Acute or subacute presentation (upon waking)
- Usually unilateral
- Frequent history of previous occurrences (usually subacute and self-limiting)
- Classic corneal symptoms
  1. Sandy, gritty sensation
  2. Foreign-body sensation
  3. "Something under upper lid"
- History of staphylococcal lid disease (subclinical, chronic, subacute, or acute)
- Visual acuity rarely effected
- Generally a painful, watery eye with or without photophobia
- Consider infectious keratitis risk factors in history

Objective

- Staphylococcal toxic (sterile) infiltrative response at the peripheral corneal margin
- Lesions are most often found inferiorly
  1. Most common at 4 and 8 o'clock positions, where inferior lid margin intersects limbus (4–8 syndrome)
  2. May also be superior or circumlimbal
- Lesions may be single or multiple, usually ranging in size from approximately 0.5 to 1.5 mm (maximum)
  1. Multiple lesions may combine into an elongated circumlimbal single appearing lesion
  2. Any combination of single, elongated and even 360° infiltrative lesions possible
- Infiltrative lesions are *always* island(s) on the corneal periphery with clear corneal tissue between distal border of lesion and limbus (interval of Vogt)
  1. Surrounding edema (when dense) may cloud interval
  2. But NaFl staining pattern will reveal lesion as a distinctly (brighter) staining "island"
- Bulbar conjunctiva produces moderate to severe superficial hyperemic, injected vessel patterns
  1. Usually greatest inferiorly
  2. Most common to have "leashes" (radiating pattern) of vessels ranging from 15 to 90° pointing directly toward infiltrated marginal corneal area
- Superficial injected conjunctival vessels often cross corneolimbal juncture (inflammatory or immune response)
  1. Produce prominent limbal arcades and ultimately superficial corneal vascularization (pannus)
  2. Chronic (inflammatory or immune) vascular response can begin to produce deeper, fine vessel tufts with terminal branching into anterior (and deep) corneal stroma (neovascularization)
- Surrounding corneal edema usually mild to moderate
  1. Produces a haze around infiltrate (especially in subacute and chronic cases)
  2. Usually 0.5- to 1-mm diameter
  3. Mostly epithelial edema, but could also involve anterior stroma (up to half-stromal thickness)
- Occasionally radiating pigmented spokes (keratomelanocytosis may be associated)
- Proximal or adjacent subepithelial infiltrates may develop secondarily
- Chronic, subacute, delayed, or undertreated lesions may produce anterior stromal (antigen–antibody) infiltration
  1. Usually result in anterior stromal focal hazes and nebula (faint opacification)
  2. May also produce leukomatous anterior stromal scar(s) (often noted in subclinical presentation)
- Rarely, staphylococcal toxins or other toxic agents may progress (by resisting immune defense mechanisms) to produce anterior stromal necrosis (tissue destruction and loss)
  1. This must be considered a "sterile ulcer," as opposed to the more common sterile infiltrate
  2. Sterile ulcer (as with infectious ulcers) is a more advanced, depressed, pale gray lesion, usually 1 to 2 mm in diameter
  3. Sterile ulcers should be treated and managed under infectious keratitis guidelines

Assessment

- Differentiate from infectious keratitis
- Rule out other peripheral corneal lesions
- Rule out sterile ulceration
  1. More advanced and intense response
  2. Loss of anterior stromal substance
  3. Infiltrate is raised lesion (on slit-lamp examination) versus depressed (ulcerative) appearance
  4. Infiltrate stains superficially (from breaks in squamous epithelial cell junctures) and clear within minutes
  5. Ulcers stain deeply (into stroma) and tend to produce an amorphous spreading pattern to stain over following minutes

Plan[30]*

- Clinical presentations *without* significant infectious risk factors
  1. For mild presentations (mild to moderate symptoms and one or few small (≤ 0.5 mm) superficial lesions

---

*See also Appendix 4.

a. Hot packs qid for 7 to 10 days
b. Gentamicin drops tid to qid for 5 to 7 days
c. Bacitracin ointment on lid margins tid to qid
d. Return check in 3 to 5 days or PRN
2. For moderate presentations, moderate to severe symptoms with 0.5- to 1-mm lesion(s)
   a. Cycloplege/dilate with 1 percent tropicamide qid
   b. Gentamicin (or tobramycin) drops q2–4h
   c. One percent prednisolone drops qid
   d. Hot packs and bacitracin ointment (as with mild)
   e. Return check 2 to 3 days or PRN
3. For severe presentations (severe symptoms and larger, suspicious-looking lesions)
   a. Cycloplege and dilate with 5 percent homatropine q5h
   b. Loading dose
      i. Delivered in-office during first visit
      ii. 1 gtt tobramycin every minute 5 ×
   c. Extended dose
      i. Delivered by patient (or advocate) at home
      ii. Three gtt tobramycin (at 1-minute intervals) hourly for 24 hours (asking patient to wake q2h throughout the night)
   d. Return check within 24 hours of initial visit
   e. Do not introduce steroids in severe presentations for the first 24 to 48 hours
      i. Risk of sterile or infectious ulcerative process, especially with any risk factors, indicates withholding early steroid use
      ii. Secondary risk of anterior stromal infiltration, causing mild peripheral scarring attributable to delayed immunosuppression preferable to risk of aggravating possible early ulcer

- Clinical presentations *with* multiple or significant infectious risk factors
  1. For mild presentations
     a. Hot packs qid
     b. Gentamicin drops q4h
     c. Bacitracin ointment on lid margins tid to qid
     d. Return check within 24 to 48 hours or PRN
  2. For moderate and severe presentations
     a. Same as for severe presentation without infectious risk factors
     b. Seriously consider culturing cornea before administering antibiotic therapy
     c. If degree of clinical suspicion is high, based on multiple, suggestive ulcerative signs, follow guidelines for infectious keratitis immediately

Follow-up

- *Without* infectious risk factors
  1. Mild conditions on return check (3 to 5 days)
     a. Stable or improving: reduce and discontinue plan within 7 to 10 days
     b. If worse, increase plan to moderate level
     c. After control and discontinued therapy, advise "staph risk-reduction program" (see Table 2–1)
     d. Prognosis: usually complete resolution with no scarring and minimal risk of reoccurrence
     e. Recheck in 6 to 12 months or PRN
  2. Moderate conditions on return check (2 to 3 days)
     a. Stable or improving: reduce and discontinue plan within 10 to 14 days
     b. If worse, increase plan to severe level
     c. After control and discontinued therapy, advise "staph risk-reduction program"
     d. Prognosis: usually complete resolution, with slight risk of recurrent staph problems
     e. Recheck in 6 months or PRN
  3. Severe conditions on return check (within 24 hours)
     a. Stable: continue for additional 24 hours
     b. Improving: introduce moderate level plan (with steroid) and reduce slowly and discontinue over 2- to 3-week period, depending on response
     c. If worse, culture (if not done initially) and introduce bacterial keratitis treatment plan
     d. After control and discontinued therapy, advise on continued risk of reinfection and need for "staph risk-reduction program"
     e. Prognosis: probable anterior stromal peripheral leucomatous scar (usually minimally apparent)
     f. Recheck in 3 months or PRN
- *With* infectious risk factors
  1. Mild conditions on return check (within 24–48 hours)
     a. Stable or improving: reduce and discontinue plan within 7 to 10 days
     b. If worse, increase to severe level plan
     c. Advise and educate patient regarding specific infectious risk factors and introduce appropriate care when indicated
     d. Prognosis: no risk of scarring and with proper care and control of risk factors, minimal risk of recurrence
     e. Return check in 3 to 6 months or PRN
  2. Moderate to severe conditions on return (within 24 hours)
     a. Stable: continue for additional 24 hours
     b. Improving: introduce moderate level plan (with steroid) and reduce slowly and discontinue over 2- to 3-week period, depending on response
     c. If worse, culture (if not done initially) and introduce bacterial keratitis treatment plan
     d. Advise and educate patient regarding specific infectious risk factors and introduce appropriate care when indicated
     e. Prognosis: probable anterior stromal peripheral leucomatous scar (usually minimally apparent) and with proper care and control of risk factors, mild to moderate risk of reoccurrence
     f. Return check within 3 months after com-

plete discontinuation of all medical therapies, or PRN

G. PHLYCTENULAR KERATOCONJUNCTIVITIS

Subjective

- Usually unilateral presentation
- Acute or subacute onset of symptoms
- Classic corneal symptoms
  1. Sandy, gritty feeling
  2. Foreign-body sensation
  3. "Something under upper lid"
- Frequently associated with staphylococcal signs and symptoms
- Visual acuity minimally affected
- Variable degrees of lacrimation and photophobia

Objective

- Phlyctenule (or phlycten) is localized, superficial, infiltrative reaction
  1. A raised, circumscribed, focal accumulation of infiltrative cells and debris
  2. Caused by superficial epithelial toxins
  3. Lesion associated with variable degrees of surrounding edema and hyperemia
- Lesions may form at any site on ocular surface
  1. On bulbar conjunctiva away from limbus, phlycten produces phlyctenular conjunctivitis
  2. When proximal to limbus, phlycten may extend onto peripheral cornea, producing phlyctenular keratoconjunctivitis
- Most common sites for limbal phlyctenules are the inferior circumlimbal areas, especially the 4 and 8 o'clock positions (4–8 syndrome)
- Usually, injected bulbar conjunctival vessels create "leash" of hyperemia pointing toward lesion
  1. Vessels may overlie corneal portion of phlycten
  2. May produce a superficial pannus onto cornea
- Occasionally (not common), multiple phlyctenules may develop simultaneously
- Size of phlyctenules vary considerably
  1. Width may range from 1 to 4 mm
  2. Extension onto cornea may range from 1 to 3 mm
- Rarely, mucopurulent discharge will be associated
- Generally, corneal surface surrounding phlyctenule will demonstrate variable degrees of toxic SPK

Assessment

- Older sources generally associate phlyctenular keratoconjunctivitis with tuberculosis
  1. Probably correct regarding worldwide distribution
  2. In industrialized, developed countries (e.g., United States), 75 percent of cases are toxic staphylococcal reactions
  3. Nontheless, rule out history of tuberculosis (TB)
- Rule out other peripheral inflammatory corneal reactions
  1. Marginal keratitis: mid-periphery (island) lesion without raised conjunctival portion
  2. Limbal infiltrates (e.g., vernal, atopic): limited to corneolimbal tissue, with no conjunctival (raised) portion
  3. Others: usually keratitic rather than keratoconjunctivitic (associated conjunctival lesion)
- Rule out noninflamed, raised corneolimbal lesions
  1. Such as pterygium, degenerations
  2. Usually insidious versus acute and not inflamed

Plan

- Topical steroids (e.g., prednisolone) in relatively high dosages (q3–4h) to "melt" infiltrate quickly and minimize risk of anterior stromal scarring
- Prophylactic gentamicin drops qid for 5 to 7 days
- For moderate to severe presentations (extensive corneal involvement), cycloplege and dilate with 1 percent tropicamide or 5 percent homatropine during acute phase
- If *Staphylococcus* likely cause, add bacitracin ointment on lids bid to qid
- Recheck within 3 to 5 days depending on steroid dosage

Follow-up

- Phlyctenule should show quick response and reversal
  1. If not, increase steroid dosage
  2. Upon improvement, continue steroid until complete reduction of raised lesion and (it is hoped) total resolution of corneal (anterior stromal) haze
- Often, permanent anterior stromal leucomatous hazy scar will persist with or without overlying pannus (and rarely, neovascularization)
- Full course of therapy may run up to 2 to 4 weeks
  1. Monitor closely during treatment for steroid complications
  2. Taper therapy once phlycten or scarring maximally reduced
- If staphylococcal toxins determined (or assumed) cause, advise and prescribe "staph risk-reduction program" (see Table 2–1)
- Recheck within 6 months or PRN

H. STAPHYLOCOCCAL SUPERFICIAL PUNCTATE KERATITIS[28] (Color Plate 55)

Subjective

- History of staphylococcal lid problems or active lid disease
- Variable age ranges

- Usually sandy, gritty corneal irritation
- Most frequently bilateral presentations
- Often a previous history of similar irritations
- Visual acuity may be decreased slightly
- Variable degrees of photophobia or lacrimation
- More frequent in dry eye (older) patients and contact lens wearers

Objective

- Variable quantity and quality (fine to coarse) SPK (punctate NaFl staining of squamous epithelium)
  1. Most frequent presentation concentrated on inferior corneal surface (to lower limbus)
  2. May also present as diffuse SPK (entire corneal surface)
  3. Frequently localized areas of SPK (greater inferiorly, especially at 4 or 8 o'clock) may become dense and confluesce into "patches" of NaFl staining (prodromal sign of toxic marginal infiltrative keratitic response)
- Broad range of bulbar conjunctival hyperemia
  1. Most common pattern is inferior injection, ranging from localized "leashes" of vessels (usually at the 4 and 8 o'clock positions) up to 180°
  2. Diffuse SPK ranges from minimally observable to grossly hyperemic (meaty red) with widely dilated, injected superficial vessels
  3. Frequently hyperemic pattern may limit itself to the lateral, nasal–temporal palpebral fissure exposed areas, producing an "angular" pattern
- Palpebral conjunctiva usually produces a mild to moderate degree of papillary conjunctivitis
  1. Papillae are slightly raised vascular tufts, poorly visualized individually when small and dense as in staphylococcal keratitis (versus giant forms in superior tarsal palpebral reactions)
  2. Presentation usually appears as a hyperemic velvety texture to the inferior palpebral conjunctiva
- Discharge is absent in the mild to moderate forms but mucopurulence will be present in keratitis secondary to hyperacute bacterial conjunctivitis
  1. Cultures are indicated in hyperacute forms
  2. Treatment should be aggressive with close follow-up
  3. Rule out risk of bacterial (versus secondary toxic) keratitis
- Active or residual staphylococcal lid signs usually present (e.g., crustation, tylosis, madarosis)
- Occasionally, corneal epithelium will produce a secondary microcystic type edema
  1. May be diffuse edematous haze
  2. May be a localized (e.g., 4–8 positions) edematous patch ranging from mild haze to dense epithelial edema or even anterior stromal edema
- Varying degrees of marginal anterior stromal scars often observed on peripheral cornea (greater inferior from old marginal infiltrative reactions

1. Mild translucent hazy spot(s) (macula scarring)
2. Moderately dense spot(s) (nebula)
3. Opaque whitish-gray spot(s) (leucomas)

Assessment

- Rule out other causes of inferior and diffuse SPKs
- Rule out infectious keratitis
  1. Especially viral keratoconjunctivitis
  2. Diagnosis by "the company the SPK keeps" (e.g., tearing, preauricular lymph node enlargement, and follicular palpebral conjunctival changes are viral "company" to a diffuse SPK)

Plan*

For Mild Presentations (Fine SPK With Mild Hyperemia)

- Ocular lubricants 6 to 10 times per day
- "Staph risk-reduction program" (with bacitracin ointment) bid to tid[31]
- Recheck in 10 to 14 days or PRN

For Moderate Presentations (Dense SPK With Hyperemia)

- Ocular lubricants 6 to 10 times per day
- "Staph risk-reduction program" (with gentamicin ointment) tid to qid
- Recheck in 7 to 10 days or PRN

For Severe Presentations (Dense, Confluescing SPK)

- Gentamicin (or tobramycin) drops combined and topical steroid (or antibiotic–steroid combination regimen) qid or q4h
- "Staph risk-reduction program" (with gentamicin ointment) qid
- Recheck in 3 to 7 days or PRN

Follow-up

- All levels of presentation should improve within 1 to 2 weeks of treatment
  1. If unchanged or advancing (SPK), reconfirm noninfectious (toxic) etiology and add steroid (if not already being used), or increase dosages
  2. After positive response, taper steroid first, and then reduce treatment plan to maintenance level
- Maintanence levels for "staph risk-reduction program"
  1. One week at bid (with antibiotic ointment)
  2. One week at hs (with antibiotic ointment)
  3. One month at hs (without antibiotic ointment)
  4. Three months at 2 × per week
- Recheck in 3 to 6 months or PRN

I. STERILE KERATITIS

1. Synonyms
   a. Hypersensitivity (immume) keratitis

---

*See also Appendix 4.

b. Infiltrative keratitis
c. Marginal infiltrative keratitis
d. Marginal keratitis
e. Marginal ulcer (misnomer)
f. Staphylococcal infiltrative keratitis
g. Sterile infiltrative keratitis
h. Sterile ulcer
i. Toxic keratitis
2. See appropriate diagnosis (per synonym)

J. SUPERFICIAL PUNCTATE KERATITIS (SPK) OF THYGESON[32]

Subjective

- Etiology unknown (viral suggested)[33]
- Greatest frequency in young adult females (age 15 to 40)
- Usually mild symptomatic reports (if at all) of transient sandy, gritty sensation
- Occasional mild to moderate photophobic reaction
- Any reports of symptoms usually remit and exacerbate over short periods of 4- to 6-week duration
- Patients begin to remain relatively asymptomatic in later years of disease process, with remission periods becoming longer and exacerbations shorter and milder
- Disease tends to self-limit over a 4- to 7-year period
- Often diagnosed during routine examination because of its asymptomatic nature

Objective

- Generally bilateral, but greater in one eye
- Diffuse SPK with slightly greater concentration in central corneal regions
  1. SPK may be fine or coarse, sparse or dense
  2. When dense, visual acuity is reduced
  3. When coarse or dense, confluescence of NaFl staining may produce large patches and spots on corneal surface
- Epithelial infiltrates (slightly raised) frequently develop with subsequent exacerbations of disease
  1. Produce negative staining patterns (i.e., break up NaFl pattern directly over epithelial surface above infiltrate)
  2. Recurrences of infiltrates often change with reactivation of keratitis
     a. Position of lesions may change
     b. Size of lesions may change
     c. Shapes of lesions may change
- Eyes tend to remain white and clear in the presence of distinct keratitis, which would normally produce a secondary conjunctival inflammatory response
- Beyond the primary SPK, eyes show no associated signs of any infectious or inflammatory disease process
  1. SPK of Thygeson "keeps no company"

2. One of the only keratites that "keep no company"

Assessment

- Rule out other causes of SPKs
  1. Bacterial
  2. Viral
  3. Sterile
- If patient wears contact lenses, rule out lens-associated causes of SPK
  1. Material-related causes
  2. Solution-related causes
  3. Mechanical, physiological, toxic causes

Plan*

- Mild to moderate SPKs may require lubrication therapy only, with close monitoring for complications
- For moderate to severe degrees of SPKs (with or without symptoms)
  1. Heavy lubrication (6 to 10 times per day)
  2. Topical steroids q2–4h for 10 to 14 days (or more)
     a. Occasionally condition may not respond to steroids
     b. Discontinue use if no response in 3 to 4 weeks
  3. Reports of viral etiology (e.g., herpes simplex, zoster) recommend use of Viroptic q3–4h for 2 to 4 weeks[33]
     a. Beware of antiviral epithelial toxicities
     b. As with steroids, if no response in 3 to 4 weeks discontinue and reconsider diagnosis, other therapies (e.g., steroids, if not previously tried), lubrication, no therapy (with close monitoring) or bandage soft lenses
  4. Soft contact lens bandaging useful in medically nonresponsive cases or symptomatic patients
- Soft contact lens wearers who present with SPK of Thygeson may be kept on lens wear (as bandage) with close monitoring (every 4 to 6 weeks or PRN)
- With any therapy of moderate to severe degree SPK, add prophylactic gentamicin or tobramycin drops bid to qid (also in conjunction with bandage lens wear)

Follow-up

- Advise and educate patient as to unkown etiology, clinical course, chronicity, risks, and prognosis of condition
- Treat moderate to severe degrees only during periods of exacerbations with patient instructed to report initial symptoms (if present) or signs (e.g., vision) of each episode

---

*See also Appendix 4.

- Without contact lens wear, recheck every 4 to 6 month or PRN
- With contact lens wear (cosmetic or therapeutic), recheck every 4 to 6 weeks or PRN

K. VIRAL KERATOCONJUNCTIVITIS

A complete discussion of viral keratoconjunctivitis begins in section VIII of this chapter

VII. Infectious Keratitis

Background Information

A. SUBJECTIVE CONSIDERATIONS

1. Symptoms are usually acute to hyperacute including corneal irritation and uveitic (deeper) pain
2. Whereas traumatic histories (injury and irritation) help differentiate etiology of superficial corneal epithelial disease (e.g., inflammatory or immune response from irritation or injury), epithelial injury is a major risk factor in the diagnosis of infectious keratitis
3. Risk-factor analysis is the most important means of early assessment of infectious keratitis
   a. Helps differentiate between early physical signs of sterile versus infectious keratitis
   b. Helps differentiate between possible causes of infectious keratitis (e.g., bacterial versus fungal)
   c. Helps determine the significance of symptoms (e.g., foreign-body sensation in a noncompliant, extended wear contact lens patient with 3-year-old lenses versus a non-lens-wearing patient)
4. Risk-factor analysis for infectious keratitis
   a. Symptom-related risk factors (in approximate order of increasing risk)
      i. Mild, nonspecific irritation
      ii. Burning sensation (toxins from microbe?)
      iii. Lacrimation
      iv. Photophobia
      v. Reduced visual acuity
      vi. History of corneal injury
      vii. Foreign body sensation
      viii. Continuing foreign-body sensation in contact lens patient after lens removal
   b. Contact lens-related risk factors (in approximate order of increasing risk)
      i. Noncompliance (e.g., regarding wear, care)
      ii. Poor hygiene
      iii. Tight-fitting lenses
      iv. Extended wear
      v. Old lenses (usually greater than 6 to 12 months)
      vi. Dirty lens surfaces
      vii. Recent lens manipulations (e.g., insertion and removal procedures)
      viii. Contaminated solutions
   c. Health-related risk factors (in approximate order of increasing risk)
      i. Diabetes
      ii. Warm climates
      iii. Staphylococcal toxins
      iv. Dry eye syndromes
      v. Immune-compromised patients, such as acquired immune deficiency syndrome (AIDS)
      vi. Postsurgical corneas
      vii. Topical steroids
      viii. Mechanical irritation (corneal trauma)
      ix. Focal epithelial defects

B. OBJECTIVE CONSIDERATIONS

1. Infectious keratitis indicates the presence of a viable infectious organism (microbe) living and proliferating both on and in the cornea
   a. Bacteria
   b. Virus
   c. Fungi
   d. Protozoa (e.g., *Acanthamoeba*)
2. Critical indication for laboratory analysis along with clinical assessment
   a. Cytology (histopathology)
   b. Cultures and sensitivities
   c. Specimens (ideally) should be taken before any treatment is rendered
      i. Often not the case because of initial noninfectious diagnosis or secondary infection
      ii. Laboratory workup still useful af-

ter commencement of therapy for differential diagnostic purposes and for resistant organisms

3. Active proliferating microbes usually render pathological effect on corneal stroma, with resultant deep keratitis reactions versus superficial epithelial keratitis, which is usually sterile (toxins rather than live organisms on cornea, with the exception of some viruses)

4. Toxic by-products (e.g., enzymes) of the active, proliferating microbial organisms (e.g., endotoxins of gram-negative bacteria: *Pseudomonas*) produce ulcer or necrotizing effect to stromal substance versus epithelial infiltrative reaction in superficial keratitis

5. Deep stromal reaction associated with infectious ulcerative keratitis produces deep (usually full stromal thickness) infiltrative or immune response to proliferating toxic (proteolytic) enzymes of offending organism

   a. Immune defense system is attempting to neutralize toxins and protect stromal tissue

   b. Because of virulence of organism and depth of reaction, immune system produces more dramatic and diffuse response than to the focal, localized, superficial toxins (usually staphylococcal exotoxins) associated with superficial keratitis

6. Most corneal ulcers tend to develop centrally, father away from the immediate influence of the immune system (probably avoiding such influence) from the vascular supply at the limbus; thus, the immune system is further obligated to produce a more disseminated, pronounced, deep infiltrative response to effect neutralization of the offending organism and protection of the stromal tissue (from further ulceration)

   a. Not to say that some highly virulent organisms can also seed peripherally on the cornea and succeed in overcoming at least the initial effects of a proximal immune system response

   b. In either case, such a pronounced, deep infiltrative or immune response produces a significantly more dramatic and disseminated clinical inflammatory reaction than that of a localized superficial epithelial infiltrative response

7. Because of this intense inflammatory reaction, occurring in response to the ulcerative process, considerable adverse associated findings to the cornea and adjacent anatomy are produced (in spite of the attempted benefits being administered by the immune defense mechanism)

   a. Lid edema and erythema

   b. Conjunctival hyperemia and chemosis

   c. Corneal
      i. Edema (epithelial and stromal)
      ii. Infiltration (deep stromal)
      iii. Neovascularization (as chronic response)
      iv. Posterior corneal keratic precipitates
      v. Folds in Descemet's membrane (striae)

   d. Anterior chamber
      i. Uveitic response (cells and flare)
      ii. Endophthalmitis (sterile hypopyon, accumulated white blood cells in chamber)
      iii. Increased intraocular pressure (secondary to angle congestion)

C. ASSESSMENT (DIFFERENTIAL DIAGNOSTIC) CONSIDERATIONS*

1. The primary diagnostic consideration is the accurate differentiation between infectious ulcerative keratitis and sterile infiltrative keratitis

   a. Definition of *ulcer(ation)*: a local defect, or excavation, of the surface of an organ or tissue, which is produced by sloughing of inflammatory necrotic tissue[34] (Fig. 4–11)

   b. Definition of *infiltration*: the diffusion or accumulation in a tissue or cells of substances not normal to it or in amounts in excess of the normal[35] (Fig. 4–12)

2. Differential diagnosis is established by three steps

   a. Careful history and risk-factor analysis (Table 4–4)

   b. Detailed physical examination (Table 4–5)

   c. Categorizing patient based on combined assessment of history, symptoms, and risk factors (subjective) relative to physical examination (objective)

---

*See also Appendices 2 and 3.

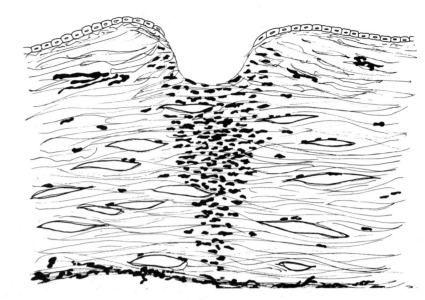

Figure 4–11.
Histopathology of corneal ulceration

3. Risk categories for infectious keratitis
   a. Low risk: few subjective or objective findings
   b. Medium risk: risk factors in the presence of suspicious physical findings
   c. High risk: significant risk factors combined with ulcerative finding(s)
4. Comparison of sterile infiltrate to corneal ulcer[36,37] (Table 4–5)

5. After establishing a definitive diagnosis of infectious keratitis, next step is to attempt to differentiate type of infectious keratitis (Table 4–6)
   a. Clinical differential sometimes difficult
   b. Laboratory workup essential (e.g., cytology, cultures, and sensitivities)
6. After establishing specific type of infec-

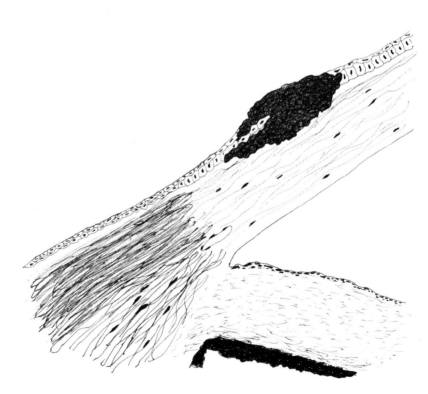

Figure 4–12.
Histopathology of corneal infiltration

TABLE 4-4. INFECTIOUS KERATITIS: SUBJECTIVE[a]

Risk	Symptom-related Risk Factors	Contact Lens-related Risk Factors	Health-related Risk Factors
Increasing risk[b]	A Mild irritation B Burning C Lacrimation — — — — — — — — D Photophobia E Reduced VA F FB sensation G FB sensation continues (or increases) after CL removal	A Noncompliance B Poor hygiene procedures C Tight fit D Extended wear — — — — — — — — E "Old" lenses F Dirty lenses G Recent manipulation H Contaminated solutions	A Diabetes B Warmer climates C Staphylotoxins D Dry eyes E Immune-compromised points — — — — — — — — F Postsurgical corneas G Topical steroids H Mechanical irritation I Focal epithelial defects

[a]History, symptoms, and risk factor analysis.
[b]Dotted lines in risk factor categories indicate Author's levels of significant concern. Risk factors below dotted lines, in combination with corneal lesion(s), should be considered as no less than moderate (to severe) presentations.

TABLE 4-5. STERILE VERSUS INFECTIOUS KERATITIS: OBJECTIVE[a]

Findings	Sterile Infiltrate		Bacterial Corneal Ulcer
Eyelids			
Edema	Minimal		Ptosis
Erythema	Faint		Crimson red
Conjunctiva			
Injection	15°–90°		>180°
Intensity	Pink to red		Crimson to violet
Exudate	Lacrimation		Mucopurulence
Cornea (day 1)			
Epithelial defect			
Size	≤ 1mm		≥2 mm
Position	≤2 mm off limbus	THE	≥3 mm in from limbus
Depth	Epithelial		≥50% thickness
Height	Raised	GRAY	Depressed
Edges	Well defined		Fuzzy
NaFl	Superficial (as "Island")	ZONE	Deep
Lucency	Nebula (haze)		Macula to opaque
Edema			
Size	>2 mm (surrounding "Island")		≥50% of surface
Intensity	Epithelial		≥50% stromal thickness
Folds in Descemet's	None		≥2
Infiltration	Superficial		Full stromal thickness
Neo/Pannus			
Area	0–30°		0–360°
Length	0–2 mm		0–4 mm
Anterior chamber			
Cells and flare	None to trace		Countable to dense
Hypopyon	None		≥1 mm
Other			
Pupil size	PERRLA		Miotic
IOP	Normal range		Usually raised
BVA	Unaffected		≤20/50

[a]Clinical signs and physical examinations.

TABLE 4–6. NONBACTERIAL INFECTIOUS KERATITIS: ASSESSMENT[a]

Differential Diagnosis	Subjective	Objective	Assessment	Plan	Prognosis
Herpes simplex stromal keratitis	Burning irritation Recurrent history (?)	Dendrite possible Stromal infiltration	Disciform Wessely ring	Antiviral agents Steroids	Bad!
Fungal keratitis	History of vegetative injury	Spores and hypha Serpiginous	Mooren's ulcer Marginal infiltrate	Natamycin Other antifungal agents	Worse!
Acanthamoeba	History of trauma Poor hygiene Solution contaminates	Localized infiltrate progressing to stromal ring ulcer	↓Usually mistaken for HSV stromal keratitis Nonresponsive	Brolene (?) Neosporin (?) Penetrating keratoplasty	Worst!

[a]Differential diagnosis (ruling out).

tious keratitis, next step is to attempt to differentiate specific category, family, genus, species, depending on infectious etiology (see specific types of infectious keratites)

D. PLAN AND FOLLOW-UP (TREATMENT AND MANAGEMENT)

1. Hospitalization or diligent home care is necessary for all forms of infectious keratitis
   a. Primary concerns are for patient compliance and cooperation with frequency, complexity, intensity, and toxic risks of indicated therapies
   b. Skilled nursing care is usually essential in proper administration of most treatment plans associated with infectious keratitis
2. The most effective method of delivering drugs in infectious keratitis is topical administration
   a. Speed of infectious or ulcerative process on the avascular cornea necessitates topical drug use in high concentration
   b. Oral and intravenous medications do not deliver effect rapidly enough or in high enough concentration (through tears, aqueous, or translimbal effects) as compared with topical agents
      i. May be used if there is significant risk of corneal perforation
      ii. Theory is to bathe posterior corneal tissue with high concentrations in aqueous
   c. Depot injections (subconjunctival or subtenons) may also be used in severe clinical presentations

3. Oral tetracycline may have some value in corneal ulceration as an anticollagenolytic agent[38]
4. Immunosuppressive agents (corticosteroids) are *contraindicated* in active infectious ulceration
   a. Immune system is serving a positive function during active ulcerative process by helping to neutralize toxins and reduce further stromal penetration
   b. Immunosuppression would reduce effect and permit increased penetration and possible perforation
   c. Notwithstanding positive functions of immune system response, deep stromal infiltrative activity potentiates permanent (full thickness) stromal scarring
      i. This is considered an unavoidable sequalae of corneal ulceration
      ii. However, until all infectious organisms and their associated toxins are neutralized and destroyed by appropriate anti-infective agents, the immune system is the singular defense mechanism working to protect the cornea
   d. Once infectious agents are neutralized (as determined by negative culturing), steroids then become *indicated* to reduce any further stromal damage and scarring
5. Unfortunately (for patient and practitioner), the most appropriate and effective therapy for most forms of infectious keratitis (in fact, any stromal infiltrative, ulcerative, or traumatic insult) usually results in permanent corneal scarring
   a. Such scarring (especially in central ul-

ceration) virtually guarantees the risk of cosmetic awareness and permanent functional (vision) loss

b. Negative sequelae of permanent cosmetic scar and functional loss (although unavoidable) are often cause for patient dissatisfaction and distress

c. Substantial potential for such negative outcomes should be considered by the primary eye care provider upon diagnosis and before treatment

   i. Explain diagnosis in clear and simple terms

   ii. Firmly advise patient of need for care

   iii. Discuss nature and goals of treatment

   iv. Carefully and clearly define the associated risks and prognosis of the condition (with and without proper care)

   v. Recommend and coordinate the most appropriate (e.g., corneal specialist) and accessible professional care for treatment and management of the patient

   vi. Contemporaneously (at that very moment) document all clinical information, care, instructions, advice, and recommendations at initial visit and all subsequent visits

Clinical Conditions

A. ACANTHAMOEBA KERATITIS[39,40]

Subjective

- A ubiquitous protozoan capable of infecting injured corneas or corneas of contact lens patients
- History usually includes some form of corneal trauma
- Exposure to stagnant water sources, swimming pools, hot tubs, and so forth, have been reported as risk factors
- Contaminated contact lens solutions have become somewhat notorious risk factors
- Pain is acute and often far more dramatic than early physical signs might suggest
- History often includes nonresponsiveness to steroid therapy or anti-infective medications[41]

Objective

- Early signs may be limited to epithelial disruption nonresponsive to standard anti-infective regimens
- Associated inflammatory reactions include anterior uveitis and scleritis

   1. Advancing conditions produce hypopyon, hyphema, and potential scleral "melt"

   2. Steroids may mitigate inflammation but may not resolve condition

- Corneal involvement advances over days to weeks with little response to standard medical regimens

   1. Epithelial and stromal edema

   2. Circumscribed stromal infiltrative or inflammatory responses

     a. Early appearances include localized stromal infiltrates or radiating infiltrates

     b. Progresses to ring infiltrate or ulcer

     c. Stromal "melt" can occur

     d. Descemtocele can lead to perforation

   3. Posterior corneal surface produces guttata-like endothelial changes

- Other associated findings vary with intensity of progressing infectious corneal involvement

   1. Conjunctival chemosis

   2. Pseudomembranes

   3. Preauricular lymphadenopathy

   4. Pseudodentrites (infiltrative)

- Degree of clinical signs, although chronic, may wax and wane in spite of treatment modalities

Assessment

- Differentiate sterile versus infectious keratitis
- Standard bacterial cultures prove negative
- Deep corneal biopsies are necessary to isolate organism
- Corneal smears under immunofluorescent microscopy with a "calcuflour" agent is considered an accurate diagnostic test[39]
- Early differential diagnosis usually difficult

   1. Often made *ex juvantia* (from lack of response to other forms of therapy)

   2. Risk factor analysis critical in early corneal infections not responding to other therapies

- Rule out all other conditions that might mimic infectious keratitis
- Most common misdiagnosis is stromal herpes simplex

Plan and Follow-up

- Consider and coordinate the most appropriate professional resource(s) for care and management
- Provide patient with proper advise and instructions
- Medical therapies generally ineffective
- Multiple therapies suggested in literature

   1. Ketoconazole (Nizoral)

   2. Miconazole (Monistat)

   3. Neomycin (Neosporin)

   4. Propamadine isethionate (Brolene)

- Adjunctive therapies include

   1. Topical steroids

   2. Bandage soft lenses

   3. Pain relievers

- Surgical intervention (corneal grafting) is usually the long-term prognosis in all cases

B. BACTERIAL KERATITIS (Color Plates 58, 59, and 60)

Background Information

1. Synonyms
   a. Bacterial ulcer
   b. Central corneal ulcer
   c. Corneal ulcer
2. Bacteria generally categorized as gram-positive and gram-negative
   a. Most common gram-positive corneal infectors
      i. *Staphylococcus* (multiple species)
      ii. *Streptococcus pneumoniae* or *pyogenes*
   b. Most common gram-negative corneal infectors (in approximate decreasing order of frequency)
      i. *Pseudomonas aeruginosa*
      ii. *Neisseria gonorrhoeae* (with venereal disease)
      iii. *Hemophilus influenzae* (common in children)
      iv. *Morax axenfeld* (higher risk in alcoholics)
      v. Others
         • *Serratia marcescans*
         • *Proteus vulgaris*
         • *Klebsiella*
         • *Escherichia coli*
         • *Corenybacterium*
3. Most common cause of all bacterial keratitis is *Pseudomonas*
   a. Greater in warmer (southern) climates
   b. Clinical "rule of thumb" is to assume *Pseudomonas* until proved (by culture) otherwise
4. Highest-risk ulcer patients are contact lens wearers[42]
   a. Risk in daily wear soft approximately 0.5 percent
   b. Risk in extended wear soft about 3.5 percent
5. Parents with children in diapers are at greater risk of infection by some gram-negative, gastrointestinal (GI) bacteria
6. Generally, *Staphylococcus* (gram-positive) tends to produce less intense and slower developing ulcers because of its exotoxic (versus endotoxic) nature
   a. *Streptococcus* and the gram-negative bacteria that produce endotoxins are more virulent corneal infectors, developing more rapidly, with hyperacute signs and symptoms and greater risk of corneal damage

   b. *Pseudomonas* is the notorious gram-negative corneal infector because of its virulent endotoxins, rapid proliferation, ubiquitous, opportunistic nature (especially in warm, moist environments) and its ability to destroy corneal stroma within minutes to hours after entering the cornea
      i. The only (minimal) "good news" about *Pseudomonas* is that it cannot penetrate an intact corneal epithelial surface
      ii. It requires a "focal epithelial defect" to enter and begin to infect and ulcerate corneal stroma

Subjective

- Unilateral, acute presentation
- History usually includes at least one (but usually multiple) risk factors
  1. Most common risk factor tends to be history of recent trauma causative of a focal epithelial defect
  2. Recent contact lens manipulations (procedures) can be considered traumatic event
- Other corneal disease states may be considered predisposing factors for ulceration
  1. Superficial keratites
  2. Marginal infiltrate (as focal epithelial defect)
  3. Dry eye–keratitis sicca syndromes
- Rate of progression of ulcer varies with bacteria (in increasing order of speed of progression)
  1. *Staphylococcus* (usually over days)
  2. *Streptococcus* (usually within 1 to 2 days)
  3. Most gram-negatives (usually within 24 hours)
  4. *Neisseria gonorrhea* (usually within 12 to 24 hours)
  5. *Pseudomonas* (within hours)
- Pain usually develops subacutely (within days) to acutely (within minutes to hours)
- Symptoms usually follow typical sequence, especially in contact lens wearers
  1. Nonspecific irritation
  2. Burning sensation (toxins of bacteria)
  3. Lacrimation
  4. Photophobia (secondary to corneal edema)
  5. Reduced vision (from edema and infiltration)
  6. Foreign-body sensation
     a. May develop early without contact lens wear
     b. With contacts (especially soft), bandaging effect can artificially reduce foreign-body sensation late into ulcerative process
  7. Continued (or increasing) foreign-body sensation upon contact lens removal or over extended period of time (hours to days)
  8. Dull, aching (inflammatory or uveitic) pain
- Evaluate carefully for all risk factors

Objective

- Eyelids
  1. *Staphylococcus* usually produces mild to moderate edema and erythema with frequent associated staphylococcal lid signs (marginal crustation, tylosis)
  2. Streptococcal and gram-negative bacteria usually produce severe lid reactions
     a. Pronounced inflammatory response
     b. Pseudoptosis
     c. Preseptal cellulitis
  3. *Hemophilus influenzae* often produces a bluish, purplish preseptal flush in acute phase
  4. *Gonorrhoeae* (and other hyperacute purulent bacteria) may accumulate discharge under a "stuck-shut" lid during sleep and present a "ballooning" lid upon waking (and examination)
     a. Separate lids slowly and carefully
     b. Purulence has tendency to projectile outward on release of lid margins
- Conjunctiva
  1. Bulbar conjunctival reaction is usually a severe crimson-violet red (violacious) hyperemia involving greater than 180°, usually 360°
  2. Chemosis ranges from mild elevation of portions or all the bulbar conjunctiva (<1 mm) to dramatic "watchglass" (bulbar conjunctiva grossly elevated and overlapping peripheral cornea) effects
  3. Strep and some gram-negatives will occasionally produce hemorrhages on the bulbar conjunctiva
  4. Palpebral conjunctiva usually produces mild to moderate papillary (velvety type) changes
  5. Amount of mucopurulent discharge varies considerably according to bacteria, intensity of infection and duration of infection
     a. Staphylococcal discharge ranges from nothing at all to moderate amounts
     b. *Streptococcus* and gram-negative bacteria tend to produce moderate to copious amounts of discharge
     c. Often, a mucous plug congests and overlies the ulcer site on the corneal surface
     d. Gonorrhea is most notorious for its hyperacute mucopurulent nature[43]
- Corneal epithelium during active ulceration
  1. Ulceration usually destroys epithelial surface (and anterior stromal substance) early in the process, producing a depressed, "excavated" lesion
     a. *Staphylococcus* tends to produce well-defined borders creating a clearly circumscribed lesion
     b. *Streptococcus* and gram-negative bacteria produce indistinct "fuzzy" edges to the ulcer
     c. Edges of ulcers frequently show a overhang effect of necrotic epithelial tissue
     d. NaFl stain will pool at the site initially and

spread amorphously into a geographic stromal pattern within minutes
  2. Ulcer is usually about 2-mm diameter or greater
  3. Position on the corneal surface varies
     a. Most common location is centralward, away from the vascular or immune effects of the limbus (synonym: central ulcer)
     b. Virulent organisms may be able to overcome such effects and seed themselves at the corneal periphery (perhaps, using a sterile infiltrate as their focal epithelial defect for entry)
  4. Rarely, additional ulcers (satellite lesions) may develop on cornea during disease process
- Corneal stroma during active ulceration
  1. Corneal edema (epithelial and stromal) usually covers more than 50 percent of the cornea and affects at least 50 percent of the stromal thickness
     a. Produces a whitish-gray corneal haze
     b. Advancing edema creates secondary fold in Descemet's membrane (striate keratitis)
  2. Infiltration occurs under and around the entire ulcer in a classic deep and dense pattern
     a. Depth is usually full-thickness stroma
     b. Density ranges from hazy to opaque
     c. *Staphylococcus* tends to demonstrate a more circumscribed pattern of infiltration, whereas other bacteria (especially *Pseudomonas*) produce diffuse whitish-gray infiltration (sometimes over the entire cornea)
     d. *Pseudomonas* has also been reported as producing ring infiltration or ulceration
  3. Highly virulent organisms, resistant bacteria (to selected antibiotics), and delayed treatment can lead to additional stromal complications
     a. Stromal abscess
     b. Descemetoceles
     c. Stromal melting
     d. Corneal perforation
- Posterior cornea during active ulceration
  1. Striate keratitis (folds in Descemet's)
  2. Keratic precipitates (WBCs on endothelium)
  3. Fibrin plaques (infiltrative or inflammatory debris)
  4. Pseudo-guttata-like formations
- Anterior chamber during active ulceration
  1. Anterior uveitic reaction (cells and flare) always present, ranging from trace reaction to dense (fibrinous) anterior chamber reaction
  2. Staph tends to produce mildest uveitic response, rarely presenting a measurable hypopyon
  3. Sterile hypopyon (endophthalmitis), accumulation of WBCs producing an opaque fluid level in the inferior aqueous, varying in height, presents in most advanced bacterial keratites
- Other associated findings during active ulceration
  1. Neovascularization may develop in varying degree in delayed or untreated corneal ulcers

2. Intraocular pressure (IOP) frequently begins to rise during active ulceration secondary to anterior angle congestion
3. Miotic pupils are often noted during acute phase
4. Visual acuity is almost always reduced significantly, usually below 20/40

Assessment

- Follow step-by-step approach
  1. Analyze risk factors
  2. Careful physical examination
  3. Categorize patient risk
- Differentiate sterile infiltrate from corneal ulcer
- Differentiate bacterial keratitis from other forms of infectious keratitis (Table 4–6)
- Cultures and sensitivities
  1. Positive laboratory workup is always reassuring
  2. Negative laboratory workup is inconclusive
  3. With negative cultures, best to rely on clinical data and presumptive diagnosis
- "Assume the worst" (Pseudomonas) until proven otherwise or correct
- Beware of three bacteria that can penetrate intact corneal epithelium (no focal epithelial defect necessary for corneal invasion and ulceration)
  1. Streptococcus (especially in children)
  2. Hemophilus influenzae (especially in children)
  3. Neisseria gonorrhoeae (venereal disease in adults and transmissible to newborns)
- Do not forget to assess less obvious risk factors
  1. Alcoholism (increased risk for moraxella)
  2. Parents of kids in diapers (increased risk of GI gram-negative bacteria)
  3. Venereal disease (increased risk of Gonococcus, Chlamydia, herpes)
  4. Systemic risks (e.g., diabetes, immunosuppressive oral medications)

Plan*

- Consider and coordinate the most appropriate professional resource(s) for care and management
- Provide patient with proper advice and instructions
- Hospitalization should be considered based on the best interest and needs of the patient determined through reasonable and prudent professional judgment.
  1. Considerations should include risk of patient noncompliance, need for supervised care, access to hospital care, and cost
  2. Medicolegal considerations are based on minimum standard of care for the given condition in that community

*See also Appendix 4.

- Cultures and sensitivities (before any treatment)
  1. Cultures (and smears for cytology, if available) should be collected from lids, conjunctiva, cul-de-sac, corneal scrapings, and (if applicable) contact lenses, solutions, and accessories
  2. Upon return of a positive culture, treatment can be adjusted or maintained, depending on results[44]
  3. But initial treatment should be intensive, broad-spectrum antibiosis with specific emphasis on antipseudomonal therapy
- Cycloplege and dilate with 1 percent atropine q2–4h or 5 percent homatropine q1–2h
- Minimum of two fortified aminoglycosides commonly used[45]
  1. Must include gentamicin and tobramycin
  2. Commercial (proprietary) concentrations usually 3 mg/ml
  3. Fortified concentrations equal 10 to 15 mg/ml
  4. Can be compounded by pharmacist or, if circumstances dictate, prepared in-office (for short course, 24-hour maximum use per preparation) by using dilute sterile injectable products as eyedrops such as tobramycin (Nebcin) and Garamycin
  5. Standard dosage every 30 minutes around the clock
- Alternative dosage regimen reported as equally effective as every 30 minutes (and useful if outpatient care indicated or necessary)[46,47]
  1. Loading dose
     a. Delivered in-office during initial visit
     b. One drop fortified tobramycin every minute 5 ×
  2. Extended dose
     a. Delivered by patient (or advocate) at home
     b. 3 gtt fortified tobramycin (at 1-minute intervals) q1–2h for 24 hours (asking patient to wake q2h throughout the night)
  3. Beware of toxicities with frequent or fortified dose levels necessary in ulcer care
- Subconjunctival and subtenons injections of aminoglycosides often provided in advancing cases of bacterial keratitis
- Oral tetracycline (as an anticollagenolytic agent) may be prescribed at 250 mg qid
- Oral and IV antibiotics are usually indicated in ulcers with significant threat of corneal perforation
- Additional oral penicillins, cephalosporins, tetracycline, erythromycin, and so forth, are indicated in venereal organisms (e.g., Gonorrhoeae)
  1. Patient should also be referred to primary physician
  2. Sexual partners must be identified and treated

Follow-up

- Reculturing should be conducted within 48 hours after commencement of therapy and every 24 hours thereafter, until negative cultures are established

1. Upon negative culture, topical steroids should be introduced at q3–4h[48]
2. If bacterial keratitis diagnosis was presumptive (i.e., without positive cultures), steroids should be withheld for minimum of 2 to 3 days

- Active ulcerative process could persist (even with full medical therapy) for weeks to months
    1. Usually a result of resistant strains to aminoglycosides used or available
    2. Resultant full-thickness stromal scarring almost ensured
    3. Corneal (stromal) melt and perforation always major risk
- Penetrating keratoplasty often required after resolution of active infectious process
- Continued patient education, advice, and counseling essential for proper patient management

C. FUNGAL KERATITIS

Background Information

1. Synonyms
    a. Fungal ulcer
    b. Mycotic keratitis
2. Tends to mimic other forms of infectious keratitis
3. Generally rare, but more prevalent in certain "risk areas"
    a. Southern and southwestern states
    b. Temperate climates
    c. Farming communities
4. Most common infectors
    a. *Fusarium*
    b. *Candida*
    c. *Aspergillus*
5. Frequently found in compromised hosts
    a. Steroid (oral or topical) users
    b. Anticancer therapy
    c. AIDS patients
6. Notorious as a lacrimal apparatus infector

Subjective

- Most common presentation includes a history of vegatative injury to the cornea (e.g., plants)
- Careful medical history useful to assess risk
    1. Use of steroids
    2. Immunosuppressive diseases
    3. Diagnosis of (or major risk factors for) AIDS
- Insidious to rapid onset of corneal symptoms

Objective

- Usually a dirty grayish infiltrate (raised)
    1. More frequently on peripheral cornea
    2. Serpiginous ("creeping") ulcerative process on corneal surface usually moving along the periphery, but may move centralward as well
- Ulcerated area has rough textured surface
- Feathered edges to ulcerated area, with branching hyphae and spores at the leading edge
- Satellite lesions are common
- Degree (width and depth) of surrounding infiltration varies with virulence of organism
- Other associated findings are relative to degree
    1. Conjunctival hyperemia
    2. Posterior corneal infiltration
        a. Folds and fibrin
        b. Endothelial plaques
        c. Immune rings (Wessely)
    3. Anterior chamber reaction
        a. Cells and flare
        b. Fibrin
        c. Hypopyon (common)

Assessment

- Laboratory diagnosis essential
- Rule out sterile infiltrative keratitis
- Rule out other forms of infectious keratitis (Table 4–6)
- Valuable differential test for serpiginous type ulceration (fungal and Mooren's ulcers) is a combined fluorescein–rose bengal staining technique
    1. Serpiginous ulcer has active (live–vital cells) leading edge and necrotic (dead–devitalized) rear edge
    2. Leading edge will stain with fluorescein only, while rear edge will stain with rose bengal

Plan and Follow-up

- All antifungal therapies (topical and systemic) include extremely toxic medications
- Consider management by corneal specialist skilled in use of antifungal drugs
- Some antifungal drugs used include
    1. Nystatin (nonophthalmic preparation)
    2. Amphotericin B (nonophthalmic preparation)
        i. Extremely toxic
        ii. Medicamentosa usually within 7 days
    3. Natamycin (only ophthalmic preparation available)
- Owing to vast number of potential fungal infective organisms, resistant strains are common and therapy and response is highly unpredictable

D. HERPETIC KERATITIS

A complete discussion of herpetic keratitis follows in section VIII, part D of this chapter

VIII. Viral Keratoconjunctivitis

Background Information

Refer to Chapter 3, section II, "Viral (and Other Folicular) Conjunctivitis, part A," Adenoviral Types, under "Background Information" for a complete discussion.

Clinical Conditions

A. NONSPECIFIC ADENOVIRAL

Subjective

- Extremely common in children and adults
- Mostly unilateral, but may show contralateral autoinoculation
- Patient rarely presents for care because of mild, usually subclinical, symptoms (e.g., mild burning or nonspecific irritation at inner canthal region)
- Duration of mild acute phase is short (3 to 5 days)

Objective

- Mild, diffuse, or regional (may be greater nasalward) superficial, bulbar pinkish injection
- Mild to moderate follicular response on inferior palpebral conjunctiva
- Eye(s) may show mild to moderate amount of hyperlacrimation
- Vision is not affected
- Corneal epithelium usually remains negative
  1. Occasionally, a fine diffuse SPK
  2. Most often only a few scattered punctata
- No preauricular lymph node enlargement or adenopathy

Assessment*

- Rule out other forms of conjunctivitis and keratoconjunctivitis
  1. Bacterial (meaty red and mucopurulent)
  2. Allergic (itching and edema)
  3. Toxic or hypersensitive (chronic versus acute)
  4. Others (by "the company they keep")
- Compare course of events (by time) to other more specific viral keratotconjunctivites (Table 4–7)

Plan†

- Usually not treated because patient never presents
- Reassure and treat supportively
  1. Warm packs bid or tid (optional)

*See also Appendix 3.
†See also Appendix 4.

2. Cold water irrigation (ad lib)
3. Lubricating drops qid
4. Decongestant or astringent drops (e.g., Vasoclear-A)

Follow-up

- For children, instruct parent or caretaker on dormant viral nature
  1. Recurrencies should be monitored
  2. Nonspecific adenoviral infection can be early reservoir for subsequent EKC virus
- Return checks not indicated, unless patient requests

B. PHARYNGOCONJUNCTIVAL FEVER

Subjective

- Pharyngoconjunctival fever (PCF) is a viral syndrome associated with adenovirus 3
  1. Also associated (to lesser degree) with other adenoviral strains
  2. Occasionally adenovirus 4 and 7
- Only ocular surface involvement with a distinct, relatively predictable systemic association
  1. Almost always a recent history of an upper respiratory condition (pharyngitis)
     a. Sore throat
     b. Congestion (throat or chest)
     c. Cough
  2. Low- to moderate-grade fever (usually 99 to 101°F)
- Most common in children 5 to 15 years of age (±3 years)
- Occasionally referred to as Beal's conjunctivitis
- Frequently called "pink eye" by patients and nurses
- May present with a recent exposure to swimming pool (or hot tubs)
  1. Called "swimming pool" conjunctivitis
  2. Adenovirus transmitted through fecal material in poorly chlorinated water
- Although most common in children, if syndrome fits (e.g., pharyngitis, fever, history of hot tub), adults should also be considered candidates

Objective

- Similar to viral conjunctivitis forms
- Usually mild to moderate viral signs
  1. Purplish-pinkish bulbar hyperemia
  2. Starts at inner canthus and spreads
  3. Tearing (serous) discharge
  4. Quick BUT (which can lead to secondary staining)

  5. Follicular palpebral changes
  6. Preauricular lymph enlargement or lymphadenopathy
■ Corneal involvement is usually mild (sometimes absent)
  1. Fine, diffuse SPK or scattered punctata
  2. Rarely, a few, small subepithelial infiltrates

Assessment*

■ Rule out other forms of conjunctivitis and keratoconjunctivitis
  1. Bacterial (meaty red and mucopurulent)
  2. Allergic (itching and edema)
  3. Toxic or hypersensitive (chronic versus acute)
  4. Others (by "the company they keep")
■ Compare course of events (by time) with other more specific viral keratotconjunctivites (Table 4-7)
■ Three helpful considerations in differentiating PCF from other viral keratoconjunctivites
  1. Ages 5 to 15
  2. It is a systemic syndrome (i.e., pharyngitis, fever)
  3. A swimming pool or a hot tub history (also in EKC)
■ Do corneal hyposensitivity ("cotton wisp") test to differentiate from recurrent herpes simplex keratitis
  1. Make cotton wisp from cotton ball or swab
  2. Firmly brush wisp over unaffected cornea and define response to patient as a 10 on a scale of 1 to 10
  3. Then brush affected cornea (using same pressure and region), and ask patient to quantify sensation on a 1 to 10 scale
  4. Response of ≤7 = corneal hypoesthesia (i.e., reduced corneal sensitivity), which is suggestive of recurrent herpes simplex keratitis
■ Laboratory workup (e.g., serotyping) is not usually done in primary clinical setting due to relative obvious clinical presentation and delay (up to 2 weeks for final viral titers) in results

Plan†

■ Advise patient of viral diagnosis
■ Explain noncurable nature of virus
  1. Benign course with no permanent damage
  2. Self-limiting course (usually about 10 to 14 days)
  3. No curative therapy, only supportive and palliative measures
  4. Possibility of contagious nature (EKC)
     a. Always assume the worst (EKC) until time and physical findings prove otherwise
     b. Instruct carefully not to rub or touch, to use of personal towels and sheets, and so forth
■ Advise patient that "this may get worse before it gets better!" (i.e., possibility of EKC)
■ Supportive, palliative measures
  1. Warm or cold (for symptom relief) packs
  2. Ocular lubricants
  3. Irrigation (ophthalmic solutions or cold water)
  4. Decongestants or astringents (optional)
  5. If systemic signs and symptoms still present, therapy for pharyngitis and fever (per physician)

Follow-up

■ Recheck in 7 to 10 days after report of first symptoms
  1. Reducing signs and symptoms indicates no EKC
  2. Increasing clinical course suggests EKC
■ If cornea involved, recheck 10 to 14 days after confirmation (at first recheck visit) of non-EKC conditions
■ Advise patient of dormant, obligate, parasitic nature of adenovirus (lies dormant in tissue) and recurrent potential with various stress factors
■ Routine follow-up or PRN

---

*See also Appendix 3.

†See also Appendix 4.

TABLE 4-7. COMPARISON OF VIRAL KERATOCONJUNCTIVITIS (BY TIME)

Time Interval (days)	Nonspecific	PCF	EKC	Herpes Simplex
1–3	Mild	Mild	Moderate	Moderate to severe
4–6	Mild	Moderate	Moderate to severe	Severe (75% dendrite)
7–10[a]	Improving	Moderate (occasional SPK)	Moderate to severe (with SPK)	Moderate (with therapeusis)
11–14	Resolved	Improving	Moderate (with supportive therapy)	Improving (with therapeusis)
14–21	Resolved	Resolved	Subepithelial infiltrates	Improving (with therapeusis)
22–28	Resolved	Resolved	Improving	Resolved (with therapeusis)

[a]Return visit during this interval usually confirms diagnosis.

C. EPIDEMIC KERATOCONJUNCTIVITIS (Color Plates 61 through 64)

Background Information

1. EKC is arguably the most common contagious clinical condition managed in primary eye care practice
   a. Highly contagious nature in its early (milder) phases causes "epidemic" spreading potential
   b. Most patients do not realize, or underestimate, communicable nature because of mild symptoms and clinical signs during early contagious phase
2. Virus transmitted by direct or indirect contact (e.g. from a contaminated towel, hand, instrument) with the infected tissues or tears
3. EKC is traditionally associated with adenovirus 8
   a. Each year new strains are presenting increasing frequency and virulence of EKC type syndromes
   b. Other EKC adenoviruses: 4, 11, 13, 19, 37[49]
4. Originally, EKC syndrome was a fairly definitive set of clinical parameters and findings
   a. Called EKC rule of 8's
      i. Adenovirus 8 most common
      ii. First 8 days (conjunctivitis stage) most contagious
      iii. Eighth day, corneal SPK presentation
      iv. Eight days later (sixteenth day), subepithelial infiltrates (SEIs)
   b. Time sequences are rough approximations
   c. With increasing numbers and virulence of EKC type adenoviruses, exceptions to the rule of 8's are becoming frequent[50]
      i. Conjunctivitis stage may be shorter than 8 days or completely absent with contagious period being prodromal or during the keratitic phase
      ii. Keratitic phase (SPK and SEI) may be immediate or within days (rather than weeks)

Subjective

- Most common viral presentation (in practice) because of intensity and duration (resulting in patient concern)

- Frequently seen as an "epidemic" (outbreak and spread within a given period of time)
- Usually a common denominator is (ultimately) recognized as potential contaminating source of environment
   1. Family
   2. Neighborhood
   3. Workplace
   4. School
   5. Hospital
   6. Eye doctor's office!
- Age range is usually 15 to 18 years or older
   1. Classic differential for PCF (usually in children)
   2. However, more virulent strains are transmissible to children under age 15 (in increasing numbers)
- Never any significant systemic signs or symptoms associated (as with the PCF syndrome)
   1. Strictly an ocular reaction
   2. Any systemic associations are probably coincidental in that adenoviruses producing EKC are not known for any substantial systemic reactions
- Classic viral-type symptoms in milder presentations
   1. Nonspecific irritation
   2. Burning sensation
- Day of presentation (for care) varies with intensity
   1. Milder, more common forms, within 5 to 10 days
   2. Virulent forms (e.g., 19, 37) within 3 to 5 days
- Degree of symptoms varies with intensity and duration
   1. Milder presentations vary from phase to phase
      a. First 8 days: mild to moderate symptoms of nonspecific irritation, burning, and photophobia
      b. Second 8 days: moderate to severe burning, photophobia, corneal irritation, and blurring
      c. After 14 to 18 days: blurring may persist or increase slightly while irritation, burning, and photophobia begin to diminish
   2. Virulent forms are highly symptomatic within days
      a. Corneal irritation may be severe in 3 to 5 days
      b. Symptoms will increase without therapy

Objective

- Vision varies with time and intensity
   1. Milder forms produce slight fluctuations during the first week from 20/20 to 20/30
   2. Second week (SPK stage) shows moderate reductions to approximately 20/40
   3. After about 16 days, reduction (secondary to SEI stage) can vary from 20/30 to 20/60 or less
   4. In virulent conditions, acuity can fall dramatically at any stage (usually within days rather than weeks) to 20/100 or less

- Most common presentation is unilateral with second eye usually infected (to lesser degree than primary) by autoinoculation during the first week
- Eyelid(s) usually mild to moderately edematous, depending on virulence of ocular viral reaction
- Early (and persisting) signs typical of viral conjunctivitis
  1. Purplish-pinkish bulbar hyperemia
  2. Starts at inner canthus (in milder forms)
  3. Tearing, serous discharge
  4. Reduced BUT (with risk of secondary exposure SPK)
  5. Follicular palpebral (inferior) conjunctivitis
  6. Preauricular lymph enlargement or adenopathy
- Bulbar conjunctival reaction varies significantly with virulence of virus
  1. Purplish-pink in mild to moderate forms
  2. Hemorrhagic changes in severe forms (11, 19, 37)
- Pseudomembranes (infiltrative cells combined with mucin and fibrin) form in more virulent presentations (Color Plates 61, 62, and 63)
  1. Mild forms show film over palpebral conjunctiva
  2. Moderate forms produce coagulates (usually inferior cul-de-sac)
  3. Severe involvement covers parts or all of the palpebral conjunctiva with dense, opaque, whitish sheets of exudative-like material
  4. All forms are adherent by fibrinous adhesions to "true" underlying mucous membranes
- Keratitis usually begins to develop after about 6 to 8 days (1 week) from initial conjunctival hyperemia
  1. Usually diffuse SPK
  2. May vary from fine to coarse punctate spots
  3. Virulent viruses will present a much faster keratitis (sometimes simultaneous with conjunctivitis)
- Subepithelial infiltrates (SEIs) usually begin to develop within 14 to 16 days or about 2 weeks (Color Plate 64)
  1. Again, virulent forms will produce keratitic complications much faster than typical syndrome
  2. SEIs are flat accumulations of infiltrative cells and WBCs (especially lymphocytes), and some surrounding edema
  3. Number from few to "countless" (with increasing virulence)
  4. Central localization is most common but may also present peripherally as well
     a. May be central and peripheral
     b. Not usually peripheral only
  5. SEIs do not stain with NaFl
     a. Secondary stain may occur in large, dense spots that disrupt overlying cells
     b. Secondary disruption of epithelial surface may result in a negative (breaking up of) staining pattern or positive staining
  6. Edges of EKC SEIs are usually indistinct

  7. Vary from pale, hazy subepithelial level spots to dense, opaque anterior stromal level leucomas
     a. Subepithelial level SEIs will blanch with or without therapy in weeks to months
     b. Anterior stromal level spots may or may not blanch over weeks to years (if ever), some resulting in translucent to opaque scars from anterior stromal fibrogenic, antigen–antibody reaction to overlying infiltrative subepithelial response
- Depending on virulence of virus and corneal involvement, secondary anterior uveitis will vary from no response to florid reactions

Assessment*

- EKC can present difficult and misleading diagnostic assessments
  1. Mild forms (or stages) that can be banal in appearance but that are nonetheless highly contagious may be underestimated or neglected
  2. Severe forms that are easily misdiagnosed and often overtreated out of concern for potential damage and progression, are usually self-limiting and in a noncommunicable stage
- Rule out bacterial, atopic, toxic keratites by the subjective and objective "company they keep"
  1. EKC is so common that it may appear in combination with other keratites
  2. As parasitic infection, it may be exacerbated with any form of ocular surface stress (e.g., disease)
- Differentiate EKC from PCF
  1. By age (PCF in 5 to 15 versus EKC in over 15)
  2. EKC has no systemic involvement versus PCF
  3. Rule of 8's usually helpful (in spite of exceptions)
- Compare course of events by time to other viral conditions (Table 4–7)
- Rule out SPK of Thygeson
  1. SPK of Thygeson "keeps no viral company"
  2. Usually asymptomatic with white eye
  3. Remits and exacerbates for years
- Rule out herpes simplex (HSV) keratitis
  1. History of recurrences (in adults)
  2. Dendritic ulcer (75 to 80 percent of time)
  3. Corneal hyposensitivity test
     a. Pronounced corneal hypoesthesia in recurrent HSV epithelial keratitis
     b. Could also be present in severe forms of EKC
- Laboratory workup (e.g., serotypes) not usually done due to well defined clinical picture over a period of time usually shorter than that necessary to establish viral titer in the laboratory

---

*See also Appendix 3.

Plan*

- All first presentation viral conjunctivitis or kerato-conjunctivitis should be treated as suspect EKC
  1. Presume a contagious, communicable infection
  2. Advise patient of contagious nature and instruct
     a. Do not touch or rub eyes
     b. Use separate towels, sheets, pillowcases
     c. If in unavoidable contact situation (e.g., work, school), discontinue activities until confirmed diagnosis or follow-up visit
  3. Advise carefully of possibility of eye and vision "getting worse before it gets better"
     a. Increased likelihood of EKC if initial presentation is "hot"
     b. Increased likelihood if "pink eye" in family or school or workplace (i.e., "it's going around")
- Theoretically, no treatment at all required for EKC
  1. All presentation will be self-limiting (through autoimmune defense mechanism)
  2. However, most EKC produces enough discomfort, inflammation (secondary to immune response) and patient concern that supportive or palliative care is indicated
  3. Moderate to severe forms require therapy for support as well as some protection against secondary tissue changes and potential scarring of SEIs areas from immune response
  4. Certainly all secondary associated reactions (e.g., as anterior uveitis) require appropriate therapy
- Pseudomembranes should be removed for patient comfort and more rapid recovery
  1. Mild forms can be brushed off with wetted cotton swabs
  2. Moderate to severe forms can be "peeled off"
     a. Anesthetize area with topical anesthetic (1 gtt every 15 seconds 4 × over pseudomembrane)
     b. Peel (from edges) slowly with jeweler's forceps
     c. Petechial hemorrhages (small conjunctival bleeds) may result from fibrin adhesions during removal (don't worry)
     d. Patient will report discomfort during procedure
  3. Irrigate tissues copiously with ophthalmic irrigator after removal
- Supportive or palliative measures
  1. Warm or cold packs, or both (q3–4h)
  2. Topical decongestants or astringents (q3–4h)
  3. Ocular lubricants (mucomimetic agents) q3–4h
  4. Irrigation with ophthalmic irrigator or cold water (q3–4h)

  5. Aspirin or ibuprofen (in lieu of contraindication)
- Use of topical antibiotics are optional but recommended
  1. No proven "prophylactic" value, as often believed
  2. However, some research supports antibiotic as a "therapeutic" measure against viral spread, penetration, duration, and recurrence
  3. In either case, antibacterial coverage on a compromised corneal surface is always clinically reassuring (better to be safe than sorry!)
- Antiviral agents (e.g., IDU, vidarabine, trifluridine) are of no value against adenoviruses
  1. Some reports of early use of trifluridine helping against EKC viruses
  2. However, treatment of early viral conjunctivitis or keratoconjunctivitis (3 to 5 days old) with a relatively toxic antimetabolite is questionable
- The use of topical steroids in EKC is a "delicate" decision
  1. Definitely not indicated in mild forms
  2. In severe forms there may be no alternative
     a. Reduces inflammation and potential scarring
     b. Makes patient more comfortable
     c. Blanches SEIs and improves vision
     d. Reduces pseudomembranous response
     e. However, as immunosuppresive on a virus
        i. Reduces immune response to virus
        ii. Steroid enhances virus with resultant increased risk for rebound and recurrent patterns of SEIs and reinfection
        iii. If HSV dormant in tissue, steroid could aggravate that condition as well
  3. In moderate degree EKC, consider pros and cons of steroid use and base decision on following criteria and judgments (individually or any combination)
     a. If VA falls below 20/40 to 20/60
     b. If SEIs appear dense (anterior stromal) with risk of fibrinogenic scarring
     c. If inflammatory response is severe enough to threaten tissue damage
     d. If significant secondary anterior uveitis develops
     e. If patient discomfort is uncontrollable by other means
- Finally, always take careful personal (and office) precautions against contagious or infectious patients
  1. Wash hands thoroughly after care with water and alcohol
  2. Clean instruments
     a. Consider postponing tonometry on infectious conditions during acute stages (unless necessary)
     b. All other instruments and equipment can also be contaminated directly or indirectly
  3. Advise office personnel to necessary precautions

---

*See also Appendix 4.

Follow-up

- Recheck in 7 to 10 days after initial presentation (unless severe or corneal presentation)
- Subsequent recheck should be based on progress or advancement of clinical course
  1. Monitor cornea at least weekly until resolution of SPK phase
  2. Monitor SEIs at least monthly until resolved or stable (anterior stromal scars)
- Release to PRN after thorough education, advice, and instruction of exacerbation
- If patient is a contact lens wearer
  1. Discontinue lens wear during acute phase
  2. Rewear (sterilized) lenses after negative corneal staining for 5 to 7 days
  3. If condition exacerbates within 1 to 2 weeks after rewear, discontinue wear, wait for 5 to 7 days, and replace lenses if hydrophilic material
  4. During exacerbation periods (secondary to aggravants or stress factors), discontinue contact lens wear during acute phase and 3 to 5 days post
     a. rewear after exacerbations
     b. Always recheck cornea before rewear

D. HERPES SIMPLEX VIRUS

Background Information[51,52]

1. Most common virus in humans (only natural host)
2. Responsible for more than 1.5 million cases of blindness in the United States per year (leading infectious cause of blindness)
3. Two forms of virus: herpes simplex virus type 1 (HSV-1) (oral) and herpes simplex virus type 2 (HSV-2) (genital)
   a. Original theory was 90 percent of HSV infections "above the waist" were HSV-1 and 90 percent "below the waist" were HSV-2
   b. Current statistic uncertain, since dramatic increases in occurrence of HSV-2 (genital herpes)
   c. Thus, ocular infections can possibly have an HSV-2 (genital) association (check history)
4. Sources of HSV infections
   a. Primary infection
   b. Recurrent infection (after primary attack)
   c. Transmission from symptomatic or asymptomatic carrier
5. Transmission is through direct contact

a. Mostly saliva and mouth contact
b. Also contact with active skin lesions (vesicles)
c. Incubation period approximately 1 week

6. Most common site of infection is mucocutaneous border of lips
   a. Classic fever blister or cold sore
   b. Route to trigeminal ganglion and ultimately eye (although far less frequent than mouth)
   c. Corneal epithelium is frequent site through this route
7. Primary HSV attacks uncommon but dramatic
   a. Mostly in children and young adults
   b. Older age ranges protected by immunity
8. Greatest risk for primary infection from 6 months of age to 5 to 10 years of age (as immunity begins to develop)
   a. Seventy percent of children infected by 5 years of age
   b. Ninety percent of these infections remain subclinical
   c. Seventy percent immune to HSV by 15 to 25 years of age
   d. Ninety percent immune to HSV by 60 years of age
9. Recurrence will occur in 25 percent of HSV infections
   a. One third will recur once or more per year
   b. Two thirds will recur once or more every 2 years
   c. Males recur 50 percent more than females
   d. Sources of infection, age, race, and so forth, are not considered factors in recurrent potential
   e. Climate may be a factor in that recurrences are more frequent in fall and winter
   f. Recurrent infection can present ocularly in spite of nonocular primary infection
10. Increasing data suggests that recurrent potential is related to the strain of infecting HSV[53]
    a. Thus, statistics work against recurrent patients
       i. Primary HSV attack: 25 percent risk of recurrence
       ii. First recurrence: 50 percent risk of recurrence

iii. Second recurrence: 75 percent risk of recurrence
iv. Third recurrence: 100 percent risk of recurrence

11. Aggravating or inciting factors for recurrence
    a. Sunlight (UV)
    b. Trauma (especially localized to ocular area)
    c. Extreme heat or cold
    d. Fever
    e. Steroids
    f. Infectious disease (systemic or ocular)
    g. Surgery
    h. Epilation

12. HSV replicates in corneal epithelium only
    a. However, substantial tissue destruction and inflammatory reaction in the stroma can be produced by the immune response to the virus
    b. Factors influencing the intensity of the host immune response (stromal ulcer) are unpredictable
       i. Genetic factors
       ii. HLAs
       iii. Atopias (familial tendencies)
       iv. Other unknown factors
    c. To what degree the host response is necessary and beneficial to viral control (in epithelium cells) versus stromal inflammation, infiltration, ulceration, and scarring is unknown
       i. Such information is key to steroid considerations in treatment
       ii. Too little steroid would permit excessive stromal destruction and scarring
       iii. Too much steroid would permit the epithelial infection to proliferate and trigger a cycle of increasing adverse clinical responses

13. Fortunately, most HSV ocular disease presents as epithelial keratitis which is relatively controllable with antiviral or antimetabolite drugs
    a. Usually no deep stromal immune reactions
    b. Occasionally, mild stromal reaction controllable with adjunctive steroid therapy
    c. Rarely, virus may show primary clinical response to the stroma (e.g., disciform keratitis) with significant and relatively uncontrollable tissue destruction

14. In summary, HSV is poorly understood with a highly varied and unpredictable clinical course

Clinical Conditions[54]

1. Primary HSV Keratitis

Subjective

- Usually infants and young children (ages 5 to 15)
  1. Rare in adults but may be increasing with increasing HSV-2 (genital) infections
  2. Autoinoculation from open genital lesion to eye
- Occasional history of 2-day to 2-week contact with infected host (with or without active lesion
- Mild to moderate fever or malaise (versus recurrent form with no systemic response)
- Usually, "red eye" is secondary issue (rarely severe) and treated prophylactically (with antibiotic drops) by attending pediatrician or primary physician
  1. Mild foreign-body sensation
  2. Mild photophobia
  3. Unilateral
  4. Burning irritation

Objective

- Skin lesions (vesicles or pustules) most prominent clinical feature
  1. Greatest in and around mouth (mucocutaneous border of lips)
  2. Often adjacent to lid margins (single or grouped)
  3. Often buried between lashes
- Lid usually mildly to moderately swollen
- Moderate to severe lymphadenopathy
  1. Preauricular node (ipsilateral)
  2. Frequently dramatic face and neck adenopathy
- Usually moderate follicular conjunctivitis
- In more severe eye involvements
  1. Bulbar conjunctival hemorrhages
  2. Pseudomembranes
  3. Phlyctenules
- Keratitis *always* epithelial (never stromal)
  1. Immature immune system precludes host immune response to stroma
  2. Conversely, immature (absent) immune response produces relative increase in viral activity in epithelial cells
- Corneal findings are fairly predictable
  1. Fine to coarse diffuse SPK
     a. Occasionally regional patches
     b. Sometimes greater inferiorly
  2. Dendrites (when present) may be quite large and multiple
     a. Attributable to poor immune protection
     b. Stain with rose bengal

3. Often multiple subepithelial infiltrates
   a. Central or peripheral
   b. Appear within 1 to 2 weeks, depending on severity of keratitis

Assessment*

- Rule out bacterial infections
  1. Staphylococcal (papillae versus follicles)
  2. Impetigo (adenopathy too pronounced)
- Rule out pharyngoconjunctival fever (PCF)
  1. Corneal involvement too severe
  2. Skin lesions (to eye or remote)
- Rule out chlamydia (no mucopurulence)
- Rule out epidemic keratoconjunctivitis (EKC)
  1. Wrong age range
  2. No rule of 8's
  3. Systemic involvement (malaise and fever)
- Rule out herpes zoster
  1. Pain not so severe
  2. Vesicles to pustules versus ulcerations
  3. Midline not respected

Plan†

- Co-manage with pediatrician or patient's primary physician
- Skin lesions should be mildly abraded (washcloth) and treated with Acyclovir ointment
  1. Dosage q4h for 21 days
  2. Alternate therapy: alcohol scrubs tid for 14 to 21 days
- Supportive systemic therapy (e.g., Acyclovir, aspirin, ibuprofen)
- Cycloplegia and dilation if indicated
- Antiviral ocular therapy
  1. Antiviral drops (only with keratitis)
  2. Viroptic
     a. q4h for first week
     b. qid for second week
     c. tid for third week
     d. bid for fourth week

Follow-up

- Recheck every 3 days, until cornea is clear
- Recheck every 5 days, until skin lesions resolve
- Be watchful for complications
  1. Bacterial or fungal (rare) superinfection
  2. Secondary preseptal cellulitis
  3. Stromal involvement
     a. Best to get corneal specialist consultation
     b. Avoid steroids
- Advise patient (or parents) on recurrence risks
- Routine rechecks or PRN

---

*See also Appendix 3.

†See also Appendix 4.

2. Recurrent HSV Epithelial Keratitis

Subjective

- History of previous attacks is most useful diagnostic tool in recurrent HSV infections
- Careful history may reveal primary HSV infection in first recurrent episodes
  1. Previous ocular involvement (mild or severe)
  2. Fever blister or cold sore
  3. Mouth ulcerations
  4. Previous (or active) vesicular skin lesions
     a. Periocular
     b. Mouth or skin
     c. Genital region
- Consider other aggravating stress factors
- Corneal pain and irritation ranges from absent to severe
  1. Usually more severe in initial recurrences
  2. Diminishes with subsequent attacks owing to increasing corneal hypoesthesia
- Variable photophobic response
- Burning irritation
- Vision reduction varies with intensity of keratitis

Objective

- General findings in all epithelial forms
  1. Always unilateral
  2. Follicular conjunctivitis
  3. Moderate to severe bulbar hyperemia
  4. Occasional bulbal conjunctival hemorrhages
  5. Occasional pseudomembranes
  6. Ipsilateral preauricular lymphadenopathy
  7. Tearing (serous) discharge
  8. Quick BUT
  9. Keratitis
  10. Secondary anterior uveitis (relative to intensity of keratitis)
- Dendriform keratitis (75 to 80 percent frequency) (Color Plate 65)
  1. Starts as dense coalescing of focal SPK
  2. Usually fine, linear branching pattern forms with overhanging, pale, flat margins
     a. Usually about 0.1 to 1.0 mm wide
     b. Varies from 1 to 2 mm, up to 10 mm long
  3. Demonstrates classic rounded endings to each linear branch (called "terminal end buds")
  4. May be single or multiple lesions
  5. Associated with surrounding SPK
  6. Located centrally or peripherally
     a. Peripheral dendrites are more resistant to treatment
     b. Thicker corneal nerve involved
  7. Stains with rose bengal
  8. Frequently a mild to moderate stromal edema surrounds dendrite
  9. Reaction usually remains superficial and localized
  10. Corneal hypoesthesia develops and increases with each recurrent attack

11. True dendritic "ulceration" of epithelium versus infiltrative forms of dendriform keratitis (Color Plate 66)
- Metaherpetic (trophic) keratopathy (less common) (Color Plate 67)
  1. Chronic "sterile" indolent ulceration secondary to epithelial (dendriform) keratitis
     a. Probably caused by damage to basement membrane and possibly live virus "embedding" in membrane
     b. Antigen–antibody (immune) response to live virus produces sterile, indolent ulcerative process and anterior stromal damage
  2. Epithelial ulcer shape is usually oval, ameboid, or geographic (amorphous shape)
  3. Edges are distinctly raised, thickened, gray borders appearing rolled or heaped
  4. Size of ulcer varies from 2 to 8 mm
  5. Usually vertically oriented in longer axis
  6. Stains brilliantly with rose bengal
  7. Produce moderate to dramatic anterior stromal response (infiltration and edema)
     a. Usually beneath and more diffuse than overlying dendrite(s)
     b. If persistent (i.e., virus "embedded" for 6- to 8-week life of basement membrane), could produce collagenolytic scarring and corneal melting
  8. Chronic nature may produce neovascularization

Assessment*

- Differentiate primary versus recurrent HSV by history, age, systemic involvement (in primary)
- Check for corneal sensitivity (decreases with each recurrent attack)
- Rule out bacterial and other possible infectious keratites (cultures, if necessary)
- Rule out other viral keratites

For Dendritic Form
- The presence of a dendrite should always raise suspicion of epithelial HSV keratitis
- However, HSV is the only condition that will produce a true ulcerative dendritic keratitis
- All other forms of dendriform keratitis are infiltrative keratites
  1. Recurrent corneal erosion
  2. Keratitis sicca
  3. SLK of Theodore
  4. SPK of Thygeson
  5. Atopic keratoconjunctivitis
  6. Vernal keratoconjunctivitis
  7. Herpes zoster ophthalmicus
- Under slit-lamp examination
  1. Ulcerative dendrite will be depressed versus infiltrative dendrite being raised
  2. Within 2 to 4 minutes after instillation, NaFl stain undermines ulcerative dendrite versus

shedding effect over infiltrative dendrite (Color Plate 66)

For Metaherpetic Form
- Differentiated from dendritic form by
  1. Shape and edges
  2. Diffuse and deeper stromal response
  3. Persistence in lieu of antiviral therapy
- Differentiated from stromal forms by
  1. Persistent NaFl and rose bengal staining
  2. Chronic epithelial involvement

Plan†

Primary Care (Table 4–8)
- Some practitioners debride all dendrites
  1. Studies indicate medical therapy equally effective with or without debridement
  2. Occasional risk of spreading virus with debridement procedure
- Treat aggressively with antiviral agents
  1. IDU (e.g., Stoxil) no longer heavily used because of increasing toxicity and decreasing spectrum of effectiveness[55]
  2. Vidarabine ointment (e.g., Vira A) and trifluridine (e.g., Viroptic) preferred drugs
  3. Viroptic arrests dendrites in 3 to 5 days versus 5 to 7 (or more) for vidarabine and IDU
  4. Long-term effects of Viroptic unknown (therefore, do not overuse!)
- Dosages
  1. Viroptic drops q1–2h for 48 to 72 hours with Vira A ointment at bedtime and patient waking as frequently as possible during night to reinstill drops or ointment
  2. Reduce to q3–4h (with ointment hs) after 3 to 5 days or upon dendrite regression
     a. Dendrites usually begin to regress to "islands"
     b. Live virus supposedly present as long as rose bengal staining persists
  3. Continue treatment for 14 to 21 days or until rose bengal and NaFl negative, tapering to qid then tid during last week of treatment
- Beware of antiviral toxicity (usually at 5 to 8 days
  1. Follicles
  2. Chemosis
  3. Fine to coarse SPK
  4. Retarded epithelial (dendritic) healing
- Cycloplege or dilate (standard dosages), if indicated
- Nonsteroidal anti-inflammatory agents (e.g., Ocufen)
- Warm packs ad lib
- Ocular lubricants qid
- Topical antibiotic drops as prophylactic (and therapeutic agents!)
  1. Research has demonstrated a possible therapeutic value of antibacterial agents as antiviral

---

*See also Appendix 3.

†See also Appendix 4.

TABLE 4–8. DAY-BY-DAY FLOWCHART FOR PRIMARY CARE MANAGEMENT OF EPITHELIAL HERPES SIMPLEX KERATITIS

Time Interval	Corneal Findings	Standard Treatment	Possible Complications	Treatment Additions and Adjustments
Day 1–2	1. Hypoesthesia 2. Coarse diffuse SPK 3. Coalescing dendrite(s)	1. Antiviral q1–2h (24 hr continuous) 2. Antibiotic cycloplege and dilate qid 3. Ocular lubricant qid 4. Warm packs ad lib 5. Aspirin ad lib	1. Secondary bacterial or fungal infection	1. Culture eye 2. Add antibiotic or antifungal
Day 3–4	1, 2 (plus) 4. Ulcerative dendrite(s)	Continue all steps 1–5	1 (plus) 2. Anterior stromal edema 3. Anterior uveitis	1, 2 (plus) 3. Cycloplege and dilate (increase) No steroids! 4. Increase hot packs
Day 5–6	1, 2, 4 (plus) 5. SPK decreasing 6. Dendrite(s) stable	Continue 2–5 (plus) 6. Antiviral q3–4h with ointment at bedtime	1–3 (plus) 4. SPK increasing[a] 5. Dendrite worsening[a]	1–4 (plus) 5. Change antiviral agent
Day 7–10	1, 5 (plus) 7. Dendrite resolving	Continue 2–6	1–5 (plus) 6. Deep stromal edema	1–4 (plus) 6. Recheck every 24 hr
Day 11–14	1 (plus) 8. Negative rose bengal	Continue 3 and 4 (plus) 7. Antibiotic bid 8. Antiviral qid 9. Patient counseling re: HSV	1–6 (plus) 7. Stromal infiltration 8. Metaherpetic ulceration	7. Refer to ophthalmologist
Day 15–21	1 (plus) 9. Cornea negative	10. D/C antibiotic 11. Antiviral tid	1, 3–8 (plus) 9. Neovascularization	8. Refer to ophthalmologist or corneal specialist
Day 22–28	1 (plus) 10. Cornea remains negative	12. D/C antivirals 13. Schedule weekly for weeks 5 and 6	1, 3–9 (plus) 10. Stromal keratitis	9. Refer to corneal specialist
Week 5–6	1 and 10	14. Recheck PRN or 6 months	Recurrence(s)	10. Dig in!

[a]Probable drug toxicity.

agents by reducing the viral "spread factor" and support of the interferon (viral inhibitor) system

2. Theory based on fact that hyaluronidase enzyme degrades mucopolysaccarides (MPS) during ocular surface infection or inflammation

3. High concentrations of hyaluronidase are produced by gram-positive bacteria (e.g., *Staphylococci*) and cell lysis during external inflammation of the eye

4. Ocular surface defense mechanism (tear mucin layer, superficial epithelial cells) and intercellular ground substance is made up of large percentage of MPS

5. During surface infection or inflammation, increased exposure of MPS substrate in the presence of high concentrations of hyaluronidase (from normal floral bacteria, e.g., *Staphylococci*) causes significant increase in the viral spread factor

6. Also, the interferon induction system (a known viral inhibitory system) produced by cellular defense mechanism is also suppressed by hyaluronidase–MPS degradation

7. Thus, combination of the two effects (i.e., increased spread factor and suppression of the interferon system) from bacterial produced hyaluronidase on MPS, supports the reasonable use of gram-positive antibacterial agents as therapeutic agents in antiviral external (ocular surface) viral infections
   a. Reverses spread of viral infection
   b. Reduces course of viral disease
   c. Increases latency of dormant virus

8. Clinical research has proved such a theory to be highly effective with HSV keratitis and believed to have similar potential in adenoviral (e.g., EKC) disease as well[56]

■ Ninety percent of all epithelial dendrites heal through primary care in 14 days or less without scarring

1. Certainly, repeated recurrences can eventually lead to mild to moderate anterior stromal hazing and scarring

2. Also, lingering dendrites (usually greater than 21 days) could produce scarring

■ *Never* introduce steroids in primary or recurrent HSV epithelial keratitis

Secondary Care (See Table 4–8)

- Consider dendriform keratitis care as secondary level care in the following situations;
  1. If dendrite is (or has been) "steroid enhanced" iatrogenically or out of necessity from stromal therapy
  2. If dendrite(s) has not responded to primary care within 10 to 14 days
  3. Advancing metaherpetic involvement
- Consider care by most appropriate practitioner
- Treatment should include (but not necessarily be limited to) any or all of the following
  1. Debridement (repeated as indicated)
  2. All primary care steps described above
  3. Different class(es) of antiviral drugs at full strength for full cycles and recycles
  4. Bandage soft contact lenses
  5. Intermittent pressure patching
  6. Heavy lubrication therapy
  7. Acetylcysteine (i.e., Mucomyst) for corneal melting
  8. Cyanoacrylate glues
  9. Investigational antiviral agents
  10. Surgery (as a last resort)
      a. Conjunctival flap
      b. Keratoplasty (guarded-to-poor prognosis)

Follow-up

- Secondary care requires close management and ongoing monitoring by the specialty provider
- Primary care should be followed closely
  1. Every 24 to 48 hours during first week
  2. Every 3 to 5 days during second week (resolving)
  3. Weekly for 2 to 3 weeks after resolution
- Contact lens rewear should be similar to approach with EKC
- Long-term management includes careful instruction to patient on recurrent nature of condition
  1. Use "red eye" criteria, not corneal pain, as patient's guideline for assessing recurrence
  2. Corneal pain will decrease (sometimes to zero) with subsequent recurrent attacks and possibly be neglected by patient
- Recheck every 6 months for 1 year and then annually or PRN

3. Stromal HSV Keratitis

Subjective

- History is usually quite apparent regarding recurrent epithelial or stromal keratitis
  1. Recurrent epithelial HSV keratitis almost always associated with stromal, interstitial form
  2. Disciform usually has no epithelial history
- Pain may vary from epithelial types
  1. Frequently corneal pain may be absent or minimal (owing to corneal hypoesthesia from multiple recurrences)

  2. Usually deep, throbbing (headache) pain caused by secondary keratouveitis
- Vision is almost always substantially reduced
  1. Loss is insidious in stromal forms
  2. Subacute loss in disciform type
- Clinical presentation usually insidious versus acute onset in epithelial responses
  1. Acute or subacute epithelial response may occur after stromal presentation
  2. In disciform, epithelial response rarely follows stromal involvement

Objective

- Intensity of all forms varies widely

Stromal or Interstitial Type

- Stromal infiltration with mild to moderate edema
  1. Deep to full-thickness infiltrates
  2. Infiltration substantially exceeds edema
- Neovascularization (usually deep stromal)
  1. Vessels may reveal active (whole blood) flow
  2. Vessels may be empty and gray in appearance ("ghost vessels")
- Patchy infiltrative response resulting in permanent scarring
- Ulcerative necrosis can develop as creamy homogeneous stromal breakdown (to abscess)
  1. Produces localized (or diffuse) areas of stromal thinning
  2. Could lead to corneal "melting"
- Wessely rings (antigen–antibody reactions) in anterior stroma are frequently seen (partial or complete infiltrative annular rings)
- Edema usually causes ground-glass appearance and corneal thickening
- Corneal endothelium is usually involved
  1. Keratic precipitates (infiltrative and pigment debris)
  2. Guttata
  3. Fibrin plaques
- Epithelial edema (diffuse and bullous) is probably a product of endothelial disruption
- Keratouveitis is always present (secondary response)
  1. Associated trabeculitis (with IOP increase) in severe cases
  2. Red blood cells (microhyphema) may be seen among cells and flare in chamber
- Descemetocele formations occur in advanced cases

Disciform Type

- Frequently presents with no history or presence of epithelial keratitis
- Usually centrally located, dense edematous (not infiltrative as in interstitial type) stromal disc
  1. Etiology of edema (versus infiltrates) is uncertain
  2. Reaction is known to be a type IV (delayed hypersensitivity) response
- Disciform type presents with a uniformly rounded

disc-shaped stromal involvement with well-defined borders (versus diffuse stromal, interstitial type)
- Disc may have a Wessely ring around it
- Fine granular infiltrates are occasionally scattered elsewhere in stroma
- Folds in Descemet's are usually apparent
- Moderate keratouveitis and KPs usually present
- No necrosis or neovascularization (as in interstitial, stromal form)
- Secondary epithelial response may occur in cases with advanced endothelial changes

Assessment*

- Most deep (interstitial) keratitis in nonsyphylitic patients is presumed HSV stromal keratitis
  1. Thus, FTA–ABS in inactive cases
     a. Indicates active versus inactive syphylitic infection
     b. Also, positive for congenital or acquired forms
  2. FTA–ABS plus VDRL in active cases
     a. VDRL indicates only active process
     b. This would confirm syphylitic involvement versus possible false-positive FTA–ABS taken alone
- Differentials beyond syphilis for stromal HSV keratitis are limited and quickly ruled out by epithelial involvement or history
  1. Rule out herpes zoster
  2. Systemic disease associations
  3. Bacterial causes
- Rule out stromal corneal dystrophies
  1. Classic triad of interstitial keratitis (i.e., infiltration, neovascularization and thinning) is not present in dystrophy
  2. Neovascularization and thinning usually absent
- Disciform keratitis is almost exclusively considered herpetic (with or without epithelial involvement
  1. Rule out herpes zoster
  2. Systemic causes
  3. Bacterial causes

Plan and Follow-up†

- Recurrent nature, guaranteed scarring (with resultant cosmetic effect and functional loss), and need for extensive, ongoing steroid therapy, with attendant epithelial risks, indicates need for appropriate corneal (specialist) care (Table 4–9)
  1. Secondary ophthalmological care
  2. Tertiary corneal specialist care
- Specialty care will probably include (but not be limited to) any or all of the following steps
  1. Topical steroids during active infiltrative periods with concomittant antiviral agents to reduce or control epithelial infection
  2. Cycloplegia–dilation when indicated
  3. Prophylactic antibiotics
  4. Lubrication therapy
  5. Penetrating keratoplasty when indicated
     a. Should be withheld for case of corneal melting and perforation risks
     b. Should not be considered strictly for cosmetic or functional reasons
     c. Guarded to poor prognosis with interstitial forms, especially with neovascularization moving centralward
- Ongoing management should be co-managed with specialist due to likelihood of recurrences
- Prognosis
  1. Poor for stromal (interstitial) forms
  2. Guarded to poor for disciform types
  3. For both, highly unpredictable, often unremitting and invariably destructive

E. HERPES ZOSTER OPHTHALMICUS (Color Plate 93)

Background Information[57,58]

1. Varicella-type virus infecting dorsal root ganglion
   a. Virus called chickenpox in children
   b. Virus called shingles in adults
2. Two possible means of contagious spread
   a. Reactivation of latent virus (in ganglion)
   b. Contact with (externally) infected host
3. Usually effects first division of trigeminal (fifth) cranial nerve
   a. Most often attacks frontal branch of nerve
   b. Can attack nasal branch or (less commonly) maxillary or mandibular branch
   c. Nasal branch gives off nasociliary branch to eye and tip of nose
   d. Vesicle on tip of nose (Hutchinson's sign) indicates nasociliary involvement and thus, higher risk of ocular involvement (HZV ophthalmicus)
4. Ocular involvement is highly variable and can mimic almost any anterior segment disease
   a. Must differentiate by history, subjective pain and accompanying lid signs
   b. Must be especially careful in differentiating HSV

Subjective

- Usually a 2-week incubation period after contact with an infected source

---

*See also Appendix 3.
†See also Appendix 4.

TABLE 4–9. CLINICAL SIGNS AND LEVELS OF CARE IN HERPES SIMPLEX KERATITIS[a]

Degree	Primary HSV Infection	Recurrent HSV Ocular Infections				
		Epithelial	Metaherpetic	Stromal	Disciform	Complications
Mild	Fever Dermatoses Lid swelling Viral conjunctivitis SPK SEI	Dermatoses Viral conjunctivitis Lymphadenopathy SPK	Dermatoses SPK	Dermatoses Dendrites SPK	Dermatoses Dendrites SPK	Drug toxicity Secondary cataract Secondary dermatosis infections Bacterial Fungal
Moderate	Malaise Lymphadenopathy Phlyctenules Conjunctival hemorrhages Pseudomembranes Dendrites	Conjunctival hemorrhages Pseudomembranes Dendrites Anterior stromal edema Anterior uveitis	Nonresponsive dendrite(s) Stromal edema Stromal scarring	Epithelial edema Endothelial guttata Keratic precipitates Wessely ring	Granular infiltrates Keratic precipitates Wessely ring Central edematous stromal disk Descemet's folds	Keratouveitis Trabeculitis Vasculitis Secondary glaucoma
Severe	Systemic reactions	Stromal infiltration Neovascularization	Indolent ulcer Stromal infiltration Neovascularization Stromal melting	Deep infiltration Endothelial plaques Neovascularization Necrosis or abscess Corneal melting	Dense edematous stromal disc Neovascularization Corneal melting	Superinfection Bacterial Fungal Hypopyon Descemetocele Corneal melting Perforation

[a]No shading indicates primary care, light shading indicates opthalmological care, and dark shading indicates corneal specialist.

- Distinctive history of severe pain associated with classic lid signs
- Patient may report history of associated systemic signs
  1. Headache
  2. Malaise
  3. Fever
  4. Chills
- Pain usually severe because of associated neuralgia, which is usually dramatic in the primary attack and remits and exacerbates chronically with or without recurrent objective signs

Objective

- Lids signs are usually prodrome to ocular involvement
  1. With vesicle at tip of nose (Hutchinson's sign), about a 75 percent risk of ocular involvement
  2. Without vesicle, risk approximately 25 percent
- All ocular signs are nonspecific and mimic many other external ocular diseases
- Usually follicular conjunctivitis presents earliest
  1. Lymphadenopathy varies from mild to severe
  2. Pseudomembranes (and true membranes) common in severe involvements
- Scleritis can develop and advance to "melting" stage
- Keratitis highly variable
  1. Diffuse SPK usually occurs early and may persist for months to years
  2. Chronic epithelial (trophic type) ulcerations are fairly common and create substantial risk of secondary infection
  3. Dendriform keratitis mimics HSV epithelial keratitis
     a. Dendrite is infiltrative versus ulcerative
     b. Dendrite has tapered endings versus "terminal end buds"
     c. Only HSV dendrites are ulcerative with terminal end buds
  4. Corneal hypoesthesia may occur (mimicking HSV) producing reduced subjective corneal irritation
  5. Interstitial (stromal) keratitis
     a. Infiltration (anterior to full thickness)
     b. Neovascularization
     c. Thinning (with risk of stromal "melting")
- Anterior uveitis almost certain with keratitis
- Hyphema occasionally associated with uveitis
- Sympathetic ophthalmia possible
- Posterior segment involvement (e.g., chorioretinitis) occasionally associated with progressive, unremitting forms
- Congestive glaucoma (trabeculitis) frequently part of advanced anterior segment involvements

Assessment*

- Because of the highly variable presentations of HZV ophthalmicus and its tendency to mimic almost any anterior segment disease, technically every anterior segment disorder must be ruled out
  1. A formidable task, except for classic HZV presentation
  2. HZV produces a definitive pattern of severe pain associated with distinctly unilateral (dramatic midline "respect") lid involvement
- Carefully rule out HSV keratitis, which is mimicked more than any other corneal involvement
  1. Pain, lid signs, and infiltrative dendrite usually most helpful differentials
  2. Beware of a secondary (overlying) HSV infection
- HZV involvement is often associated with systemic immunosuppressive diseases and cancers
  1. Evaluate history and risk factors carefully
  2. Medical workup may be useful with risk factors

Plan

- Medical, dermatological, and ophthalmic specialists (depending on severity) are indicated with HZV
- Treatment ranges from supportive therapies to tertiary procedures based on severity of condition
- Supportive therapies
  1. Warm or cold packs
  2. Domeboro packs
  3. Alcohol therapy (on skin for mild involvements to "oral" for pain relief to retrobulbar injection for severe cases)
- Topical prophylactic (and therapeutic antibiotics)
- Topical steroids (with advancing corneal involvement)
  1. Do not use too early, but don't consider steroids contraindicated for epithelial varicella infection (versus HSV epithelial infection)
  2. If steroid used, continually re-evaluate HSV risk
- Cycloplegia—dilation based on uveitic reactions
- Use topical antiviral agents in dendriform keratitis, if steroids are being used
  1. May suppress dormant HSV aggravated by steroids
  2. May have marginal effect on varicella virus
- Oral antiviral agents have a positive effect on HZV course both objectively and for pain relief
  1. Acyclovir (Zovirax) 250 to 500 mg qid
  2. IDU and vidarabine also reported to have positive effects
- Nonsteroidal anti-inflammatories useful for pain relief (i.e., aspirin or ibuprofen)
- Vitamin B reported helpful by many patients (placebo?)
- Oral steroids (from 30 to 60 mg) useful in more advanced cases (should be administered with physician's co-management)
- Narcotic pain control often indicated
- Oral immunosuppressive (anticancer) medications used both experimentally and clinically in severe cases
- Corneal melting and perforation risks treated nonsurgically whenever possible

*See also Appendix 3.

1. Bandage soft contact lenses
2. Cyanoacrylate adhesives

Follow-up

- HZV is notorious for its persistence and recurrence
  1. Destructive nature accentuated with each attack
  2. Pain is often unrelenting with and without clinical activity
- Risk of permanent corneal damage is directly proportional to severity of condition, overall ocular signs, and stromal involvement

- HZV presents a poor postoperative (keratoplasty) surgical risk (e.g., chronic inflammation, graft rejection)
  1. Preferable to postoperative complications, often a neovascular and pannus overgrowth is allowed to develop
  2. Alternative would be conjunctival flap
- Advise patient carefully on all aspects of disease
  1. Recurrent, chronic nature
  2. Postherpetic neuralgia
  3. Permanent scarring risks
  4. Highly variable, ongoing ocular complications
- Recheck eye every 6 months or PRN

IX. Miscellaneous Keratitis*

A. ACNE ROSACEA (Color Plates 68 and 92)

Background Information[59,60]

1. Syndrome of unknown etiology involving the skin and eyes (ocular rosacea)
2. Very common anterior segment disease, frequently misdiagnosed or undiagnosed
   a. Misdiagnosed because findings treated as separate entities rather than as part of a syndrome (defined as a predictable collection of clinical entities)
      i. Fifty-seven percent of patients with excised chalazia were found to have acne rosacea
      ii. Twenty percent of patients develop ocular signs first
      iii. Fifty-three percent develop skin lesions first
      iv. Twenty-seven percent develop eye and skin signs simultaneously
   b. Eye signs need not be proportional to skin manifestations and vice versa (either may predominate)
3. Often mimics (and is misdiagnosed as) staphylococcal blepharitis and blepharoconjunctivitis
   a. Frequently associated with overlying staphylococcal involvement
   b. Additional signs (i.e., syndrome) becomes diagnostic
4. Etiology unknown, but many theories
   a. Bacterial (especially staph)

---

*In alphabetical order.

b. Climatic exposure (e.g., sun, wind, heat, cold)
c. Psychosomatic (anxiety, depression, neurosis)
d. Gastrointestinal disorder (dietary)
e. Disorder of vasodilation (vasomotor disturbance)
f. Sebaceous gland abnormalities (hypertrophy, stagnation)
g. Demodex folliculorum

Subjective

- Usually no previous family or personal history of full syndrome (combined eye and skin involvement)
- Greatest frequency in 30- to 60-year age range
  1. Early skin signs most common in females
  2. Overall syndrome slightly greater in females
- Most common in patients with fair complexions
- Appears to be more frequent in Scotch–Irish descendants and in those of northern European origin
  1. But can be found in all patients
  2. Being reported with increased frequency in black races (previously believed rare)
- Histories of recurrent lid manifestations (i.e., "styes" or recurrent chalazia and hordeoli, chronic marginal blepharitis, especially resistant to standard therapy)
- Symptoms are usually synonymous with level of involvement and associated complications
  1. Blepharitis stage may produce only cosmetic concerns
  2. Conjunctival stage usually produces burning and nonspecific irritation (typical of conjunctivitis)
  3. Keratitis produces classic corneal symptomatology

- Suspicion and ultimate diagnosis is possible only with careful history and uncovering of active or inactive combination of classic eye and skin signs

Objective

- Mild to moderate ocular (or skin) manifestations are far more common than severe involvements
  1. Chronic blepharitis: mild (and most common ocular) manifestation
  2. Blepharoconjunctivitis: moderate manifestation
  3. Blepharokeratoconjunctivitis: moderate to severe
  4. Lids are always involved, either alone, with conjunctiva, or with conjunctiva and cornea
- Specific ocular manifestations (in approximate increasing order of occurrence)
  1. Chronic marginal blepharitis (mimicking *Staphylococcus*)
  2. Telangectatic vessels (on lid margins, mimicking seborrheic blepharitis)
  3. Chalazia and hordeoli (usually recurrent)
  4. Plugged meibomian gland orifices (milia) without inflammation
  5. Meibomianitis (inflammation of meibomians)
  6. Conjunctival hyperemia
     a. Tends to produce a 360° superficial (nonuveitic) circumcorneal flush
     b. Occasionally associated with tearing/serous discharge
  7. Prominent limbal arcades (also 360° pattern)
  8. Peripheral SPK (usually fine to moderately dense)
  9. Tear film disorders (frothing, quick BUT)
  10. Pannus (360° pattern, usually 1 to 2 mm onto cornea)
  11. Neovascularization (360° anterior stromal)
  12. Epithelial edema (peripheral and diffuse)
  13. Microcysts (peripheral and diffuse)
  14. Peripheral epithelial basement membrane changes
      a. Maps–dots–fingerprints
      b. Differ from other typical EBM changes in their peripheral (versus classic central) location
      c. Tend to produce recurrent corneal erosions
  15. Ill-defined subepithelial infiltrates (peripheral)
  16. Peripheral (to diffuse) anterior stromal infiltration and hazing
  17. Anterior uveitis (acute or chronic)
  18. Peripheral corneal thinning (with no significant risk reported for perforation)
- Specific dermatological (skin) manifestations (in approximate increasing order of occurrence)
  1. Erythematous "flushing" of skin
     a. Confined to limited "flush areas" only
        i. Cheeks
        ii. Forehead
        iii. Nose
        iv. Chin
        v. Neck
     b. Aggravated by certain substances, elements
        i. Alcohol and certain ingested foods and drink (variable among patients)
        ii. Wind, heat, cold, sunlight, airborne elements
        iii. Anxiety, stress, excitment, depression
  2. Telangectasia
     a. Prominent, dilated superficial capillary vessels on skin surface
     b. Limited to "flush areas"
  3. Papules
     a. Small (approximately 1 to 3 mm) raised, red skin nodules
     b. Limited to "flush areas"
  4. Pustules (usually small and noninflamed)
  5. Sebaceous gland hypertrophy
     a. Thickened, irregular, erythematous skin texture
     b. Limited to "flush areas"
  6. Rhinophyma
     a. Concentration of all skin findings with thickened, swollen tissue encompassing an area ranging from the tip of the nose to the entire nose
     b. Sometimes called the "W. C. Fields look"

Assessment*

- Mimics many lid and anterior segment disorders[61]
- Key to definitive diagnosis is "syndrome" findings
  1. Eye and skin findings
  2. Manifested simultaneously or one part of syndrome present (eye or skin) with positive history of other components
  3. If other components not (yet) manifested, diagnosis may be difficult, if not impossible (initially)
- If any of classic clinical signs of rosacea are treated as individual entities and do not respond to standard therapies, consider rosacea diagnosis
  1. Especially in 30- to 60-year-old patients
  2. Especially with increased risk factors
     a. Fair complexion
     b. Northern European heritage
- If clinical signs are too vague and confusing, ultimate definitive diagnosis should be considered by a dermatologist

Plan†

- Primary treatment for rosacea syndrome with ocular manifestations is oral tetracycline
  1. Dosage: 250 mg qid for 3 to 4 weeks
  2. Alternative drug (if tetracycline contraindicated)
  3. Erythromycin in similar dosage and duration

---

*See also Appendix 3.
†See also Appendix 4.

- Specific ocular complications should be treated according to standard, appropriate therapies
    1. Topical tetracyclines (or erythromycins) may or may not have any substantial value if used without oral counterpart (especially in moderate to severe involvements)
    2. Topical steroids are definitely indicated (and usually do provide significant benefits) in corneal complications and other inflammatory complications (e.g., uveitis)
- In severe conditions (with significant skin involvement), patient should be urged to seek dermatological consultation and care
- Advise and educate patient carefully on unknown etiology of disease and chronicity of complications

Follow-up

- Most patients will respond initially to oral (and, if indicated, topical) medications over the 1- to 4-week dosage period
    1. If nonresponsive, additional 2 to 4 weeks indicated
    2. Unfortunately, some patients may not respond
    3. Nonresponsive patients should receive close ocular and dermatological management by specialist
- Responsive patients often (more than 50 percent of the time) reactivate within approximately a 6-month to 2-year period and require retreatment
    1. About 50 percent of remaining patients will continue to reactivate intermittently for extended periods
    2. Some patients will require low-dose maintenance regimens for indefinite periods to control frequent recurrences
    3. Most patients will eventually self-limit (usually by age 50 to 60)
- Patients with chronic mild to moderate lid involvement should be maintained on standard anti-staph lid care procedures (see Fig. 2–2)
- Severe cases (with extensive ocular and eye involvement) and nonresponsive cases should be co-managed with dermatologist or patient's primary physician

B. CHLAMYDIAL (ADULT INCLUSION AND INCLUSION BLENORRHEA)

Background Information

1. Trachoma family organism (TRIC)
2. Called inclusion conjunctivitis in adults and inclusion blenorrhea in newborns
3. Incubation period of approximately 4 to 12 days
4. Produces combined viral and bacterial signs
5. Similar to viruses, organism is an obligate intracellular parasite (with dormant recurrent potential)
6. More benign clinical course than trachoma
7. An oculogenital disease[62]
    a. Transmitted eye to eye or hand to eye
    b. From infected mother to baby (2 to 6 percent of newborns)
    c. Nonchlorinated swimming pools (reported in Europe)
    d. Associated with hot-tub use
8. Frequency increasing dramatically with "sexual revolution"

Subjective

For Adult Inclusion Conjunctivitis
- Sexually active adults (especially from age 15 to 25) are prime candidates[63]
- History of prolonged (2- to 4-week) bacterial conjunctivitis signs and symptoms
- Nonresponsive or remitting and exacerbating with use of standard topical antibiotic therapies
- Mild to moderate corneal irritation
- Unilateral presentations more common than bilateral
- No significant visual loss or disturbance (in mild to moderate forms)
- History of nongonococcal genitourinary (or urethral or urinary) tract infection
    1. Discharge with negative culture for *N. gonorrhoeae*
    2. Patient often denies active infection but may admit to recent history of discharge

For Neonatal Inclusion Blenorrhea
- Most frequent cause of conjunctivitis in infants
    1. Usually 5 days to 5 weeks old
    2. Incubation period produces delay in clinical manifestation
- Usually positive history of maternal infection
- Risk of birth canal transmission from infected mother is greater than 20 percent
- Baby frequently presents an associated pneumonia-like upper respiratory infectious (URI) syndrome

Objective

For Adult Inclusion Conjunctivitis[64]
- Incubation (dormancy) period of 1 to 3 weeks
- Bacterial-like signs
    1. Papillary changes on palpebral conjunctiva
    2. Mild to moderate mucopurulent discharge (less on waking)
    3. Meaty red bulbar hyperemia (usually without hemorrhagic changes)
    4. Diffuse SPK (usually greater superiorward)
    5. Corneal signs may linger and ultimately self-limit within 6 to 12 months (without scarring)
- Viral-like signs
    1. Dramatic follicular conjunctivitis (greatest in inferior cul-de-sac)

2. Occasional conjunctival chemosis
3. Preauricular lymph enlargement (usually non-tender)
4. Occasionally pseudomembrane formations in more severe presentations
5. Diffuse SPK (greater superiorward) of variable density and degree
6. EKC-like subepithelial infiltrates (greater superiorward and peripherally)

- Secondary anterior uveitis usually develops in the cases with more advanced corneal involvement
- Occasionally patient may report an associated ipsilateral otitis media (earache on same side)

For Neonatal Inclusion Blenorrhea

- Similar signs to adult form
- Follicles and corneal infiltrates take longer to develop (6 to 8 weeks) owing to immature immune system
- Laboratory workup (done more frequently in infants than in adults) will reveal cytoplasmic inclusion bodies from conjunctival scrapings
- May show systemic involvements in prolonged disease (usually URI-type responses)
- Prolonged, untreated corneal involvement could lead to pannus and permanent scarring

Assessment*

- Laboratory assessment (of conjunctival scrappings) should be considered in infants or severe cases
  1. Attempting to isolate cytoplasmic inclusion bodies
  2. Difficult laboratory procedure (especially for nonophthalmic labs) with frequent false negatives

For Adult Inclusion Conjunctivitis

- Rule out bacterial keratoconjunctivitis
  1. Usually history most significant differential (i.e., sexually active adult with active or history of recent urinary tract involvement)
  2. Nonresponsive to standard topical antibiosis and chronicity usually suggestive in risk categories
- Rule out viral keratoconjunctivitis
  1. Again, history significant
  2. Chronicity of acute or subacute phases of chlamydial infection substantially longer than viral (EKC) syndromes

For Neonatal Inclusion Blenorrhea

- Rule out gonococcal infection
  1. Best done through culturing (patient and mother)
  2. Gonorrhea tends to produce immediate (day 1 or 2) clinical response versus delayed (5 days or greater) chlamydial reaction
- Rule out viral etiologies (uncommon in newborns)

Plan†

For Adult Inclusion Conjunctivitis

- Oral tetracycline (1 to 2 g/day for 15 to 30 days)
- Topical tetracycline (Achromycin) qid for 10 days
- Avoid tetracycline in pregnant females and even in women of child-bearing age (who may be uncertain or unaware of early pregnancy)
  1. Documented risk of discoloration of developing calcium (e.g., teeth) tissue
  2. Substitute sulfa drug or (preferably) erythromycin orally and topically

For Neonatal Inclusion Blenorrhea

- Co-manage patient with pediatrician or primary physician
- Definitely no use of tetracycline (same reasons as stated above)
- Sulfa or erythromycin topical and oral alternative per pediatric indications

Follow-up

- Patients, mothers of patients, and sexual partners must be advised and counseled as to venereal disease
- All patients and associated parties should be advised of the need for medical care
- Clinical signs of conjunctivitis may take 2 to 3 months to resolve completely (with treatment)
- Corneal findings (SPK and subepithelial infiltrates) may persist for 6 to 12 months
- Monitor clinical findings every 2 to 4 weeks until complete resolution
  1. Withhold contact lens rewear for 2 to 4 weeks after resolution of acute clinical presentation
  2. If reinfection occurs with lenses, discontinue temporarily and replace lenses on rewear
  3. Monitor rewear closely if subepis persist
- Advise patient on dormant obligate parasitic nature of organism and risk of recurrences

C. SUPERIOR LIMBIC KERATOCONJUNCTIVITIS (SLK) (Color Plate 69)

Background Information[65]

1. Disease originally described by Theodore in 1963 (frequently called SLK of Theodore)
2. Etiology unknown
3. Frequently (up to 50 percent) associated with hyperthyroidism
4. In early 1980, similar condition began to be reported as a complication of soft contact lens wear
   a. Initially thought to be SLK of Theodore

---

*See also Appendix 3.

†See also Appendix 4.

b. Now considered different disease for three reasons
    i. Multiple clinical differences
    ii. Directly related to thimerosol use
    iii. Caused by soft lens, whereas SLK of Theodore is, in fact, treatable with soft lenses
c. Separate entity termed "contact lens-related SLK" (CL–SLK)

Subjective

- Generalized ocular irritation and discomfort
- Symptoms and frequency of SLK of Theodore slightly more prevalent in women
- Most common age range is 20 to 50 years of age
- CL–SLK tends to present as increasing intolerance to lens wear
- SLK of Theodore tends to remit and exacerbate over 5- to 10-year period

Objective

- Mostly bilateral presentations, with one eye usually more advanced than the other
- Lid spasms frequently associated
- Prominent superior bulbar hyperemia
  1. Usually follows "corridor" pattern from insertion of superior rectus muscle to corneolimbal juncture (especially in SLK of Theodore)
  2. Occasionally, chemosis develops over injected area and along limbal border
- Superior tarsal palpebral papillary changes
  1. Range from fine (in CL–SLK) to dense (in SLK of Theodore)
  2. Not large "giant" papillae as in vernal or GPC
- Fine superior SPK pattern
  1. When abundant, will coalesce to patches
  2. Demonstrates positive NaFl and rose bengal stain
  3. Often associated with prominent limbal arcades and developing pannus
- Occasional dendriform infiltrates (pseudodendrites)
- Superior subepithelial infiltrates may form in chronic or severe presentations
- Filament formations may occur on superior cornea
- CL–SLK may produce anterior stromal hazing
  1. Usually in perilimbal zone
  2. Reported as far "south" as superior pupil border*

Assessment[†]

- Rule out GPC
  1. More dramatic, larger "giant" papillae
  2. Usually less bulbar conjunctival involvement

3. Usually less (if any) corneal involvement
- Rule out vernal keratoconjunctivitis
  1. More frequent in younger males
  2. Tranta's dots on superior limbus
- Differentiate SLK of Theodore from CL–SLK

	SLK of Theodore	CL–SLK
1. Age	Middle age	Any age
2. Sex	Women greater	Equal
3. Systemic	Hyperthyroidism	None
4. Symptoms	Irritation	Lens irritation
5. Bulbar conjunctivitis	Superior hyperemia	Superior hyperemia
6. Tarsal conjunctivitis	Dense papillae	Fine papillae
7. Limbus	Chemosis	Chemosis
8. Cornea	Superior SPK Pseudodendrites SEIs Filaments	Superior SPK Pseudodendrites SEIs Stromal haze

Plan[‡]

For SLK of Theodore

- Disease is usually self-limiting over 5 to 10 year period
- In moderate to severe presentations, topical steroids qid for 10 to 14 days often effective for subjective and objective signs
  1. Sometimes steroids have little to no effect
  2. Do not overuse (i.e., beyond 2 to 3 weeks)
- In mild to moderate cases, Opticrom qid for 3 to 4 weeks[66]
- Severe cases may require advanced therapies
  1. 0.5 percent silver nitrate painted onto superior conjunctiva and tarsus often effective (reasons uncertain)
     a. Relief usually for about 4 to 6 weeks, then recurrence likely
     b. Careful with application (do not touch cornea)
     c. Irrigate copiously after about 3 to 5 minutes
  2. Cryotherapy used in very severe cases
- Moderate to severe levels of the disease may also be treated with large diameter bandage soft contact lenses (see Chapter 7)

For CL-SLK

- Terminate all thimerosol-preserved solutions
- Temporarily discontinue soft lens wear (during acute, symptomatic stages)
  1. Resolution on removal may be rapid to very slow

---

*Personal communication with David Lamberts, M.D., 1987.
†See also Appendix 3.

‡See also Appendix 4.

2. Do not rewear lenses until all symptoms relieved

For Both Types of SLK (Adjunctive Therapies)
- Cold packs
- Oral nonsteroidal anti-inflammatories (as prostaglandin inhibitors) in lieu of contraindications
  1. Aspirin (3 g/day)
  2. Ibuprofen (400 mg qid)
- Oral antihistamine–decongestants
- Cromolyn sodium or topical steroids (1 percent prednisolone qid) for relief of inflammatory response and pain[66]

Follow-up

- Patients with SLK of Theodore should be advised of 5- to 10-year chronicity with remitting and exacerbating clinical episodes
- CL–SLK patients should be monitored closely (every 3 months) after initial episode and contact lens rewear
  1. Resolution of signs and symptoms may extend into months or years
  2. Rewear must be withheld to symptom-free status
  3. If rewear with persistent corneal signs (e.g., SPK), monitor every 4 to 6 weeks, until complete resolution
- If signs or symptoms exacerbate in CL–SLK upon rewear of original lenses, change lens design and material (to rigid gas permeable)

D. TRACHOMA

Complete discussion in Chapter 3, section II.

E. VERNAL KERATOCONJUNCTIVITIS

Subjective

- Seasonal disease presenting mostly in warmer weather
- Young males (age 12 to 30, slightly greater in blacks) at highest risk
- Usually a family or personal history of allergies
- Disease has a remitting and exacerbating history with a self-limiting nature usually within 5 to 10 years after initial attack
- Primary, overriding presenting symptom is itching with secondary corneal foreign-body sensation
- Patient usually reports burning and photophobia

Objective

- Mostly bilateral presentations
- Frequently associated with secondary lid congestion and a pseudoptosis
- Discharge is characteristically thick, ropy, whitish-yellowish strands of dense mucus
  1. Covers superior tarsus and conjunctiva

2. Spreads over cornea
3. Accumulates at inner canthus
- Generalized bulbar hyperemia
- Giant papillary ("cobblestone") conjunctivitis on the superior tarsal plate
- Most common corneal involvement is superior SPK
  1. Usually fine and scattered in upper third corneal region
  2. Increases in density at limbal area (from about 10 to 2 o'clock position)
- Occasional filamentary formations (superiorly)
- Disease presents numerous limbal forms with mild to severe subjective and objective presentations
  1. Mild forms will demonstrate small to moderately sized limbal follicles or infiltrates of a circumlimbal nature ranging from 1 to 3 mm in length with little corneal involvement
    a. Called limbal vernal infiltrate or follicle
    b. Conjunctival injection usually limited to leash of vessels associated directly with limbal infiltrate
    c. Usually no severe conjunctival or corneal involvement
  2. More advanced, generalized forms of vernal keratoconjunctivitis frequently present a limbal form of disease called Tranta's dots
    a. Found most commonly on superior limbus
    b. Puffy, white, round dots about 1 to 2 mm in size
    c. May be flat or slightly raised (in more advanced disease)
    d. Accumulations of eosinophils from type I immune response

Assessment*

- Rule out atopic keratoconjunctivitis (year-round versus seasonal vernal presentations)
- Rule out SLK (usually a milder, less symptomatic presentation)
- Rule out GPC[67]
  1. Less symptomatic
  2. More related to cause (e.g., soft lenses) versus seasonal allergic response
  3. Clinically less severe
- Rule out infectious causes (by seasonal nature and itching)

Plan†

- All forms (mild to severe, generalized to limbal) respond dramatically well to topical steroids
  1. Preferable concentration and dosage is 1 percent prednisolone (or equivalent) q2–4h for 5 to 7 days

---

*See also Appendix 3.
†See also Appendix 4.

2. Lesser concentrations are usually effective over longer period
3. Duration may have to be prolonged in severe cases
4. Taper steroids to lowest maintenance dose and continue low (maintenance) dose for 4 to 6 weeks
   a. Maintenance dose can be as low as 1 gtt 3 ×/week
   b. Less than maintenance dose will result in exacerbation of disease
   c. After 4 to 6 weeks, attempt to further taper to 0
- Other adjunctive therapies (with steroids)
  1. Cold packs
  2. Oral antihistamines–decongestants
  3. Cromolyn (Opticrom) may be introduced during steroid taper and as (possible) substitute for maintenance steroid
     a. Cromolyn is not effective as initial therapy
     b. May or may not work in maintenance, but worth a try versus long-term steroid use
  4. Oral nonsteroidal anti-inflammatory agents may have some value during acute and subacute phases[68]

Follow-up

- Milder generalized (and vernal) forms usually respond very quickly and completely to steroids within 1 week
  1. Mild generalized forms may or may not require maintenance regimens (with steroids or Opticrom)
  2. Limbal vernal forms do not require maintenance regimens beyond initial steroid for 5 to 7 days (then complete taper)
- Patients with more severe forms should be carefully advised of the chronic nature of their disease with remissions and exacerbations over extended period of years (5 to 10 ?)
  1. Severe disease may not remit completely, even with maintenance steroids
  2. Rarely, patient may require additional immunotherapy (e.g., desensitizations, immunosuppressive agents)
- Advise patients in remission to report symptoms upon exacerbation or recheck annually
- Best never to allow open-ended use or self-prescribing (restarting) steroid therapy without recheck visit

X. Irritations and Injuries*

A. ABRASIONS (Color Plates 72, 73, and 74)

1. Superficial Epithelial Abrasions

Subjective

- Usually a direct history of an acute nature
  1. Trauma to ocular surface
  2. Transient foreign body (with patient reporting it "still in the eye")
     a. Usually particulate matter
     b. Frequently fiberglass history (trouble)
- History and symptoms may be insidious (indirect)
  1. Mechanical factors
     a. Embedded lid (tarsus) foreign matter
     b. Trichiasis or entropion
     c. Contact lens edge (soft or hard), trapped foreign matter, surface problem
  2. Physiological factors (usually delayed reactions)
     a. Contact lens related edema
     b. Epithelial basement membrane disorder (greater in AM)
     c. Other epitheliopathies, dystrophies, degenerations

- One eye generally moderately to severely uncomfortable and occasionally mildly photophobic
- Classic corneal symptoms reported
  1. "Sandy, gritty" feeling
  2. Foreign-body sensation (thinking foreign body still present in eye)
  3. "Something under my upper lid" (sensation resulting from transferred pain during blink)
- In nonacute presentations, always pursue other historical data
  1. Ocular and medical history (including oral medications)
  2. Dry eye syndromes

Objective

- Visual acuity often reduced slightly owing to diffuse corneal edema
- Examine lid margins and eyelashes
  1. Trichiasis or entropion
  2. Infectious (toxic) conditions (e.g., *Staphylococcus*)
  3. Cicatrix (scarring), colobomas, lid position
- Usually moderate bulbar conjunctival hyperemia
- May show mild circumcorneal flush (with or without anterior chamber reaction)
- Corneal (squamous) epithelium will stain with NaFl

*In alphabetical order.

1. Superficial punctate keratitis (SPK) or foreign-body tracking (FBT)
2. Staining usually light, diffuse, and of variable pattern
3. No pooling or deep staining (basement membrane)
- On the basis of history, discrete particles may be found
    1. On corneal surface
    2. In cul-de-sac or at inner canthus
    3. Embedded on inferior or superior (more common) palpebral conjunctiva and tarsus
- Topical anesthetic relieves pain entirely
    1. Effective within seconds
    2. Lasts for about 15 to 20 minutes
    3. Continued "dull aching" pain is sign of secondary uveitic reaction
- In physiological edematous reactions
    1. Corneal may show diffuse epithelial edema with squamous epithelial breakdown (SPK)
    2. In dense conditions, patchy staining or entire corneal staining may occur

Assessment

- Determine definitive cause from direct and indirect history
- Rule out risk of secondary (or primary) corneal infection, ulceration
- Examine palpebral conjunctiva (especially superior tarsus) for embedded foreign matter
    1. Single evert superior lid and examine tarsus under slit lamp or loupe
    2. Double-evert superior lid and examine superior cul-de-sac
    3. Lavage tissue while lid double-everted
    4. Swab all noncorneal tissues gently with wet cotton tip and reirrigate superior and inferior cul-de-sacs and inner canthus
- Embedded fiberglass may not be visible and may require "blind" swabbing, possibly for multiple days if foreign body sensation persists
- Evaluate contact lens materials, fit, design
- Examine corneal tissue (bilaterally) for map, dot fingerprint changes and other epithelial or endothelial involvements
- Rule out secondary anterior uveitis

Plan*

- Eliminate, modify or treat direct or indirect cause(s) of abrasion
    1. Remove any foreign matter by irrigation or swabbing
    2. Epilate offending lashes in trichiasis or refer entropion for surgical repair (seek oculoplastic surgeon if possible)
    3. Modify or refit hard or soft contact lenses
    4. Manage epitheliopathies accordingly

*See also Appendix 4.

- Prophylax corneal surface once in-office with aminoglycoside ointment (e.g., gentamicin or tobramycin) after irrigation, swabbing, and reirrigation (if administered)
    1. In mild to moderate involvement, continued use of antibiotic is optional
    2. In moderate to severe involvement (dense SPKs), aminoglycoside drops or ointments may be continued qid for 48 to 72 hours or until complete corneal resolution
- Give patient (or prescribe) mucomimetic lubricating drops (or ointment) q3–4h starting 2 hours after office visit
- Warm packs should be used q2–4h during first 6 to 12 hours after injury
- With epithelial edema (alone or with mechanical or physiological squamous abrasions)
    1. Hypertonic saline drops q3–4h for 2 to 3 days
        a. Two percent or 5 percent drops (Adsorbonac)
        b. Refrigerate during use to reduce sting
    2. Five percent ointment at bedtime (e.g., #128 by Muro)
- Aspirin or ibuprofen (in lieu of contraindications) for pain relief during the first 12 to 24 hours
- Squamous epithelium heals within 6 to 12 hours with no risk of re-erosion
    1. Thus, no pressure patching is necessary
    2. Advise patient to relax, keep eyes closed, and try to sleep following superficial abrasive (mechanical or physiological) injury or irritation
- Advise patient that discomfort "will probably get worse before it gets better" over the first 12 to 24 hours (especially after topical anesthetic wears off)

Follow-up

- Recheck cornea or contact patient between 18- to 24-hour period following initial examination
- With or without compliance, squamous epithelial defects should be well healed within that period
- If FBT still present, foreign body (or other cause) is still present and requires retreatment
- If retreatment required for any reason, check corneas every 24 hours until complete subjective and objective resolution
- Reschedule patient PRN or for routine care

2. Deep Epithelial Abrasions (Nonpenetrating)

Subjective

- Usually a distinct history of a "gouging" or lacerating-type traumatic incident tangential (versus perpendicular or blunt) to the ocular surface
    1. Fingernail in eye
    2. Flying leaves or other firm materials
    3. Springing tree branches or twigs
    4. Paper cuts to eye
    5. Mascara brushes

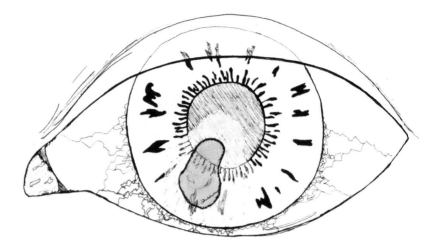

Figure 4–13.
Geography of small corneal abrasion. Approximately 20 percent of inferonasal cornea (4mm x 2mm); approximately 25 percent of pupillary zone (2mm x 2mm).

- Patient reports moderate to severe pain and photophobia
- Subjective symptoms may be disproportionate to objective findings
  1. Sometimes severe injury yields moderate ("stoical") subjective response
  2. Sometimes mild to moderate injury yields severe response with associated nausea, vomiting, psychogenic reactions

Objective

- Lid spasms ipsilateral (or bilateral) are usually dramatic
- Lid edema and erythema vary from mild to moderate
- Vision is reduced, sometimes significantly (20/200 or less) due to epithelial disruption and edema
- Bulbar conjunctiva is moderate to severely hyperemic with segmental or circumferential limbal flush (from secondary anterior uveitis)
  1. Cells and flare may not be visible through disrupted corneal surface
  2. Usually reduced IOP in abraded eye (by 3 to 6 mm compared with uninjured eye) confirms secondary uveitic reaction

- Corneal and other ocular signs vary with degree of epithelial involvement, individual patient reactions and duration of abrasion
- Generally abrasion can be evaluated (and managed) based on four basic abrasion criteria
  1. Geography: Determine and diagram approximate location and percentage of corneal surface and pupillary zone involvement (Figs. 4–13 and 4–14)
  2. Depth
     a. Determine and diagram (roughly) the layer(s) of corneal epithelial involvement and approximate diameter of each of three layers
        i. Squamous
        ii. Basal cells
        iii. Basement membrane
     b. Basal epithelial cells tend to produce a hazy, grainy, more irregular NaFl pattern than the deeper, smoother, more continuous basement membrane (EBM) pattern
     c. EBM also appears brighter (in fluorescence) due to pooling and pH differential between basal cells and basement membrane itself (Figs. 4–15 and 4–16)
  3. Edge quality: Determine the degree (and ap-

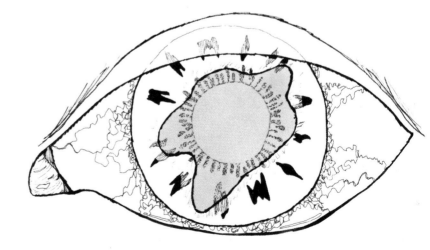

Figure 4–14.
Geography of large corneal abrasion. Approximately 35 to 40 percent of central cornea (6mm x 5mm); 100 percent of pupillary zone.

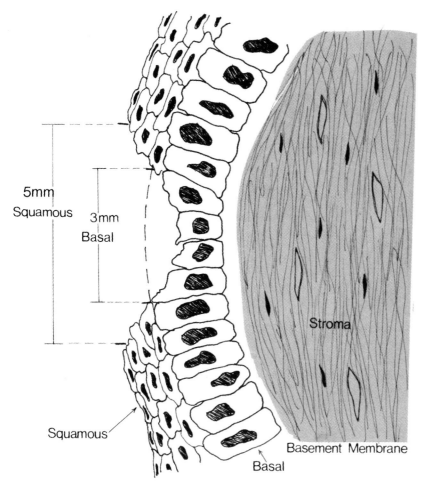

5mm
Squamous

3mm
Basal

Squamous

Basal

Basement Membrane

Stroma

Figure 4– 15.
Depth of corneal abrasion (basal cell layer)

proximate dimensions) of loosening of squamous epithelial edges and any resulting "epithelial flaps or tags," which should be incorporated into the overall "geography" of the abrasion (Fig. 4–17)

  a. No need to remove or trim epithelial flaps

  b. Epithelial healing produces sluffing off of the dead epithelial tissue without assistance

  4. Edema: Determine approximate diameter, intensity, and depth of surrounding edematous reaction to epithelium and stroma and record and diagram in overall diagram (including all four abrasion criteria) (Fig. 4–18)

■ Consider using color code from Table 1–4 with Figures 4–15 through 4–18

Assessment

■ *Rule out penetration or perforation* of the cornea (Color Plate 77)

  1. Corneal penetration equals stromal entry

  2. Corneal perforation equals full-thickness entry and puncture

■ *Subjective indications* (for penetration or perforation)

  1. Sharp or pointed items abrading in a perpendic-

ular (versus tangential) manner (e.g., pencils, pine needles)

  2. Lacerating wounds (e.g., knife, scissors)

  3. High-velocity "projectiles" (anything!)

■ *Objective indicators* (for penetration or perforation)

  1. Appearance of stromal channel (grayish-white at site of entry or maximal abrasion

  2. Endothelial disruption directly behind abrasion

  3. Foreign material in aqueous, on iris, lens capsule, in lens, vitreous or on fundus

  4. "Wrinkled" cornea or flat anterior chamber

  5. Seidel's sign (percolation effect)

    a. Instill fluorsecein

    b. With patient in slit lamp, ask to squeeze blink tightly and then release

    c. Observe point of maximal abrasion for signs of "oozing" of NaFl dye (indication of aqueous leakage through corneal perforating wound)

  6. IOP may be temporarily reduced in corneal perforation due to aqueous loss

■ *Assessment* of risk for penetration or perforation

  1. Good history is most important

  2. Good slit lamp is second most important

  3. Recognition and appreciation for the extraordinary strength and resistance of Bowman's

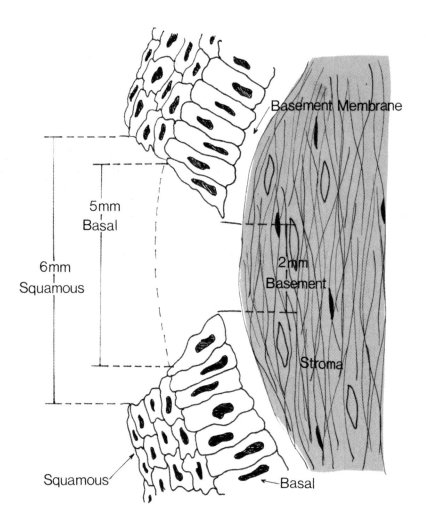

Basement Membrane

5mm
Basal

6mm
Squamous

2mm
Basement

Stroma

Squamous

Basal

Figure 4–16.
Depth of corneal abrasion (basement membrane)

layer (condensed stroma) will help toward accurate assessment of penetration risk
- *Plans* for penetration or perforation
  1. Penetration without perforation
     a. Nonsurgical treatment is similar to deep epithelial abrasion
     b. However, scarring is guaranteed with risk of cosmetic awareness and permanent visual loss
     c. Ophthalmological consultation is indicated (if for only medicolegal considerations)
  2. For corneal perforation
     a. Surgical repair should be conducted ASAP by a corneal specialist, if available
     b. Specialty care will include (but may not be limited to) cyanoacrylate glues, bandage soft lenses, topical antibiotic, and systemic antibiosis to reduce risk of intraocular infection
     c. Do not pressure patch perforations for transportation to specialist (use Fox metal shield for protection)

- Use abrasion criteria to evaluate extent, degree, and intensity of deep epithelial abrasions
- Carefully assess associated reactions to deep corneal abrasions (Table 4–10)
  1. Determine variables (usual versus sometimes versus rare)
  2. Rule out secondary traumatic anterior uveitis (usual to sometimes)
  3. Rule out secondary corneal ulcer (rare)
  4. Adjust treatment plan appropriately, per Care code for deep corneal abrasion (Table 4–11), to cover all associated reactions
- Gross assessment of corneal abrasion (when complete instrumentation is not available, such as outside office setting) can be made by simple transillumination of the cornea with flash light or collimated light source
- Finally, measure and include in final assessment and advice to patient, a prospective of the expected rate (time) of healing, prognosis, and (notwithstanding the ominous clinical appearance and dramatic subjective discomfort of a deep abra-

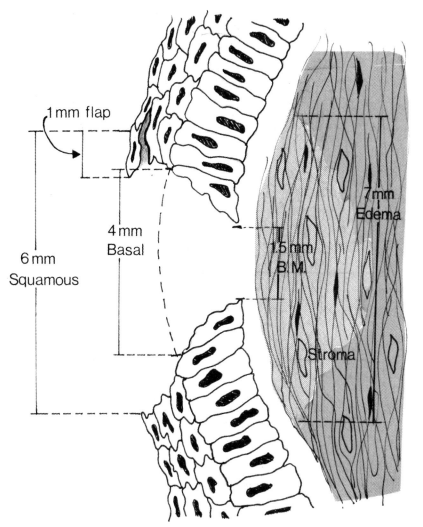

Figure 4–17.
Epithelial "flap"

sion) the classic (predictable) physiological occurrences in the normal healing pattern (Fig. 4–19)
1. During first 6 to 24 hours, squamous epithelium slides over wound area
2. During 1 to 3 days surrounding (remote) basal

epithelial cell mitosis pushes new cells into wound site (filling defect)
a. Conjunctival transdifferentiation of migrating conjunctival epithelium may also occur in larger abrasions[69,70]

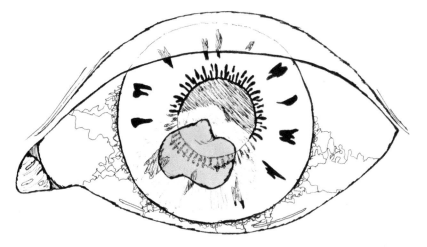

Figure 4–18.
Overall "abrasion criteria" diagram. Approximately 15 percent of inferonasal cornea (3mm x 4mm); approximately 25 to 30 percent of pupillary zone (3mm x 2mm); approximately 3mm x 1mm superior edge epithelial flap; approximately 7mm x 7mm surrounding epithelial edema.

TABLE 4–10. ASSOCIATED REACTIONS IN DEEP CORNEAL ABRASION

Clinical Features[a]	Frequency	Care Code[b]
Reduced visual acuity	Usual	8
Discomfort	Usual	1,2,4,8
Photophobia	Usual	3
Lid spasms	Usual	2
Tearing	Usual	8
Exudate	Rare	8,10
Lid edema	Usual	2
Conjunctival edema	Sometimes	2,5
Corneal edema	Usual	2,5
Superficial hyperemia	Usual	2,3,8
Circumcorneal flush	Sometimes	2,3,4,6
Anterior stromal infiltration	Sometimes	2,5
Deep stromal infiltration	Rare	2,5,7,(9?),10
Endothelial infiltrates	Rare	2,5,7,(9?),10
Folds in Descemet's	Rare	8,(9?),10
KPs	Sometimes	2,3,4,6,7
Cells and flare	Sometimes	2,3,4,6
Fibrin in chamber	Sometimes	2,3,4,6,7,10
Hypopyon	Rare	8,9
Constricted pupil	Sometimes	
Dilated pupil	Sometimes	
Irregular pupil	Rare	8,(9?),10
Elevated IOP	Rare	(9?),10
Reduced IOP	Usual	

[a]Intensity will vary on a case-by-case basis.
[b]See Table 4–11 for care code explanation.

b. Usually produces slower healing rate
3. During days 3 and 4, mitosis directly at wound site completes full-thickness healing and, if needed, begins to regenerate new basement membrane (for 6 to 8 weeks)[71,72]

Plan*

■ Follow day-by-day deep corneal abrasion protocol (Table 4–12)
   1. Should be administered only after evaluation of abrasion according to abrasion criteria
   2. Consider associated reactions (Table 4–10)
      a. Treat associated reactions according to "Care code" (Table 4–11)
      b. Care code may require adjustments or substitutions to following day by day protocol

Day 1 (Day of Initial Presentation)

■ Obtain best correctable vision (BVA) with spectacle lenses or pinhole
■ Examine carefully under topical anesthetic
   1. use "Abrasion Criteria"
   2. Check associated reactions (Table 4–10)
   3. Multiple anesthetic drops may be applied (every 15 to 20 minutes, 2 or 3 ×) if necessary for examination purposes, but *never let patient take topical anesthetic drops for home use!*
■ Lavage thoroughly with ophthalmic irrigating solution to reduce risk of secondary fungal infection (especially in vegetative injuries)

*See also Appendix 4.

TABLE 4–11. CARE CODE FOR DEEP CORNEAL ABRASION

Care Code Number	Drug, Procedure, Advice[a]	Recommended Dosages

1	Four-step pressure patch procedure
	   Lavage with irrigating solution
	   Dilate and cycloplege with 5% homatropine
	   Instill broad-spectrum antibiotic ointment (e.g., gentamicin) in inferior cul-de-sac
	   Apply pressure patch (see Table 4–13)
		24-hr duration X PRN

	Soft lens bandage alternative	Extended wear (24 hr)
2	Warm compresses	q2–4h
3	Dark glasses	PRN
4	Aspirin or ibuprofen (in lieu of contraindications)	2 tabs q4h X 2–3 days
5	5% hypertonic saline (ointment and drops)	1 qtt q3–4h and ointment at bedtime
6	Cycloplege and dilate (with 5% homatropine or 0.25 percent scopolamine)	1 X q24h with patch or tid until uveitis resolves
7	1% prednisolone or FML (with family history or diagnosis of glaucoma)	q4h until uveitis resolves
8	Advise and counsel patient (on immediate and long-range prognosis)	At each visit or PRN by phone
9	Refer to ophthalomologist	ASAP
10	Monitor closely	q24h

[a]Drugs, procedures, advice, and recommended dosages may vary with the degree and intensity of each presentation.

TABLE 4–12. HEALING OF DEEP CORNEAL ABRASIONS (DESCRIPTION AND RATE OF HEALING)[a]

	Subjective	Objective	Assessment	Plan
Day 1	Moderate to severe pain persists Moderate photophobia	Edema may be little improved (or worse) Edges show mild reduction in instability and flapping (≈10%) Depth shows mild to moderate reduction in staining (≈20%) Geography usually shows reduced diameter (≈30%)	For expected norms, follow Day 2 "Abrasion Protocol" For significant variations, refer to "Associated Reactions" in Table 4–10	Follow appropriate steps in "Abrasion Protocol" or "Care Code" (Table 4–11)
Day 2 or 3	Mild irritation may persist Photophobia reduced or absent	Edema persists (±25% improvement) Edge instability significantly reduced (≈50%) Depth shows significant reduction in deep staining (≈75%) Geography dramatically reduced (≈80%)	For expected norms, follow Day 3 or 4 "Abrasion Protocol" For significant variations, refer to "Associated Reactions" in Table 4–10	Follow appropriate steps in "Abrasion Protocol" or "Care Code" (Table 4–11)
Day 3 or 4	Patient comfortable No photophobia or other symptoms	Edema begins significant drying (>60%) Edges stable with resolving infiltrative ring (80–90%) Depth completely filled with no deep staining remaining Geography shows completely covered abrasion area	For expected norms, follow "Deep Abrasion Protocol" For significant variations, refer to "Associated Reactions" in Table 4–10	Follow appropriate steps in "Abrasion Protocol" or "Care Code" (Table 4–11)

Improvement	Day 1 Abrasion Criteria				Day 2 or 3 Abrasion Criteria				Day 3 or 4 Abrasion Criteria			
(%)	Edema	Edges	Depth	Geography	Edema	Edges	Depth	Geography	Edema	Edges	Depth	Geography
10												
20												
30												
40												
50												
60												
70												
80												
90												
100												

[a]Exceptions to these descriptions and rates include the following: diabetic patients (usually three to five times longer to heal), significant damage to basement membrane (≈6 to 8 weeks or more for total repair), and abrasions greater than 50 to 75 percent of geography (usually three to five times longer to heal).

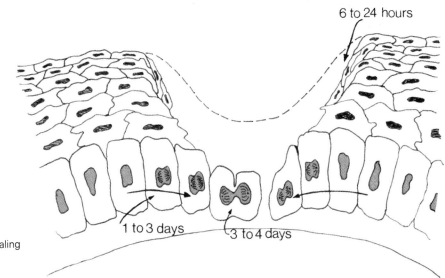

6 to 24 hours

Figure 4– 19.
Deep epithelial abrasion healing process

1 to 3 days

3 to 4 days

- Dilate and cycloplege with 5 percent homatropine
  1. To reduce risk of secondary uveitis
  2. Observe adequate dilation before patching or discharging patient
  3. Add more dilating drops if necessary
- Instill broad-spectrum antibiotic ointment in eye
  1. Aminoglycoside (e.g., tobramycin) preferable
  2. Nonaminoglycoside (e.g., Polysporin) OK in clean, low (pseudomonal) risk abrasions
- Pressure patch firmly (Table 4–13)
  1. Not indicated in mild to moderate abrasions
  2. Indications in moderate to severe abrasions
     a. Noncompliant patient (rubbing eye)
     b. Loose epithelial edges (e.g., flaps)
     c. Exposed basement membrane
     d. Extremely large (≥ 4 to 6 mm) abraded area
  3. Soft contact lens bandage may be used as an alternative to pressure patching in deep abrasions with mild to moderate basement membrane exposure (less than 3 to 6 mm)
     a. Use thin, large-diameter, mid- to high water material or collagen lens (Bio-Core)
     b. Fit plano to minimal power
     c. Approximate keratometry from opposite eye
     d. Prophylax with gentamicin drops (over lens) bid to qid
     e. Manage same as with pressure patch
     f. Benefits include increased comfort, less secondary edema, continued visual use, and, in some cases, more rapid healing rate[68]
- Advise aspirin (2 tabs 5 × daily or 3 g/day) or ibuprofen (400 mg qid) in lieu of contraindications
  1. For analgesia
  2. As anti-inflammatory (prostaglandin inhibitor) against secondary uveitic risk
  3. Contraindications
     a. GI problems
     b. Anticoagulation risks

     c. Known aspirin toxicity
     d. Advanced kidney disease
     e. Children under age 12
- Vitamin B complex may enhance epithelial regeneration (uncertain as to clinical value in corneal abrasion)
- Counsel patient on immediate and long range prognosis
  1. Risk of secondary uveitis (25 to 50 percent), even with prophylactic dilation, nonsteroidal anti-inflammatory agents
  2. Stress importance of leaving patch (or soft lens bandage) on to promote proper heal versus recurrent erosion
- Reschedule patient for 24-hour recheck (absolute!)

Day 2 (24 Hours After First Presentation)
- Remove pressure patch or soft lens bandage
- Obtain BVA
  1. Use same method as day 1
  2. May be worse than day 1 because of increasing edema
- Evaluate patient's subjective discomfort
  1. Without topical anesthetic gives corneal response
  2. With topical anesthetic gives indication of secondary uveitic pain (i.e., "dull, aching")
- Compare all objective findings with day 1 findings
- If secondary uveitic signs present
  1. Continue dilation and aspirin or ibuprofen
  2. Introduce steroids only in severe (3+) reactions[73]
- Reinstitute day 1 treatment if indicated
  1. Severe discomfort
  2. Minimal healing of basal epithelial cells
- If patch or lens not reapplied
  1. Introduce warm packs q2–4h
  2. Hypertonic saline (drops q2–4h and ointment at bedtime)
  3. Reschedule for 24 to 48 hours

TABLE 4–13. APPLICATION OF A PRESSURE PATCH

Materials Needed

Balanced ophthalmic irrigating solution in "squirt" bottle, e.g., Blinx (Barnes Hind), Dacriose (Cooper), Eye Stream (Alcon)

Broad-spectrum antibiotic ointment, e.g., Garamycin (Alcon), Polysporin (Burroughs-Wellcome), Tobrex (Alcon)

Preshaped gauze eyepads, e.g., Curity, Johnson & Johnson, White Cross

Hypoallergenic, one-inch paper, plastic, or cloth adhesive tape, e.g., Micropore (paper), Dermiclear (plastic), Dermicel (cloth) (my preference for adhesion and ease of use is Dermiclear)

Application of Patch

After conducting all ocular preparatory procedures

    Have patient rest back of head against firm headrest

    Close both eyes with normal pressure and keep closed

    Clean and dry skin of mid-forehead and cheek lateral to ipsilateral eye

    Push back loose hair from forehead and face (Beards are a tough break!)

From side view, assess depth of orbit and prepare two to four pads as single unit (stack)

Fold one pad in half (lengthwise) and place it over closed lid (cotton balls, folded tissues, or gauze pads can also be used) (wet folded pad slightly for improved molding)

Place two to four pads (unit) over folded pad at slight angle (downward temporally) to cover orbit area maximally

Using 6- to 7-inch strips of tape, start first strip at mid-forehead, and angle directly over mid length of pads (on eye)

Pinch skin of cheek upward (toward eye) and pull end strip of tape tightly over cheek (below level of ear); remember to hold strip already applied to mid-forehead

Tape down first strip to cheek skin and release; if strip is tight, it should cause folding of lateral skin toward pads

Starting again at mid-forehead, apply a second 6- to 7-inch strip at a slightly upward angle from first strip

Contour this second strip over the superior edges of the pads such that all are covered by the strip as it passes over the pads; a slight curve will be necessary (and beneficial) in achieving this coverage

Apply the end of the second strip tightly and firmly onto the skin of the cheek (at a slight downward angle) partially covering the end of the first strip

Apply a third 6- to 7-inch strip in a similar manner as the second strip but in a downward direction to cover the lower edges of the pads.

Finally, add one more (fourth) 6- to 7-inch strip over the same course as the first strip (mid-length of pads); use this strip to cover the inner edge of strips 2 and 3 as they curve over the surfaces of the pads; Apply tightly and firmly to the cheek over ends of other 3 strips

Removel of Patch

Instruct patient ("forcefully") to leave patch in place (no temporary removals) for 24-hr period

Patch should be removed by a practitioner, preferably the same person who applied the patch

Remove tape gently to avoid added irritation to skin (adhesive removers are usually not needed)

    Allergic reactions may appear as mild red erythematous patches under and around taped areas

    Prolonged taping (i.e., retaping for 2 to 3 days straight) often yields mild to moderate skin irritation which will respond to 0.5% hydrocortisone creams, cold packs or will self-limit without care

Upon ocular examination after removal of a pressure patch, a frequent sequela of the patching (beyond the healing abrasion) may be the development of a mild to moderate striat keratitis secondary to mechanical folding of the cornea and Descemet's membrane; resolution of this normal response is usually rapid (48 to 72 hours) and requires no treatment

Value of Pressure Patch

Decreased subjective discomfort

Immobilizes eyelids, reducing risk of blink loosening edges of abrasion

Creates warm environment to promote healing

Presses regenerating basal layer epithelial cells down firmly onto basement membrane

Reduces potential of formation of subepithelial pockets of edema

Tarsal plate (inside of upper lid) provides smooth surface for squamous epithelial sliding to re-establish smooth epithelial surface

Provides protective shield over injured eye against further irritation (e.g., patient touching eye or inadvertently rubbing it during sleep)

Day 3 or 4

- Obtain BVA
- Re-evaluate subjective and objective status versus days 1 and 2
- Reconsider anterior uveitis therapy if indicated
  1. If no worse or better than day 2, reduce or discontinue dilation, aspirin, ibuprofen
  2. If worse, continue dilation, and add 1 percent prednisolone (or FML) q4h

Follow-up

- All abrasion criteria will improve on a day-to-day basis, except edema
  1. Usually increases over first 24 to 48 hours
  2. Will not begin to decrease until patch is discontinued (possibly faster with soft lens)
  3. Often produces stromal hazing and temporary secondary striate keratitis (usually will resolve within 1 week after discontinued patch)

- Continue warm packs for about 1 week
- Continue hypertonic drops for 2 to 3 weeks (tid)
- Continue hypertonic ointment at bedtime for 4 to 6 weeks
- Advise patients on short- and long-term risks of recurrent corneal erosion[74]
  1. Instruct on early symptoms (AM syndrome)
  2. Stress value of 6 weeks of postabrasion hypertonic ointment at bedtime
  3. Explain importance of therapy to decrease (but not eliminate) risk
- Beware of patients lost to follow-up in early stages of abrasion protocol
  1. Mild to moderate cases may not require aggressive follow-up management
  2. Moderate to severe cases should be followed closely and contacted if noncompliant (Table 4–12)

B. BLUNT (CONCUSSION OR CONTUSION) INJURY[75]

Subjective

- A wide variety of causes
  1. Sports injuries (e.g., racket sports, baseball)
  2. Punch in the eye
  3. Blast injuries (to the closed lid)
  4. Industrial, domestic, or automobile accidents
  5. Birth trauma
- Discomfort and general subjective response vary with nature and degree of injury
- Usually associated with decreased vision and pain
  1. Vision loss secondary to edema and uveitis
  2. Pain associated with inflammation and occasional secondary acute glaucoma
- Frequently, presentation is out of concern and fear

Objective

- Many common associated findings
  1. Ecchymosis ("black eye")
  2. Subconjunctival hemorrhage and chemosis
  3. Corneal abrasion (and sometimes laceration)
  4. Corneal edema
  5. Secondary anterior uveitis
  6. Others
- All ocular tissues may be involved
- Caused by birth trauma (forceps delivery or birth canal trauma)
  1. Usually produces vertical folds or tears in Descemet's membrane
  2. Left eye far more frequently involved than right due to typical left occiput birth presentation
  3. Often seen in later life (during general examination) with mild to significant visual reduction
  4. More severe cases show permanent stromal haze
- Cornea (and other tissue) damage varies with nature and degree of injury

Mild Corneal Injury

- Epithelial and anterior stromal edema
- Mild epithelial staining
- Pigment deposits scattered on endothelium

Moderate Corneal Injury (as for Mild, plus)

- Deep stromal edema
- Folds (or lattice pattern) at Bowman's layer
- Folds in Descemet's membrane (straite keratitis)
- Blood staining on posterior cornea (secondary hyphema)
- Disruption of endothelium
- Substantial reduction in VA

Severe Corneal Injury (as for Mild and Moderate, plus)

- Translucent or opaque cornea because of dense, full-thickness edema
- Tears in Descemet's membrane
- Ruptures in corneal stroma (perforation unlikely)
- Hemorrhaging into corneal stroma
- Gross disruption and pigmentation of endothelium

Assessment

- With all blunt (contusive) injury, noncorneal ocular injury must always be ruled out, including (but not limited to) following possibilities
  1. Anterior segment
     a. Iridoplegia (mydriasis or miosis)
     b. Cycloplegia
     c. Hyphema
     d. Iridodialysis (angle recession)
     e. Traumatic cataract
     f. Luxation or dislocation of crystalline lens
     g. Vossius ring
  2. Posterior segment
     a. Choroidal rupture
     b. Retinal hemorrhage
     c. Preretinal hemorrhage (intravitreous)
     d. Retinal edema (commotio retinae or Berlin's edema)
     e. Macular hole
     f. Retinal tears or detachment
     g. Papillitis
     h. Optic nerve avulsion
     i. Ruptured globe
  3. Glaucoma (secondary)
- Determine degree (mild, moderate, or severe) of corneal involvement

Plan

- Treat all ocular involved tissues and structures appropriately
- Mild to moderate corneal involvement is usually self-limiting and resolve with or without treatment
  1. Warm packs q2–4h for 3 to 5 days
  2. Hypertonic saline drops q3–4h and ointment hs
  3. Reassurance of patient

- Severe corneal involvements should be managed by most appropriate available eye care practitioner
  1. As with mild to moderate involvement, self-limit and self-resolving nature with or without therapy
  2. Greater risk of permanent corneal damage (stromal scarring) because of dense edema and ruptured membranes (Descemet's and stromal tissue)
  3. With significant scarring risk, aggressive medical or surgical therapies may (or may not) be of additional value
     a. Lowering IOP
     b. Cauterization techniques
     c. Penetrating keratoplasty

Follow-up

- Recheck all blunt trauma cases within 1-week period
  1. Monitor initial damage (resolution or advances)
  2. Recheck all tissues and structures again
- If cornea improving, reduce dosages and recheck once again within 1 week
- If no improvement, continue treatment and recheck in 2 to 3 days
- If patient returns with increased complications, seek corneal consultation (from corneal specialist)

C. BURNS

Background Information

1. Lids and associated blink (menace) reflex tends to protect the ocular surface and cornea from many burns
   a. Lid tissue suffers major portion of damage
   b. Measured as first-, second-, and third-degree tissue damage (see Chapter 2)
2. Ocular surface burns classified in three categories
   a. Thermal (or heat related)
   b. Radiation (by tissue absorption)
   c. Chemical (toxic or hypersensitive reactions)
3. Thermal burns to the cornea usually produce an eschar
   a. Focal superficial burn causing "charring" of epithelial cells creating a whitish-gray (sometimes raised mass) corneal surface lesion
   b. Underlying stromal usually completely spared
   c. Common causes include heated particles or objects
      i. Cinders
      ii. Match heads

     iii. Heating instruments (e.g., soldering irons)
     iv. Hair "curling" irons
   d. Eschar is removed by standard foreign-body procedures and treated subsequently as a routine deep corneal abrasion
4. Radiation burns to cornea are most commonly related to ultraviolet (UV) light sources (i.e., sunlight, sun lamps and welding arcs)
   a. Produce focal or diffuse SPKs varying from mild to dense
   b. Treatment and management is similar to standard infectious superficial keratitis care
5. Chemical burns to the eye are considered true ocular emergencies (i.e., care within minutes to save vision)
   a. Three categories should be considered clinically
      i. Aromatic compounds (benzene ring chemicals)
         - Benzene
         - Turpentine
         - Paint thinners
         - Gasoline
      ii. Acids (pH <7)
         - Battery acid
         - Acids containing heavy metals (far more dangerous than other forms)
      iii. Alkali (pH >7)
         - Ammonia compounds (e.g., cleaning agents, fertilizers)
         - Lye (sodium hydroxide, drain cleaners)
         - Lime (mortar, cement, plaster)
         - Magnesium hydroxide (flares, sparklers, firecrackers)
         - Chlorine (Chlorox, pool chlorines)
   b. Other agents can also produce toxic or hypersensitive-type chemical reactions to ocular surface
      i. Petroleum products
      ii. Household cleaners
      iii. Detergents, soaps, aerosols
      iv. Tear gas, mace
   c. All chemical agents will produce variable degrees of damage to the ocular surface based on the amount of substance entering the eye and its concentration
      i. Amounts will determine localized versus diffuse involvement

ii. Concentrations will dictate degree and depth of penetration of burn

d. Amounts and concentrations for all chemicals have an effect on their immediate ocular surface reaction, beyond which rapid neutralization begins to occur for all substances, *except alkali*

i. Besides initial (amount and concentration) reaction, alkali continues to penetrate through its collagenolytic reaction for hours to days after initial contact

ii. Collagenolytic response can result in unrelenting ulceration, melting, and permanent stromal scarring or perforation

iii. Reaction is directly proportional to pH (greater pH equals greater tissue damage)

6. Chemical burns to the cornea require accurate assessment, quick action, and careful clinical management to protect the ocular tissue and the visual function

Subjective

- Usually an emergency phone call (hopefully) will be the first encounter with the patient
  1. Patients delaying immediate care to travel to an office or hospital may have allowed additional, irreversible damage to occur
  2. Care is required virtually within seconds to potentiate maximal potential clinical benefits
- History must include certain facts
  1. When and how accident happened?
  2. What was the substance or chemical?
  3. How much got in the eye?
  4. What specifics are available on the product?
  5. What has been done so far?
- Common causes of ocular (corneal) burns include (but are not limited to)
  1. Accidents in or around the house
  2. Industrial accidents
  3. Agricultural accidents
  4. Car battery explosions
  5. Radiation causes (e.g., arc welding, sun lamps)
  6. Thermal (heat)-related injuries
- Common substances include (but are not limited to)
  1. Chemicals (aromatics, acids, alkali)
  2. Aerosols (e.g., hair sprays, deodorants)
  3. Cleaning compounds and disinfectants
  4. Swimming pool chemicals
  5. Bleaches
  6. Sulfur particles of match heads (when striking)
  7. Cinders or hot ashes from fires
- Patient symptoms include classic corneal irritation
- Discomfort may range from mild to severe

Objective

- Immediate first aid should be administered STAT (emergently) assuming worst possible objective picture (before examination)[76]
  1. Must be based on history alone
  2. Examination should follow first aid and preliminary determinations of nature of substance involved

Mild Involvement

- Lids may be more involved than eye itself
- Conjunctival hyperemia and chemosis about 1 to 2+
  1. May show subconjunctival hemorrhages
  2. Mild circumcorneal flush may be present
  3. No pale ischemic patches should be present
- Corneal epithelium may stain in varying degree
  1. Iris features clearly visible through cornea
  2. May show diffuse band or inferior SPK pattern
  3. Confluent patches of stain (small or large)
  4. Diffuse, hazy epithelial edema
- Anterior chamber usually quiet or trace cells

Moderate Involvement

- Lid tissue frequently more involved
- Conjunctival tissue is grossly hyperemic and chemotic
  1. Circumcorneal flush more obvious
  2. One (or more) small (less than 3- to 4-mm diameter) patches of ischemia may be noted perilimbally or randomly placed
     a. These patches signify cauterization of superficial conjunctival vessels secondary to focal patch of highly concentrated chemical (e.g., granule, crystal)
     b. Ischemic patches represent partial loss of blood supply (and nutrition) to anterior segment
- Corneal involvement distinct
  1. Iris features are hazy when viewed through cornea
  2. Deep epithelial staining (usually diffuse or greater inferiorly)
  3. From 25 to 50 percent of epithelium may "melt"
  4. Deep stromal edema producing hazy cornea
- Anterior chamber reaction with or without raised IOP

Severe Involvement

- Dramatic clinical presentation
- Lids (and face) may show extensive involvement
- Diffuse conjunctival chemosis often present
- There may be a paradoxical white eye (with a distinct history of chemical burn and advanced corneal findings)
  1. This paradoxical finding may be a partial or diffuse ischemia (from a high concentration chemical)
  2. Do not be deceived by white eye appearance
  3. Calculate degree of burn by corneal involvement

4. Diffuse ischemia is a serious risk potentiating anterior segment necrosis
- Cornea is usually translucent to opaque
  1. Iris features are barely visible or obscured
  2. Dense, deep stromal edema
  3. From 50 to 100 percent of epithelium may "melt" away
  4. Occasionally with alkali burns, corneal findings may appear as moderate degree on initial presentation and progress to severe during first 3 to 5 days after injury
     a. Thus, history of alkali burn with even moderate-level corneal involvement should be considered severe in clinical approach
     b. Corneal damage by any other chemicals (other than heavy metal acids and alkalis) will demonstrate maximal damage within hours
- Anterior uveitis almost assured (but not visible through dense corneal edematous haze)
- IOP may be significantly raised, especially during the 24 to 48 hours after injury

Assessment

- All differential considerations should be postponed in favor of immediate first aid (refer to "Plan," below)
- Initial assessment begins with careful history
- After proper first aid, objective evaluation will determine mild, moderate, or severe involvement
- A pH evaluation (with standard pH paper applied to the tear meniscus) sometimes helps in determining need for continued irrigation after patient arrives for care

Plan*

- Immediate first aid for all burn patients begins with instruction over the phone as follows:
  1. Get name and telephone number
  2. After brief history (as described in "Subjective," above), obtain as much information about chemical involved
     a. Label information (e.g., brand, generic, or chemical name)
     b. Patient's knowledge of substance or chemical
  3. Instruct patient on copious and continuous lavage (irrigation) with ophthalmic irrigator or water
     a. Form lateral trough around eye with paper towels
     b. Anesthetize ocular surface with topical anesthetic drops (optional)
     c. Pull lids away from eyeball and irrigate upper and lower fornices, and then inner canthus
  4. Neutralizing agents (acidic or basic) are not indicated

5. Irrigating bottles or balanced or buffered commercial saline solutions are OK, but not necessary
6. Any means of getting copious amounts of readily available neutral solutions (i.e., water) in the eye is the best approach
   a. Sink faucets
   b. Shower nozzles (get in the shower)
   c. Hoses (outdoors)
   d. Industrial irrigating apparatus
7. Delays greater than 3 to 5 minutes or discontinuation sooner than 20 to 30 minutes (minimum) reduces prognosis significantly
8. Tell patient you will call them back in 20 to 30 minutes and reinforce urgency of irrigation procedure
- If substance or chemical is unknown to patient, immediately contact your local or regional emergency service (e.g., 911) or a poison control center
  1. Always keep number available
  2. Identify yourself as a health professional with emergent patient need
  3. If no service available in your area, investigate alternatives (in advance of emergency situation)
- Give emergency service all facts available and ask for assistance with the following information
  1. Nature of substance or chemical (if unknown)
  2. Suggested first aid measures beyond irrigation
- After receiving necessary information, or within 20 to 30 minutes, recontact patient
- Get update on subjective condition
- See patient or have patient seen immediately
  1. Best to see patient in office
  2. Avoid hospital emergency rooms unless you are to see patient or unless qualified optometrist or ophthalmologist is on site (or on call) at emergency facility
- Upon objective evaluation of condition
  1. Consider most appropriately trained eye care practitioner based on level of involvement
  2. Ideally, and when assessible
     a. All severe chemical burns as well as moderate alkali burns should be managed by a corneal specialist
     b. Moderate acid and aromatic burns and mild alkali burns should be managed by properly trained O.D.s or ophthalmologists
     c. Mild burns are treatable at the primary care level
- Treatment steps for mild to moderate (nonalkaline) chemical burns to the cornea
  1. First aid (as described above)
  2. Direct lavage of corneal epithelium to dislodge and clear any occult particles, granules
  3. Swab superior and inferior cul-de-sacs with wet cotton swab to dislodge and clear any embedded particles (reirrigate after swabbing)
  4. Tobramycin (Tobrex) ointment q2h to qid
  5. Cycloplege or dilate with 5 percent homatro-

*See also Appendix 4.

pine qid (in moderate cases or when indicated for secondary uveitic reaction)
6. Steroid (1 percent prednisolone or 0.1 percent dexamethasone) qid for 5 to 7 days and then taper off
7. Warm packs qid
8. *No* pressure patching or therapeutic bandage soft lenses
9. Recheck in 24 hours

■ Severe chemical burn (including moderate alkali burn) to the cornea usually requires advanced ophthalmic care, often in a hospital setting
1. All previously described therapies
2. Oral and intramuscular pain relievers
3. Oral antiglaucoma medications (e.g., carbonic anhydrase inhibitors) for secondary IOP increases
4. Collagenase inhibitors (e.g., acetylcysteine)
5. Soft contact lens bandage for epithelial control
6. Surgical therapies (e.g., keratoplasty, flaps)

Follow-up

■ Singular goal of treatment is to get epithelium to successfully close and cover (nonstaining) cornea
■ Recheck cornea every 24 hours in moderate to severe cases until epithelium shows pronounced healing
■ Recheck mild to moderate cases every 3 to 5 days until complete healing occurs
■ Always taper steroids after 5 to 7 days in burns (especially alkali) to minimize ulceration risks
■ Continue tobramycin cover (with tapering dosages) until negative staining
■ Prognosis
1. Complete resolution for all mild chemical burns within 1 to 2 weeks
2. Resolution of moderate (nonalkaline) burns within 2 to 4 weeks (usually)
3. Moderate alkali burns may take 3 to 6 weeks with risk of mild permanent stromal haze and VA loss
4. Severe burns frequently run an unrelenting course of corneal decompensation with significant risk of secondary ulceration, infection, scarring, and perforation
5. Other complications in chemical burns to cornea
a. Symblepharon
b. Entropion
c. Keratitis sicca
d. Neovascularization and pannus
e. Chronic anterior uveitis
f. Chronic glaucoma
g. Phthisis bulbi

D. DRY EYE–KERATITIS SICCA-TYPE SYNDROMES (Color Plates 70 and 71)

Subjective

■ Common syndrome in older (postmenopausal) women

■ Almost always bilateral (one eye may be more irritated or more involved than second eye)
■ Most common symptom is mild to moderate, mid to late day superficial irritation (corneal type)
1. "Sandy, gritty feeling"
2. Foreign body sensation
3. Nonspecific ocular surface "dryness" or discomfort
■ Patients tend to define times, places, and specific factors that aggravate symptoms
1. Arid (dry) conditions (especially with wind)
2. Airborne irritants
a. Dust
b. Smoke (e.g., especially cigarettes, cigars)
c. Fumes (and pollution)
d. Fine particles (e.g., fabrics, threads, spores)
3. Air-conditioning (with dehumidification) and home heating systems
4. Bright lights
5. Extended near work (staring syndrome)
6. Chlorinated swimming pool water
■ Occasionally a family history associated
■ Sometimes associated with common medications
1. Antihistamines (especially OTC chlorpheniramine)
2. Decongestants
3. Diuretics
4. Atropine-based compounds
5. Oral steroids
6. Birth control pills (uncertain)
7. Alcohol-based medications (or plain old "booze")
■ Dermatological conditions
1. Seborrhea
2. Variable dermatites
3. Eczema
4. Psoriasis
5. Rosacea[61]
■ History of other ocular conditions or contact lenses
1. Lagohthalmos
2. Blepharitis
3. Meibomianitis
4. Soft or hard contact lenses
■ General systemic conditions
1. Collagen vascular diseases (especially rheumatoid)
2. Infectious or inflammatory diseases
3. Cancers (especially lymphoma)
4. Kidney disease
5. Sjögren's syndrome
6. Neurotropic responses (Bell's palsy)
7. Thyroid (exposure) conditions
■ Nosocomial (hospital related) causes often reported
1. Secondary to primary cause of hospitalization
2. Discontinuation of eye care during hospital stay
■ Patient may report "paradoxical" wet eye problems

1. Dry eye stimulates trigeminal reflex
2. Stimulates excess reflex aqueous tearing

Objective

- No discharge present
  1. Excess dryness leads to reflexive aqueous tearing ("paradoxical" wet eye)
  2. Occasional mucoid or lipid buildup in inferior cul-de-sac
- Generally a low-grade, angular-type bulbar hyperemia
- Nonspecific papillary (palpebral) conjunctivitis
  1. Typical of allergic and bacterial conjunctivites
  2. Usually less "velvety" appearing (appears dryer)
- Lid margin and inferior fornix tear menisci may be reduced (<0.5 mm) or absent
- Mucoid debris (lipids, dessicated epithelial cells) may accumulate on the ocular surface or in the aqueous tear film or meniscus
  1. Meniscus may demonstrate "frothy" appearance
  2. Not uncommon to have both froathing and debris
- Most typical clinical sign in dry eye–keratitis sicca syndromes is SPK staining greatest in the band region of cornea and conjunctiva (exposed area of cornea and conjunctiva in palpebral fissure region)
  1. Cause of cellular disruption is process called squamous cell metaplasia (cell differentiation)
  2. Area stains with NaFl (disrupted cell junctures) and rose bengal (devitalized necrotic cells and cell wall destruction)
  3. Rose bengal stain is specific for keratitis sicca cell devitalization (drying) (refer to first page of Color Plate section for Figure 4–20 showing rose bengal stain)
- On corneal surface, debris can form filaments producing a condition called filamentary keratitis
  1. Helix of mucin and dead epithelial cells
  2. Lengths range from 0.5 mm to ≥ 4 to 5 mm
  3. Proximally adherent to corneal epithelium with distal end moving with each blink
  4. Blink causes pull on corneal epithelium with resultant foreign-body sensation (moderate to severe)
  5. Some other causes of filamentary keratitis
     a. Atopic keratoconjunctivitis
     b. Herpes zoster ophthalmicus
     c. Recurrent corneal erosions
     d. Staphylococcal keratitis
     e. SLK
     f. SPK of Thygeson
     g. Toxic keratites
     h. Vernal keratoconjunctivitis
- Occasional dellen formations (Gaule spots)
- Positive "tear breakup time" (BUT) may be one of the most diagnostic considerations if done accurately[77]
  1. Wet NaFl strip with saline or tap water

2. Instill in inferior cul-de-sac or superior bulbar conjunctiva
3. Do not touch or manipulate lids
4. Have patient take two to three regular blinks first
5. Then evaluate NaFl pattern for breakup points after 1 to 2 seconds, but under 10 seconds
   a. Instantaneous breakup should be noted as "negative staining"
   b. Negative staining diagnostic for epithelial surface abnormalities (epitheliopathies such as EBMD) versus actual tear film disorders
6. Positive BUT equals random patterns of breakup points in less than 10 seconds but more than 1 second
- Schirmer testing is quite variable with a high probability of false-negative results (strip wets attributable to reflex tearing of other stimuli in true disease state)
- Other findings to note in dry-eye diagnosis
  1. Chronic conjunctivitis
  2. Blepharitis and blepharoconjunctivitis
  3. Meibomianitis
  4. Corneal epithelial abnormalities

Assessment*

- Rule out all stimulating causes of dry eye syndrome[78] (from Subjective)
  1. Aggravants
  2. Medications
  3. Systemic causes
  4. Ocular problems
  5. Contact lenses
- "Attempt" (often difficult) to classify dry eye according to traditional (Holly and Lemp) system[79]
  1. Lipid layer (prevents evaporation) abnormalities
     a. Caused by infectious blepharitis and meibomianitis
     b. Bacterial toxins cause rupture of tear film and secondary epithelial problems
  2. Aqueous layer (thickest layer) deficiencies
     a. Lacrimal and accessory gland abnormalities
     b. Sjögren's syndrome (dry eye, dry mouth, and arthritis)
     c. Drug related
     d. Neurological
  3. Mucin layer (most important protective layer) deficiencies
     a. Goblet cell (conjunctival) abnormalities
     b. Vitamin A deficiencies
     c. Drug related
     d. Stevens–Johnson syndrome (erythema multiforma)
     e. Conjunctival diseases and disorders
  4. Lid resurfacing (Marangoni effect) disorders
     a. Blepharitis (e.g., tylosis)
     b. Lagophthalmos

---

*See also Appendix 3.

  c. Colobomas (lid notching)
  d. Keratinized lid margins
  e. Trichiasis
  f. Entropion or ectropion
- Most common differential diagnosis is between dry-eye syndromes and epithelial basement disorders
  1. Morning syndrome versus late-day symptoms
  2. Map–dot–fingerprint configurations intraepithelial versus band-region SPK pattern
  3. Negative staining versus positive BUT
- Because of prevalence of both conditions (EBMD and dry eye–keratitis sicca-type syndromes), combined disease conditions (especially in high-risk and older age ranges) is very possible
  1. Nonresponsiveness to lubrication therapy (for presumed dry eye conditions) should indicate trial of hypertonics (for possible EBMD)
  2. Combined therapies may also be indicated from time to time for symptomatic and physical relief

Plan*

For Mild to Moderate Symptoms (PM or Chronic)
- Lubricating eyedrops 5 to 10 × per day
  1. Mucomimetic agents most preferable lubricant to stabilize tear film and protect epithelium
     a. Absorbotears (Alcon)
     b. Hypotears (Cooper)
        i. Hypotonicity reduces tear osmolality
        ii. Probably too short-lived to produce significant clinical effect
     c. Tears Naturale (Alcon)
     d. Tears Plus (Allergan)
  2. Vitamin A agents (Vit-A-Drops) useful in reducing squamous cell metaplasia[80]
     a. Effective in "healing" corneal surface
     b. Best used initially and followed by lubricant as preventive
- Recheck patient in approximately 2 weeks

For Moderate Conditions
- Use mucomimetics and vitamin A drops q1–2h
- Add longer-acting tear substitutes based on degree
  1. Ointments (bid to qid)
     a. Lacrilube (Allergan)
     b. Duotears (Alcon)
     c. Hypotears (Cooper): nonpreserved ointment
  2. Lacriserts (Merck Sharp & Dohme)
     a. Methylcellulose, time-released pellets of 12- to 24-hour duration
     b. Insert pellet in inferior cul-de-sac
     c. Trigger pellet with 0.5 percent methylcellulose drop for maximal effect
     d. Procedure difficult for patient and pellet often produces discomfort and dislodges

  3. Possible adverse effects from ointments and Lacriserts
     a. Blurred vision
     b. Irritation (and pellet dislodging)
     c. Difficulty with instillation for ointment procedure
     d. SPK
- Recheck patient within 1 week

For Severe Conditions
- All moderate therapies at maximal levels
- Bandage contact lens therapy (see Chapter 7)
  1. Use low to medium water lenses
  2. Daily wear (because of increased risk of infection)
  3. Monitor patient closely (every 6 weeks or PRN)
  4. Add therapeutic drops over bandage lenses
- Additional therapies available through anterior segment specialists
  1. Punctal occlusion (collagen plugs or laser)[81]
  2. Conjunctival flap surgical procedures
  3. Lacrimal gland stimulating drugs
     a. Cholinergic–parasympathomimetics
     b. Sympathomimetics
- Other therapies to reduce tear loss
  1. Swimmer's goggles
  2. "Saran Wrap" coverings
  3. Lid taping procedures
  4. Rubber eye cups
  5. Punctal occlusion (temporary or permanent)

Follow-up

For Mild to Moderate Conditions
- If no improvement after 2 weeks
  1. Question patient on compliance and retreat for 2 to 3 weeks if noncompliant
  2. If patient compliant, upgrade treatment
- If improvement (subjective and objective)
  1. Advise patient carefully
  2. Taper therapy to minimal maintenance dosages
  3. Recheck every 4 to 6 months or PRN

For Moderate to Severe Conditions
- If no improvement after 1 week
  1. Reconfirm compliance and continue therapy for additional week if necessary
  2. If compliant, add additional or alternative therapies (primary or secondary level procedures)
- If improvement noted
  1. Taper therapies (slowly) to maintenance level
  2. Advise patient carefully
  3. Monitor closely (every 3 months) or PRN

Patient Advice Regarding Dry Eye–Keratitis Sicca Syndromes
- Have any ocular abnormality checked immediately due to increased risk for secondary infection
- Explain chronic (noncurative) nature of underlying disease (if applicable) and primary care treatment goals of protection and prevention of complications

---

*See also Appendix 4.

- Therapy must be continued in lieu of symptoms
- Overuse of drops may produce preservative reactions
- Avoid irritating or "triggering" causes of symptoms and physical changes
- Diligently comply with all professional instructions

E. FOREIGN BODIES (Color Plates 75 and 76)

Subjective

- Usually obvious history of foreign body entering eye
- Patient's discomfort ranges from mild to very severe
- History should confirm "when, how, how much (multiple particles), and where" accident occurred
  1. Also careful determination of what kind of matter entered eye
  2. Was entry of a "high-velocity" (penetrating) nature or a "soft entry" (embedded superficially)
  3. Industrial versus domestic accident?
- Common histories
  1. Objects falling into eye (e.g., rust off muffler while working under car, or fiberglass from ceiling tile)
  2. Wind blown particle(s)
  3. Grinding wheel projectile or particle(s) from a hammered surface
  4. Discrete matter rubbed in and embedded
- Frequently history of entry is 24 to 72 hours earlier
  1. Symptoms tend to increase or become annoying
  2. Metallic foreign bodies (with resultant rust ring and basement membrane or anterior stromal staining) are most common delayed presentations

Objective

- Distinct appearance of immovable, embedded particle (or multiple particles) on corneal epithelium
- Frequently a surrounding whitish-gray surrounding area of edema or dense infiltrates (Coat's white ring) or hemosiderosis (rust ring)
- Associated foreign-body tracking (FBT) may be present
- Lid spasms and hyperlacrimation (common) usually make initial assessment difficult (before topical anesthetic)
- Foreign body (FB) may be raised above epithelial surface or flush (and often covered) with epithelium
- Other ocular signs similar to those "associated reactions in deep corneal abrasion" (Table 4–10) are usually present relative to degree of involvement
- Occasionally, endothelium may show a faint to pronounced infiltrative ring directly behind site of FB (called annular keratopathy of Payreau)

1. Secondary immune or infiltrative response to trauma (including FB, abrasion, or contusion injury)
2. Will resolve within days after FB removal

Assessment

- Most important to rule out penetration or perforation (as discussed in section X of this chapter "Irritations and Injuries," part A, "Abrasions," level 2, "Deep Epithelial Abrasions," "Assessment")
- Determine epithelial depth of FB
  1. By history
  2. By slit-lamp optic section (parallelepiped)
  3. By preliminary removal techniques (irrigation)
- Rule out (by history and physical exam) multiple particles
  1. On cornea
  2. On conjunctiva, cul-de-sacs, and lids
  3. Evert and double-evert eyelids
- Evaluate associated reactions and risks
  1. Anterior uveitis
  2. Infectious keratitis (bacterial, fungal ulcer)
  3. Check associated reactions in deep corneal abrasion (Table 4–10)

Plan and Follow-up*

- Stromal (penetrating) FBs should be assessed and treated as penetrating or perforating abrasion or laceration
  1. Probability of permanent scarring and visual loss
  2. Specialty consultation indicated
- Superficially embedded epithelial foreign matter amenable to noninvasive (nonsurgical) removal is best treated by properly trained, accessible primary level practitioners
  1. All foreign matter must be removed completely from the corneal epithelium to relieve symptoms and protect eye from potential risks of infection or scarring
  2. All secondary associated reactions should also be treated to relieve and protect patient
- Topical anesthetic drops should be administered in-office (only) every 30 to 60 seconds for 1 to 2 minutes before examination and any removal procedure
  1. Usually provides optimal anesthesia for approximately 15 to 20 minutes
  2. If examination and procedural care exceeds length of effective anesthesia, additional dosage(s) are safe and indicated
- Many time-tested techniques and tools are widely used for nonsurgical removal of corneal foreign bodies
  1. Nonsurgical (noninvasive) being defined as no tissue incision, excision, resection, ablation, or cutting procedures involved in the techniques

---

*See also Appendix 4.

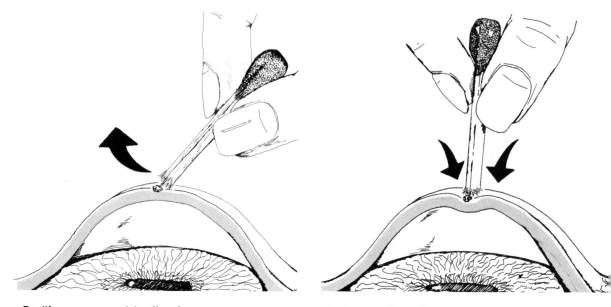

Do lift or sweep particle off surface.   Don't press down directly on particle.

Figure 4–21. Matchbook technique

2. Commonly performed by nonsurgical primary level practitioners as well as trained nonprofessional medical personnel (e.g., emergency medical technicians, military medics, athletic trainers)
- "Do's and Don'ts" of a dozen of the most commonly used superficial corneal FB removal procedures
    1. Matchbook technique (Fig. 4–21)

a. For removal of superficial FBs outside an office setting (e.g., at home, outdoors)
b. Rip a fresh paper match from a matchbook without touching the ripped, serrated end
c. This untouched end is perfect for lifting (by capillary action) small superficial particles off the corneal surface
d. No specific followup treatment is indicated
2. Forced irrigation technique (Fig. 4–22)

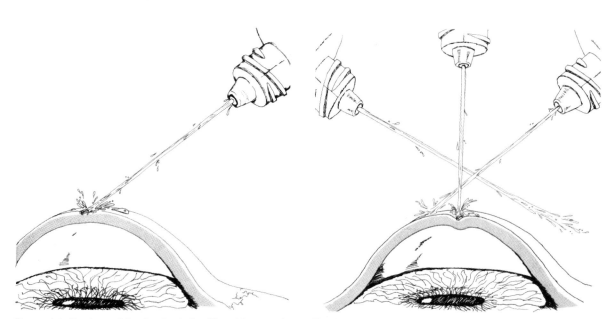

Do squirt all edges of foreign body for 10 to 15 seconds each.   Don't squirt directly down, over the top, or miss area of foreign body completely.

Figure 4–22. Forced irrigation technique

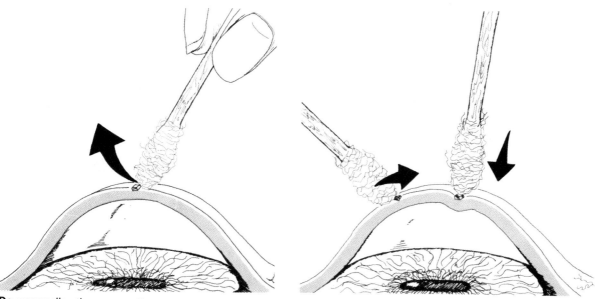

Do sweep directly over small area.

Don't press down on foreign body or sweep over too much corneal surface.

Figure 4–23. Sweeping swab technique

a. For removal of superficial FBs in or out of office

b. Use balanced ophthalmic irrigating solution in plastic squeeze (squirt) irrigating bottle (e.g., Blinx, Dacriose, Eye Stream)[76]

c. Direct a high-powered stream at edge of FB

d. Treatment may include prophylactic antibiotic ointment 1 × (in-office) and ad lib lubricants and warm packs for 12 to 24 hours

3. Sweeping swab technique (Fig. 4–23)
   a. For removal of superficial FB when nothing else is available
      i. Not a highly preferable technique because of its secondary disruption of excess epithelium (from oversized tip)
      ii. No harm done, but . . .
   b. Wet cotton-tipped swab with saline or water and pick (usually "sweep") FB off surface

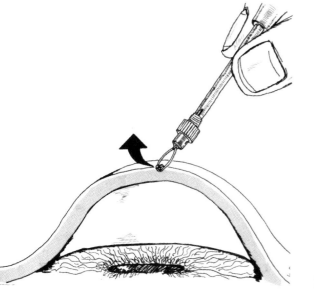

Do tease edges all around until foreign body lifts off completely.

Don't be hesitant and miss cornea completely or press down directly on foreign body.

Figure 4–24. Bailey loop technique

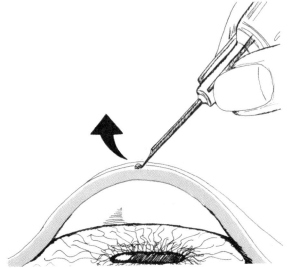

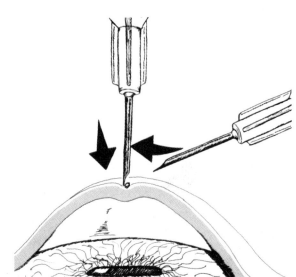

Do approach foreign body edge tangentially and then lever and lift edges.

Don't approach cornea with "perpendicular plunge", but conversely, don't be so tentative as to miss foreign body completely.

Figure 4–25. Needle technique

c. Treatment is (optional) antibiotic 1 × and ad lib lubricants and warm packs for 12 to 24 hours

4. Bailey loop technique (Fig. 4–24)
   a. For removal of partially embedded FBs partially removed by someone with "heavy hands" or who was concerned with penetrating Bowman's layer with sharp instrument (highly unlikely with proper technique)
   b. Also good technique for removal of FBs in children who cannot sit still or who may move during procedure
   c. Use Bailey nylon loop in aggressive, teasing movements at edges of FB (penetration virtually impossible with this technique)
   d. Postprocedure treatment per abrasion protocol

5. Needle technique (Fig. 4–25)
   a. For removal of partially or deeply embedded FBs
   b. Use common commercially available hypodermic needles (18-, 20-, 22-, or 25-gauge and lengths 5/8, 1 1/2, or 2 inches)
   c. No syringe needed, although some do use needle without detaching at base)
   d. Hold needle directly on shaft or at small plastic or metal flange
   e. Use point of needle to lift edges or loosen overlying cells
   f. Use side of beveled tip to loosen, lift, and lever entire FB for final removal
   g. Avoid snagging basement membrane when using sharp point (usually produces tugging feel, as if snagging canvas and may produce some transient striate lines)

h. Procedure can also be used to remove rust rings (after removal of metallic FB)
i. Postprocedure treatment per abrasion protocol

6. Cockburn curve technique
   a. For removal of partially or deeply embedded FBs
   b. Observe back side of bevel on point of hypodermic needle before removing it from its hard plastic jacket (standard casing for needle)

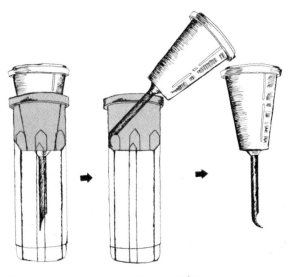

Figure 4–26. Cockburn curve procedure

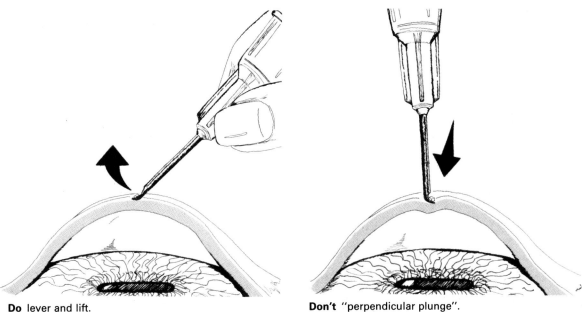

Do lever and lift.

Don't "perpendicular plunge".

Figure 4–27. Cockburn curve technique

c. Upon removing needle from jacket, drag the back side of the bevel firmly up the side wall causing it to bend in an inward, curved fashion (Fig. 4–26)

d. This curved bend provides a safer method of using a hypodermic needle with minimal risk of snagging basement membrane, and almost no risk of penetration

e. Procedure is similar to "needle" technique described above (Fig. 4–27)

7. Golf club spud technique (Fig. 4–28)

a. For removal of partially or deeply embedded FBs

b. Commonly used procedure (perhaps more than needles) because of its ease and safety

   i. Curved tip of spud creates a natural lifting and levering effect while protecting against snagging of basement membrane or penetration

   ii. Sharp edges and cupped shape of spud help loosen and lift FB

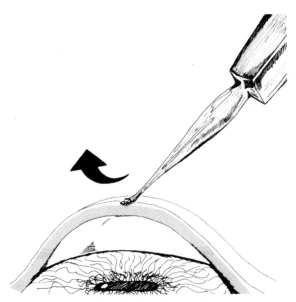

Do get under foreign body and scoop it out.

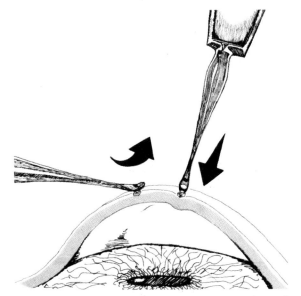

Don't scrape over top of foreign body or press down directly.

Figure 4–28. Golf club spud technique

c. Limiting factor of spud is relatively large size of head (versus needle tip) for small FBs
d. May take some extra epithelium because of size
e. Follow-up per abrasion protocol
8. Jeweler's forceps technique (Fig. 4–29)
a. For removal of partially or deeply embedded FBs
b. Easy and efficient procedure for large, deep FB that needs a great deal of edge teasing and lift
   i. Often FB remains partially embedded or adherent during edge lifting

ii. Working on one edge and other edge(s) binds back down into epithelium
c. Jeweler's forceps can first be used with tip closed (creating sharp, needle-like tip effect) to loosen and lift edge(s)
d. With edge raised above epithelial surface, forceps are then opened and used to grasp and lift FB off cornea
e. Follow-up per abrasion protocol
9. Rust ring removal technique[82] (Fig. 4–30) (Color Plate 78)
a. For removal of hemosiderotic cell staining or rust rings with particles embedded in epithelium
b. Hemosiderosis (oxidizing of metallic FB in epithelium, i.e., rusting) occurs within 2 to 48 hours after embedding
c. Often, patient is not seen soon enough (frequently, even beyond the 48-hour mark), and significant hemosiderosis occurs
   i. Slight benefit in delay is necrosing, softening effect to rust ring permitting easier removal (sluffing off with very gentle manipulation)
   ii. However, care should not be delayed purposely for such effect
   iii. Delays also lead to further staining of basement membrane and potential scar to Bowman's (stromal) layer
d. All hemosiderotic epithelial cells or oxidized particles (from FB) must be removed to avoid chronic weakening, irritation, re-erosion of epithelium, and risk of infection
e. However, staining of basement membrane and Bowman's layer from prolonged

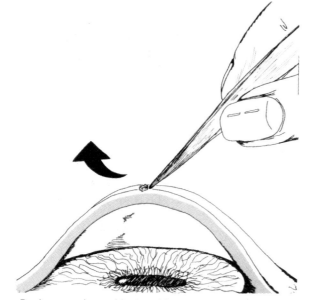

Do loosen edges with closed forceps and lever upwards.

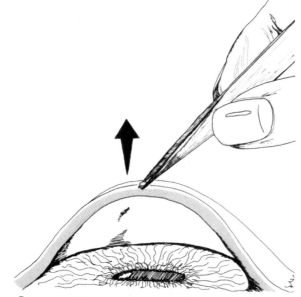

Do grasp with opened forceps and lift off.

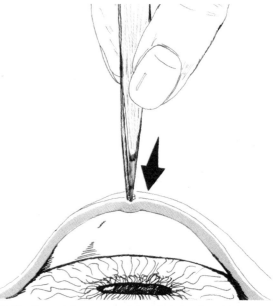

Don't attempt to grasp embedded foreign body with opened forceps without loosening edges first.

Figure 4–29. Jeweler's forceps technique

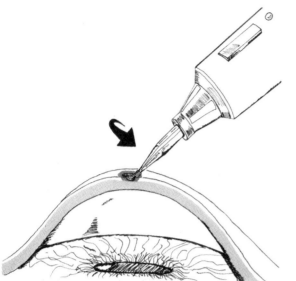

Do lightly drill epithelium down to basement membrane in circular motion.

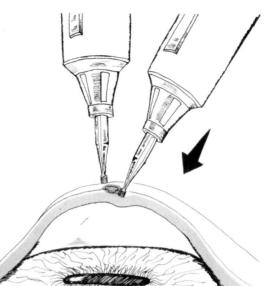

Don't press down too lightly while drilling, or, conversely, press down too firmly, producing snagging or ripping of basement membrane.

Figure 4–30. Rust ring removal technique

(greater than 48-hour) exposure to oxidation can produce permanent rust ring

  i. Awareness of basement mebrane or Bowman's layer involvement usually apparent during procedure as "canvas" texture versus gelatinous (epithelial cell) consistency

  ii. Basement membrane staining need not be removed in lieu of regeneration of new (clear) membrane within 8 to 12 weeks versus "ripping" membrane to remove stain and produce potential of chronic recurrent corneal erosion (RCE) syndrome

  iii. Scraping Bowman's layer will result in leukomatous scar usually larger and more dense than ring stain

  iv. Permanently stained Bowman's (stroma) will not produce adverse effects described for epithelial cells

  v. Thus, it is best not to attempt removal of hemosiderotic stains from basement membrane or Bowman's layer

f. Power drill(s) (using fine to coarse burrs) are used to "chew up" stained epithelial cells and oxidizing particles after metallic FB itself is removed from corneal surface

  i. Medium to fine burr preferable

  ii. Coarse burrs (on drill) tend to destroy extra epithelium and may even snag basement membrane or Bowman's with resulting striae or leucoma

g. Limiting factor with power drills (minimized with "Alger brush") is "humming" sound, which tends to alarm an already apprehensive and "shakey" patient

  i. Reassure patient as best as possible

  ii. Certainly, never show the drill (nor any "ominous" looking instruments)

h. Follow-up per abrasion protocol

10. Alger brush removal technique (Fig. 4–31)

a. All indications, contraindications, and adverse effects same as with all power drills

b. Procedure same as with standard power drill

c. Difference with Alger brush is centrifugal force mechanism, which functions to stop drill if too much downward pressure is exerted onto cornea during procedure

  i. Thus, risk of basement membrane or Bowman's snagging or ripping is minimized

  ii. Penetration risk is almost entirely eliminated

d. Adverse effect continues to be the patient apprehension created by the "drilling" sounds

11. Hand-held burr technique (Fig. 4–32)

a. Used to reduce patient apprehension in rust ring removal (with power drills and Alger brush) and associated drill sounds

b. Hold coarse dental burr between tips of fingers, and spin it as its held directly on rust ring and hemosiderotic epithelium

c. Requires a fairly steady hand but works quite effectively with no drill sounds

d. Principle and procedures remain exactly the same as with power drill or Alger brush use

12. Magnetic technique

a. The use of magnetized instrument to lift metallic FB off corneal surface

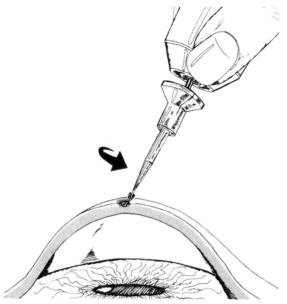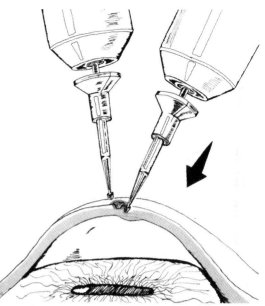

Do lightly drill epithelium down to basement membrane in circular motion.

Don't press down too lightly while drilling, or, conversely, press down to firmly, causing centrifugal force of drill to shut off automatically.

Figure 4–31. Alger brush removal technique

b. Hand instruments made with blunt magnetic end for removal of superficial, non-embedded FBs

c. Generally works poorly unless more sophisticated, expensive electromagnets (used surgically for intraocular FBs) are employed

d. For in-office, nonsurgical, primary care of superficial FBs, magnetic techniques are

not contraindicated, but certainly are inefficient, given the large array of simple highly effective alternative procedures

■ Other considerations in corneal removal of FB
  1. Use left and right hands for opposite eyes if possible
    a. If not, use dominant hand and cross over face when necessary

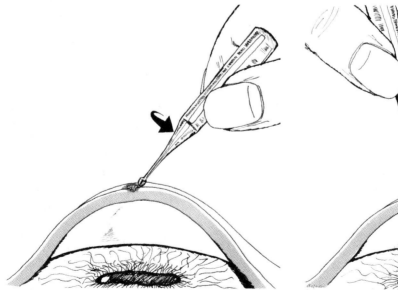

Do roll burr between thumb and index finger while pressing lightly on epithelium.

Don't press down too lightly while drilling, or, conversely, press down too firmly, producing snagging or ripping of basement membrane.

Figure 4–32. Hand-held burr technique

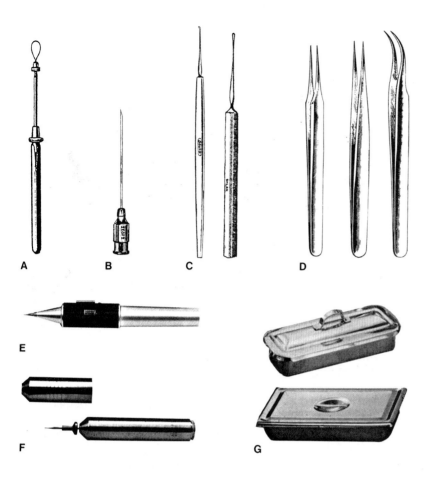

Figure 4–33.
Common instruments and accessories for foreign body removal. **A.** Bailey loop. **B.** Hyperdermic needle. **C.** Golf club spuds. **D.** Jeweler's forceps (assorted shapes and sizes). **E.** Battery-powered drill. **F.** Alger brush. **G.** Assorted instrument trays.
(Courtesy of West Coast Optical, Bradenton, Florida.)

   b. Have patient turn head as much as possible in slit-lamp head rest to minimize interference from patient's nose

2. Slit-lamp hand rests are available to stabilize hand during procedure

   a. Head rest can be lowered to point where examiner's elbow can rest (and be stabilized) on instrument table

   b. Fingers (on instrument hand) can be stabilized by resting fourth and fifth on patient's face

3. Instruments used are readily available through ophthalmic instrument companies and direct from surgical instrument wholesalers

   a. Storz: highest quality and very expensive

   b. Sklar: high quality and less expensive

   c. Wexler: high quality and less expensive

   d. Others also available

4. Instrument maintenance and cleaning (Fig. 4–33)

   a. Keep in a stainless steel tray of Zephiran HCl 1:750 (benzalkonium chloride) with antirust tablets (change weekly)

   b. Instruments can also be stored dry and rinse before use with Zephiran or alcohol

      i. Rinse Zephiran or alcohol off thoroughly with water or saline before use

      ii. Reclean and dry instruments for storage

   c. Heat sterilization (autoclaving) and sterile wrapping for storage is ideal procedure

F. RECURRENT CORNEAL EROSION SYNDROME (Color Plates 79 and 100)

Background Information[83,84]

1. Review Background Information for epithelial basement membrane (EBM)

2. Any damage to EBM or Bowman's layer causes weakening or loss of adhesions between epithelium and (anterior) stroma

3. These adhesions are produced by a sticky collagen layer on the anterior face of Bowman's layer and with finger-like projections (hemidesmosomes) off the basement membrane into the epithelium

4. Basal epithelial cells require at least 6 to 8 weeks or more to regenerate or repair EBM

5. Persistent, chronic adverse (e.g., dystrophy, diabetes) stimuli with or without acute (or subacute) trauma to cornea can produce prolonged, loose, weak adhesions resulting in unstable corneal epithelial layer

6. Finally, any injury, irritant, or aggravant to the EBM will leave it unstable, weak, and vulnerable to recurrent breakdown (erosion) and re-erosion for its regenerating period of at least 6 to 8 weeks or more and, if permanently damaged, possibly indefinitely

Subjective

- Two classic histories associated with recurrent corneal erosion syndrome (RCE)
  1. Secondary to corneal injury
  2. Spontaneous (patient denying history of injury)
- Symptoms are typical of corneal irritation and tend to be moderate to severe
  1. "Sandy, gritty" irritation
  2. Foreign body sensation
  3. Lid spasms
  4. Photophobia
- Most presentations occur upon waking (morning or AM syndrome)
  1. Probably secondary to increased edema during sleep (with lids closed and tear evaporation reduced)
  2. Combination of loose epithelial junctures (edema) and disrupted EBM (causing unstable epithelium) aggravated by dry lid opening
- Usually a unilateral presentation (associated with history of recent, or perhaps old, ipsilateral injury)
  1. Occasionally presentation may be bilateral with one eye usually worse than other
  2. History may or may not reveal underlying associated disease process (e.g., dystrophy, diabetes)
  3. Specific disease or trauma history often lacking making diagnosis exclusively physical and presumptive
- Recurring nature is definitive historical information
  1. Recurrencies could be proximal to injury or recurrent after extended (weeks to months) delay
  2. Recurrencies may be frequent (e.g., daily) or infrequent (monthly or less)
  3. Acute phase of recurrencies may be minor (mildly symptomatic and self-limiting) to dramatically acute, painful, and disabling
- When history directly associated with acute injury
  1. Symptom duration may be days to years
  2. Injury is usually of a tangential, cutting nature versus perpendicular (blunt) type (e.g., FB)
     a. Paper cut
     b. Fingernail injury
     c. Sprung tree branch or twig
     d. Glancing type injuries to corneal surface
- When history is spontaneous without associated injury
  1. Careful questioning critical for subtle clues
  2. Usually chronic, low-grade irritation (unilateral or bilateral) with intermittent acute episodes
  3. Medical history significant

4. Active medication history valuable
5. Family history of similar problem (dystrophy?)

Objective

- Milder presentations show typical corneal abrasion signs (with associated reactions)
  1. May be as mild as SPK reactions
  2. Often, morning syndrome symptoms may persist longer than observable physical signs
- Re-erosions (abrasions) secondary to injury generally occur in same corneal area as original abrasion
  1. Recurrence may be mild SPK in area
  2. Generally (unfortunately) re-erosion is equal or (more frequently) worse than original abrasion
- Recurrent erosions in the area of Hudson–Stahli's line tend to recur more frequently[85]
- Moderate to severe recurrent erosions tend to show certain classic characteristics (may be diagnostic in absent, vague, or suspicious histories
  1. Generally produce inproportionate amounts of associated edema
  2. Edema often produces (immediately or during slow healing) a brownish haze to the involved epithelium (brawny edema)
  3. Abraded area tends to create loose edges with moderate to large epithelial flaps commonly forming
  4. Healing rate is generally slower than the normal rate for a similar abrasion
- Centralward location and tendency towards dense secondary edema produce substantial visual disturbances[86]
- Physical exam and evaluation should be similar to abrasion criteria used for deep corneal abrasions

Assessment*

- Initial history should determine injury versus spontaneous nature to RCE
- If injury involved, precise nature and time of original episode should be documented, especially if original care for initial episode was provided by another practitioner
- If RCE is spontaneous (i.e., no associated injury, proximal or remote), history and examination must differentiate the following possibilities of syndrome
  1. Corneal dystrophy (check for bilateral signs and check other family members)
     a. Epithelial basement membrane disorders
        i. Most common cause of spontaneous RCE syndrome
        ii. Examine both eyes (and family members) carefully for maps, dots, fingerprints
     b. Endothelial dystrophies (i.e., Fuchs')
  2. Diabetes mellitus (cause of chronic basement membrane problems)

---

*See also Appendix 3.

- RCE syndrome is not uncommon in postoperative patients (e.g., cataracts, retinal detachment surgery, refractive surgical procedures)
  1. May be from secondary epithelial trauma or endothelial disruption and resultant secondary edema
  2. Good reason to evaluate endothelium carefully before referring for elective ocular surgeries
     a. Poor endothelium (e.g., dystrophy, low count secondary to age degeneration) significantly increases risk of postoperative RCE
     b. Good ophthalmic surgeon will usually do endothelial count before surgery
  3. Radial keratotomy has shown almost a 20 percent increase in permanent (greater than 6- to 12-week regenerative period) EBM changes thus increasing risk of RCE syndrome as long-term sequelae of the procedure[25]

Plan

- Acute presentations of RCE are treated according to normal and customary care for corneal abrasions
  1. Evaluate abrasion criteria
  2. Treat associated reactions (Table 4–10) according to care code for deep corneal abrasions (Table 4–11)
  3. Follow abrasion protocol
- Healing rates for RCE tend to be 1 to 2 days slower than rate charts (Table 4–12) for nonerosion deep abrasion
- Management for moderate RCE (25 to 50 percent of cornea or more than one to two recurrences), same as acute presentations (described above), plus
  1. Warm packs (after patch) q4h for 2 to 3 weeks
  2. Hypertonic drops (after patch) q4h for 4 to 6 weeks
  3. Hypertonic ointment (after patch) tid for 8 to 12 weeks
  4. Recheck monthly for 4 to 6 months
- Management for severe RCE (greater than 50 percent of cornea or chronic recurrences) same as moderate (above), plus[87]
  1. Mechanically debride any loose epithelial flaps
     a. Use 1 to 2 drops of topical anesthetic every 15 to 30 seconds for 2 to 3 minutes to soften epithelium and anesthetize cornea
     b. Use wetted cotton swab, spatula, spud, or jeweler's forceps
     c. Remove flaps by pulling or sweeping edges toward center of abraded area
     d. Do not pull flaps directly upward or outward
     e. Remove all flaps down to tight, firm edges
     f. Procedure will increase overall geography of abrasion (possibly by 50 to 100 percent)
     g. Avoid chemical (toxic) methods of debriding (e.g., chelating agents, EDTA, alcohol, ether)

2. Bilaterally patch patient for (maximum) 48 to 72 hours
   a. Bilateral patching will completely immobilize eyes
   b. Follow pressure patching protocol, primarily for eroded eye (Table 4–13)
   c. Repatch daily for 2 to 3 days (maximum)
      i. Any additional patching beyond 72 hours will probably be nonproductive due to advancing edema (secondary to patching)
      ii. If cornea not resolving within 72 hours, bandage soft lens should be considered
   d. Counsel and reassure patient carefully regarding bilateral patching procedure
      i. Patient usually apprehensive and concerned over procedure
      ii. Educate to reasons for bilateral patch
      iii. Should also advise in advance of possible need to retreat (repatch)
3. An alternative to extended pressure patching or after successful or unsuccessful patching therapy soft contact lens bandage therapy may be administered[88]
   a. Fit involved eye (both eyes optional) only after resolution of acute inflammatory reaction(s) (i.e., red eye involvement)
   b. In chronically re-eroding corneas (with or without bandage lens wear), an intensive course of hypertonic ointment (q2–3h) for 1 week prior to lens wear (or rewear) may improve prognosis of soft lens bandaging
   c. Extended wear for at least 8 to 12 weeks
      i. Provides comfort and protection
      ii. Extended wear affords constant protection (especially against AM syndrome)
      iii. 8- to 12-week period permits regeneration of new basement membrane without interference of re-erosions
   d. Fit thin lens design of medium to high water
   e. Fit plano or low-powered lens
      i. Do not fit high-powered lens with thick center or edge
      ii. Aphakes must be monitored closely
   f. Lens should be fit loose but stable
   g. Hypertonic drops can be used over lens (if not irritating) tid to qid
   h. Prophylactic gentamicin or tobramycin drops should be used
      i. qid for first 3 to 4 weeks
      ii. tid for second 3 to 4 weeks
      iii. hs for duration of extended wear
      iv. Maintain qid with any positive staining
   i. Patient should be instructed to remove lens upon any discomfort or injection and call immediately
   j. Recheck patient weekly for first 3 to 4 weeks and then biweekly for duration of bandaging
4. Approximately 75 percent of all bandaging is successful after first therapy (for 8 to 12 weeks)

a. Exacerbations or early discontinuations will require additional therapeutic period
b. Some patients may require multiple periods
c. Almost all will heal eventually

Follow-up

■ If standard approaches to acute presentations prove unsuccessful (re-erosions), attempt more intensive therapeutic regimen or introduce preventive measures, such as protective shields during sleep (for sleep recurrences) and instructions on no rubbing

■ After successful intensive therapy (prolonged care, debridement, extended lens bandaging), continue hypertonic drops and ointments (hs) for 3 to 6 months

■ RCE syndrome will usually heal if underlying cause is properly diagnosed and remediated (if possible)
   1. If condition is chronic, patient must be instructed on preventive measures and advised of need for indefinite continuation of procedures

2. Patient can be reassured that preventive measures will reduce and preclude risks of recurrences and permanent visual loss

■ Constant patient advocacy and reassurance is critical in the successful long-term management of the RCE syndrome due to multiple factors
   1. Prolonged (chronic) nature of syndrome
   2. Pain and discomfort associated and resultant willingness of patient to comply if properly educated and instructed
   3. Patient's constant fear and apprehensions
      a. About permanent vision loss
      b. About lifelong recurrences of severe pain

■ Finally, there is significant value (especially for patients) in a positive attitude towards RCE in spite of seemingly endless course of syndrome
   1. Explain to patient that most, if not all RCE, eventually heals or is controllable without visual loss
   2. Helps patient feel a little better, gives hope and willingness to cooperate and comply
   3. Helps doctor "stay with" a tough disease and treatment regimen to a usual rewarding conclusion

XI. Self-assessment Questions

1. A corneal diameter of 13 mm or greater (megalocornea) should raise suspicion of:
   a. Reduced IOP
   b. Increased IOP
   c. Dystrophy
   d. Degeneration

2. Which of the following anterior chamber cleavage syndromes carries the greatest risk of secondary glaucoma?
   a. Posterior embryotoxon
   b. Axenfeld's anomaly
   c. Reiger's syndrome
   d. Peter's anomaly

3. The following are all classic clinical characteristics of corneal dystrophy, *except:*
   a. Unilateral presentations
   b. Central location
   c. Single-layer involvement
   d. No associated ocular or systemic disease

4. Central crystalline dystrophy is the condition demonstrating an exception to what classic clinical characteristic of corneal dystrophy?
   a. Central location
   b. Bilaterality
   c. No associated ocular or systemic disease
   d. Single layer involvement

5. Perhaps the most painful associated reaction from Fuch's endothelial dystrophy is:
   a. Guttata
   b. Stromal edema
   c. Bullous keratopathy
   d. Bedewing

6. Dellen is a peripheral corneal dry spot produced most frequently by any form of:
   a. Infection
   b. Dystrophy
   c. Degeneration
   d. Adjacent raised lesion

7. Among the clinical signs in epithelial basement membrane disorders, which is the least common?
   a. Maps
   b. Dots
   c. Maps and dots combined
   d. Fingerprints

8. Among the clinical signs in epithelial basement membrane disorders, which is the most common?

a. Maps
b. Dots
c. Maps and dots combined
d. Fingerprints

9. Treatment for the morning syndrome associated with epithelial basement membrane disorders includes all of the following, *except:*
   a. Antibiotics
   b. Lubricants
   c. Hypertonic saline
   d. Soft contact lenses

10. The most common distribution of *Staphylococcus*-related superficial punctate keratitis (SPK) is:
    a. Inferior
    b. Superior
    c. Band region
    d. Diffuse

11. Which of the following is *not* simply an exotoxic staphylococcal response to the cornea?
    a. Phlyctenular keratoconjunctivitis
    b. Bacterial corneal ulcer
    c. Superficial punctate keratitis (SPK)
    d. Marginal keratitis

12. Marginal keratitis is characterized most distinctly as:
    a. A subepithelial infiltrate
    b. A limbal ulcer
    c. An "island" lesion on the peripheral cornea
    d. A central lesion

13. Whereas phlyctenular keratoconjunctivitis is most frequently associated with *Staphylococcus* in industrialized countries, on a worldwide basis its greater association is with:
    a. Sarcoidosis
    b. Syphilis
    c. Tuberculosis
    d. Viral disease

14. A differentiating characteristic of staphylococcal corneal ulcer from other bacterial ulcers is:
    a. Anterior chamber reaction
    b. Circumscribed lesion
    c. Dense stromal infiltrates
    d. Deep bulbar injection

15. Alcoholic and nutritionally deficient patients are at higher risk for what specific form of bacterial corneal ulcer?
    a. *Streptococcus*
    b. *Pseudomonas*
    c. *Moraxella*
    d. *Hemophilis influenzae*

16. All of the following bacteria can penetrate intact corneal epithelium, *except:*
    a. *Pseudomonas*
    b. *Streptococcus*
    c. *Gonococcus*
    d. *Hemophilis influenzae*

17. Staphylococcal corneal ulcer has been surpassed as the most prevalent bacterial ulcer in the United States by:
    a. *Streptococcus*
    b. *Chlamydia*
    c. *Gonococcus*
    d. *Pseudomonas*

18. Fungal keratitis must be seriously considered with what specific subjective presentation?
    a. Contact lens wear
    b. Chronic conjunctivitis
    c. Systemic disease
    d. Vegatative corneal injury

19. Inclusion (chlamydial) keratoconjunctivitis is a diagnostic challenge because of its features that mimic signs of bacterial and
    a. Viral disease
    b. Fungal disease
    c. Allergic disease
    d. Granulomatous disease

20. All of the following clinical signs are typical of viral infection, *except:*
    a. Burning sensation
    b. Follicles
    c. Mucopurulence
    d. Quick BUT

21. Pharyngoconjunctival fever (PCF) is traditionally found most frequently in what age range?
    a. 5 to 15 years
    b. 20 to 40 years
    c. 40 to 80 years
    d. Any age

22. Besides adenovirus 8 in epidemic keratoconjunctivitis (EKC), the traditional rule of 8s includes:
    a. Infectious during first 8 days
    b. Subepithelial infiltrates on or about eighth day
    c. Superficial punctate keratitis on or about day 16
    d. Eight recurrences per year

23. Another rule of 8 in EKC includes:
    a. Infectious during first 16 days
    b. Subepithelial infiltrates for 8 weeks
    c. Superficial punctate keratitis on or about day 8
    d. Eight recurrences per year

24. Acne rosacea can produce a large array of ocular complications, the most common of which is
    a. Dacryostenosis
    b. Blepharitis
    c. Central corneal ulcer
    d. Chronic uveitis
25. Superior limbic keratoconjunctivitis has been associated with each of the following, *except:*
    a. Contact lens wear
    b. Thimerosol
    c. Sarcoidosis
    d. Hyperthyroidism
26. The percentage of the general population infected (and immune) to herpes simplex virus by age 60 is approximately:
    a. 0.1 percent
    b. 1 percent
    c. 10 percent
    d. 90 percent
27. The judicious use of topical steroids in herpes simplex keratitis should be limited to:
    a. Epithelial forms
    b. Stromal forms
    c. Primary forms
    d. Never!
28. Herpes simplex virus can produce each of the following clinical presentations, *except:*
    a. Superficial punctate keratitis (SPK)
    b. Ulcerative dendrites
    c. Infiltrative dendrites
    d. Disciform keratitis
29. Which of the following antiviral agents is considered most effective in epithelial herpes simplex keratitis?
    a. Cromolyn sodium (Opticrom)
    b. Trifluridine (Viroptic)
    c. Vidarabine (Vira A)
    d. IDU (Stoxil)
30. The healing rate of superficial squamous corneal epithelium begins within:
    a. 2 hours
    b. 6 hours
    c. 12 hours
    d. 24 hours
31. Deep corneal abrasions (down to basement membrane) heal over a 2- to 4-day period by a process of:
    a. Squamous cell sliding
    b. Basal cell sliding
    c. Sliding and mitosis
    d. Mitosis alone

32. Some easy clinical examination techniques to rule out corneal penetration or perforation include each of the following, *except:*
    a. Geographic width of abraded area
    b. Seidel's (percolation) effect
    c. Stromal channeling
    d. Endothelial disruption
33. Essential elements included in pressure patch therapy include:
    a. Prepatch irrigation
    b. Prophylactic antibiosis
    c. Re-examination in 24 hours
    d. Prepatch tonometry
34. Ocular contusion injury is usually associated with any of the following, *except:*
    a. Corneal edema
    b. Superior SPK
    c. Hyphema
    d. Angle recession
35. Besides central retinal artery occlusion, the only other true ocular emergency requiring treatment within minutes to save eye and vision is:
    a. Acid burn
    b. Radiation burn
    c. Thermal burn
    d. Alkaline burn
36. Hemosiderosis (rust rings) usually do not require treatment when they are:
    a. Peripheral
    b. Staining of Bowman's layer
    c. Epithelial (squamous or basal)
    d. Central
37. While dry eye syndrome is a common occurrence in many patients, the candidate at greatest risk is:
    a. A young female
    b. An older female
    c. A young male
    d. An older male
38. Effective therapies for dry eye–keratitis sicca-type syndromes include each of the following, *except:*
    a. Vitamin A drops
    b. Vitamin C drops
    c. Mucomimetic agents
    d. Soft contact lenses
39. Filamentary keratitis can be found in all of the following, *except:*
    a. Recurrent corneal erosion (RCE) syndrome
    b. Vernal keratoconjunctivitis
    c. Dry-eye–keratitis sicca-type syndromes
    d. Disciform herpetic keratitis

40. Severe recurrent corneal erosion (RCE) syndrome is effectively treated with:
    a. Steroids
    b. Soft contact lenses
    c. Keratoplasty
    d. Chemical chelation

For answers, refer to Appendix 6

REFERENCES

1. Shields MB, Buckley E, Klintworth GK, et al: Axenfeld–Reiger syndrome. A spectrum of developmental disorders. Surv Ophthalmol 29:387, 1985
2. Waring GO, Rodriguez MM, Laibson PR: Anterior chamber cleavage syndrome. A stepladder classification. Surv Ophthalmol 20:3, 1975
3. Thurschwell LM, Michelson MA: Axenfeld's anomaly and related disorders. J Am Optom Assoc 57:360, 1986
4. Waring GO, Rodriguez MM, Laibson PR: Dystrophies of the Bowman's layer, epithelium and stroma. Surv Ophthalmol 23:71, 1978
5. Waring GO, Rodriguez MM, Laibson PR: Endothelial dystrophies. Surv Ophthalmol 23:147, 1978
6. Dangel ME, Kracher AP: Anterior corneal mosaic in eyes with keratoconus wearing hard contact lenses. Arch Ophthalmol 102:888, 1984
7. Presberg SE, Quigley HA, Forster RK, et al: Posterior polymorphous corneal dystrophy. Cornea 4:239, 1985/86
8. Winder AF: Relationship between corneal arcus and hyperlipidemia is clarified by studies in familial hypercholesterolemia. Br J Ophthalmol 67:789, 1983
9. Kaufman ME: Bullous keratopathy. Contact Lens Association of Ophthalmology 10:232, 1984
10. Physician's Desk Reference: Dradell, NJ, Medical Economics, 1986
11. Krachmer JM, Feder RS, Belin MW: Keratoconus and related non-inflammatory thinning disorders. Surv Ophthalmol 28:293, 1984
12. Williams R: Acquired posterior keratoconus. Br Ophthalmol 71:16, 1987
13. Cockburn DM: Wilson's disease (hepatolenticular degeneration). Clin Exp Optom 70:20, 1987
14. Guerry D: Fingerprint lines in the cornea. Am J Ophthalmol 33:724, 1950
15. Cogan DG: Microcystic dystrophy of the corneal epithelium. Trans Am Ophthalmol Soc 62:213, 1964
16. Dohlman CH: The function of the corneal epithelium in health and disease. Invest Ophthalmol 10:383, 1971
17. Brown NA, Bron A: Superficial lines and associated disorders of the cornea. Am J Ophthalmol 81:34, 1976
18. Collin HD: Clinical conditions affecting the basement membrane of the corneal epithelium. Aust J Optom 60:234, 1977
19. Williams R, Buckley RJ: Pathogenesis and treatment of recurrent erosion. Br J Ophthalmol 69:435, 1985
20. Shoch DE, Stock EL, Schwartz AE: Stromal keratitis complicating anterior membrane dystrophy. Am J Ophthalmol 100:199, 1985
21. Rose GE, Lavin MJ: Pathogenesis of recurrent corneal erosion: A further etiological factor. Trans Ophthalmol Soc UK 105:453, 1986
22. Kutzner MR, Morgan JF: Irregular astigmatism in patients with anterior membrane dystrophy. Am J Ophthalmol 19:266, 1984
23. Werblin TP, Hirot LW, Stark WJ, et al: Prevalence of map-dot-fingerprint changes in the cornea. Br J Ophthalmol 64:401, 1981
24. Alvarado J, Murphy C, Juster R: Age-related changes in the basement membrane of the human corneal epithelium. Invest Ophthalmol 24:1015, 1983
25. Nelson J, Williams P, Lindstrom RL, et al: Map–fingerprint–dot changes in the corneal epithelial basement membrane following radial keratotomy. Ophthalmology 92:199, 1985
26. Groden L, Brinser J: Outpatient treatment of microbial corneal ulcer. Arch Ophthalmol 104:84, 1986
27. Mondino BJ, Laheji AK, Adams SA: Ocular immunity to staphylococcus aureus. Invest Ophthalmol 28:560, 1987
28. Catania LJ: Contact lenses, staphylococcus, and crocodile O.D. International Contact Lens Clinics 14:3, 1987
29. Catania LJ: Sterile infiltrates versus infectious keratitis: Worlds apart. International Contact Lens Clinics 14:9, 1987
30. Cantania LJ: The bug stops here!. International Contact Lens Clinics 14:12, 1987
31. Catania LJ: Staphylococcal risk reduction program. International Contact Lens Clinics 14:6, 1987
32. Tabbara KF, Ostler HB, Dawson C, et al: Thygeson's superficial punctate keratitis. Ophthalmol 88:75, 1981
33. Nesburn AB: Effects of topical trifluridine on Thygeson's superficial punctate keratitis. Ophthalmol 91:1188, 1984
34. Dorland's Illustrated Medical Dictionary, ed 26. Philadelphia, WB Saunders, 1981
35. Critchley M, Medical Dictionary, ed 2. London, Butterworths, 1980
36. Morrison S: Grading corneal ulcers. Am J Ophthalmol 8:537, 1975
37. Maske R, et al: Management of bacterial corneal ulcers. Br J Ophthalmol 70:199, 1986
38. Perry MD, Golub LM: Systemic tetracyclines in the treatment of non-infected corneal ulcers: A case report and proposed new mechanism of action. Am J Ophthalmol 17:742, 1985
39. Shovlin JP, DePaolis MD, Edmonds Se, et al:

Acanthamoeba keratitis: Contact lenses as a risk factor. International Contact Lens Clinics 14:10, 1987

40. Moore MB, McCulley JP, Luckenbach M, et al: *Acanthamoeba* keratitis associated with soft contact lenses. Am J Ophthalmol 100:396, 1985

41. Auran JD, Stan MB, Jakobiec FA: Acanthamoeba keratitis: A review of the literature. Cornea 6:1, 1987

42. Weisman BA, Remba MJ: Results of the extended wear contact lens survey of the contact lens section of the AOA. J Am Optom Assoc 58:3, 1987

43. Ullman S, Roussell TJ, Culbertson MD, et al: *Neisseria gonorrheae* keratoconjunctivitis. Ophthalmology 94:525, 1987

44. Baum J, Jones DB: Initial therapy of suspected microbial corneal ulcers. Surv Ophthalmol 24:97, 1979

45. Gilbert ML, Osato MS, Wilhemus KR: Comparative bioavailability and efficacy of fortified topical tobramycin. (abst) Invest Ophthalmol 13:175, 1987

46. Groden L, Brinser J: Outpatient treatment of microbial corneal ulcer. Arch Ophthalmol 104:84, 1986

47. Glasser DB, Gardner S, Ellis JG, et al: Loading doses and extended dosing intervals in topical gentamicin therapy. Am J Ophthalmol 99:329, 1985

48. Kenyon KR: Decision-making in the therapy of external eye disease: Non-infected corneal ulcers. Ophthalmology 89:44, 1982

49. Keenlyside RA, Hierholzer JC, D'Angelo LJ: Keratoconjunctivitis associated with adenovirus #37. J Infect Dis 147:191, 1983

50. Kemp MC, Hierholzer JC, Cabradilla CP, et al: The changing etiology of EKC. J Infect Dis 148:24, 1983

51. Binder PS: Herpes simplex keratitis. Surv Ophthalmol 21:313, 1977

52. Oh JO (ed): Herpesvirus infections. Surv Ophthalmol 21:81, 1976

53. Stroop WG, Schaefer DC: Severity of experimentally reactivated herpetic eye disease is related to neuro-virulence of the latent virus. Invest Ophthalmol 28:229, 1987

54. Sundmacher R: Clinical aspects of herpetic eye disease. Curr Eye Res 6:183, 1987

55. Klauber A, Ottovay E: Acyclovir and IDU treatment of herpes simplex keratitis. Acta Ophthalmol 60:838, 1982

56. Romano A: Bacterial enzyme in viral infections: A new concept. Metab Pediatr Syst Ophthalmol 6:361, 1982

57. Cooper M: Epidemiology of herpes zoster. Eye 1:413, 1987

58. Womack LW, Liesegange TJ: Complications of herpes zoster ophthalmicus. Arch Ophthalmol 101:42, 1983

59. Browning DJ, et al: Ocular rosacea in blacks. Am J Ophthalmol 101:441, 1986

60. Browning DJ, Proia AD: Ocular rosacea. Surv Ophthalmol 31:145, 1986

61. Lemp MA, Mahmood MA, Weiler HH: Association of rosacea and keratoconjunctivitis sicca. Arch Ophthalmol 102:556, 1984

62. Insler MS, Anderson AB, Murray M: Latent oculogenital infection with chlamydia trachomatis. Ophthalmology 94:27, 1987

63. Ronnerstam R, Persson K, Marssan H, et al: Prevalence of chlamydial eye infection in patients attending an eye clinic, a V.D. clinic and in healthy persons. Br J Ophthalmol 69:385, 1985

64. Bialasiewicz AA, John GJ: Evaluation of diagnostic tools for adult chlamydial keratoconjunctivitis. Ophthalmology 94:532, 1987

65. Carpel EF: Superior limbic keratoconjunctivitis, Arch Ophthalmol 102:666, 1984

66. Carfino J: Treatment of superior limbic keratoconjunctivitis with topical cromolyn sodium. Ann Ophthalmol 19:129, 1987

67. Collin HB: Vernal and giant papillary conjunctivitis. Parts 1, 2, 3. Aust J Ophthalmol :64, 1981

68. Acheson JF, Joseph J, Spalton DJ: Use of soft contact lenses in an eye casualty department for primary treatment of traumatic corneal abrasions. Br J Opthalmol 71:285, 1987

69. Danja S, Friend J, Thoft RA: Conjunctival epithelium in healing of corneal epithelial wounds. Invest Ophthalmol 28:1445, 1987

70. Tseng SCG, Farazdaghi M, Rider AA: Conjunctival transdifferentiation induced by systemic vitamin A deficiency in vascularized rabbit corneas. Invest Ophthalmol 28:1497, 1987

71. Khodadoust AA, Silverstein AM, Kenyon KR, et al: Adhesion of regenerating corneal epithelium. Am J Ophthalmol 65:339, 1968

72. Kuwabara JA, Perkins DG, Cogan DG: Sliding of the epithelium in experimental wounds. Invest Ophthalmol 15:4, 1976

73. Srinivasan BD: Corneal reepithelialization and anti-inflammatory agents. Am Ophthalmol Soc 80:758, 1982

74. Weene L: Recurrent corneal erosion after trauma: A statistical study. Am J Ophthalmol 17:521, 1985

75. Canavan YM, Archer DB: Anterior segment consequences of blunt ocular trauma. Br J Ophthalmol 66:549, 1982

76. Catania LJ: Ease the ocular accident load. Optom Mgmt J 19:39, 1983

77. Prause JV, Norn M: Relationship between blink frequency and break-up time? Acta Ophthalmol (Copenh) 65:19, 1987

78. Kaufman ME: Keratitis sicca. Int Ophthalmol Clin 24:133, 1984

79. Holly FJ, Lemp MA: Tear physiology and dry eyes. Surv Ophthalmol 22:69, 1977

80. Tseng SCG, Maumanee AE, Stark WJ, et al: Topical retinoid treatment for various dry eye disorders. Ophthalmology 92:717, 1985

81. Willis RM, Folberg R, Krachmor JH, et al: Treatment of aqueous-deficient dry eye with remov-

able punctal plugs: A clinical and impression-cytologic study. Ophthalmology 94:514, 1987

82. Sigurdsson M, Hanna I, Lockwood AJ, et al: Removal of rust rings, comparing electric drill and hypodermic needle. Eye 1:430, 1987
83. Weene L: Recurrent corneal erosion after trauma: A statistical study. Am J Ophthalmol 17:521, 1985
84. Galbavy EJ: Recurrent corneal erosion. Int Opthalmol Clin 24:107, 1984
85. Williams R, Buckley RJ: Pathogenesis and treatment of recurrent erosion. Br J Ophthalmol 69:435, 1985
86. Levenson JE: Visual loss in anterior membrane dystrophy. Am J Ophthalmol 101:615, 1986
87. Kenyon KR: Recurrent corneal erosion: Pathogenesis on therapy. Int Ophthalmol Clin 19:169, 1979
88. Kaufman HE, Baldone JA: Soft contact lenses and clinical disease. (Letter.) Am J Ophthalmol 95:851, 1983

ANNOTATED REFERENCES

Barraquer JI, Binder PS, Buxton JN, et al: Symposium on Medical and Surgical Diseases of the Cornea. Transactions of the New Orleans Academy of Ophthalmology. St. Louis, CV Mosby, 1980
Transcripts of presentations by leading authorities on general care and new concepts regarding diseases and abnormalities of the cornea. Includes panel discussions on controversial issues in various areas of corneal care.

Duane DD, Jaeger EA (eds): Clinical Ophthalmology, Vol IV: External Disease. Philadelphia, Harper & Row, 1987
Chapters on standard approaches and new methods of care regarding corneal disease. Some chapters are excerpted from previous texts of corneal experts.

Duke-Elder WS: Diseases of the Outer Eye. Systems of Ophthalmology, Vol VIII, Part II. St Louis, CV Mosby, 1975
Most comprehensive work on all congenital, developmental, anomalous and disease entities of the cornea.

Grayson M: "Diseases of the Cornea, ed 2. St. Louis, CV Mosby, 1983
Classical descriptions and approaches to the diagnosis and management of all major corneal conditions. Second edition includes more recent information on some topics versus author's original text.

Leibowitz HM (ed): Corneal disorders: Clinical Diagnosis and Management. Philadelphia, WB Saunders, 1984
Clinically oriented approach to most major and common corneal disorders and diseases. Prominent expert clinicians as contributors with extensive illustrations and clinical discussion.

Olson RJ (ed): Common corneal problems, in International Ophthalmology Clinics. Boston, Little, Brown, 1984
Extensive presentations on major categories of common corneal problems by experts in specific areas. Covers fundamental basis, clinical considerations, and developments in each category.

Smolin G, Thoft RA (ed): The Cornea: Scientific Foundations and Clinical Practice, ed 2. Boston, Little, Brown, 1987
Two-part book, one presenting scientific principles of infection, inflammation, immunologic concepts, and so forth, applied clinically in second part regarding care of the cornea. Excellent approach presented by prominent corneal experts in each area.

Tabbara KF, Hyndiuk RA (ed): Infections of the Eye. Boston, Little, Brown, 1986
Three sections include basic concepts, diagnostic ocular microbiology, and clinical management. As with the Smolin and Thoft text, it presents excellent approach regarding infectious diseases of the cornea.

5

Diagnoses of the Anterior Chamber, Iris, and Ciliary Body

I. Background Information on Uveitis

A. DEFINITION

1. Inflammation of all or part(s) of the uveal tract
2. Parts include iris, ciliary body, and choroid
3. Associated tissues, such as cornea, vitreous, and retina, may also be involved

B. CLASSIFICATION

1. Clinical
   a. Acute (versus chronic) uveitis

183

    i. Important clinical management consideration
    ii. Sudden onset
    iii. Associated with moderate to severe pain
    iv. Expected duration of 6 weeks or less

b. Chronic (versus acute) uveitis
    i. Usually slow, insidious development
    ii. Often lasting greater than 6 weeks
    iii. Recurrent episodes
- First and second presentations (less than 6 weeks) considered acute
- Third (acute) presentation reclassifies condition as chronic–recurrent uveitis requiring complete medical evaluation

2. Anatomical classification

a. Anterior (main category considered in this chapter and most prevalent in clinical practice)
    i. Iritis
- Inflammation of iris
- Usually acute

    ii. Iridocyclitis
- Inflammation of iris and ciliary body
- Most common form of anterior acute uveitis

    iii. Pars planitis
- Also termed cyclitis or peripheral uveitis
- Inflammation of ciliary body or pars plana area

b. Posterior uveitis (almost always chronic)

c. Disseminated or diffuse uveitis (always chronic)

3. Pathological classification

a. Granulomatous
    i. Tends to produce mutton fat keratitic precipitates (KP) and iris nodules
    ii. Frequently chronic, but could vary

b. Nongranulomatous
    i. Usually acute but may be recurrent (chronic)
    ii. May produce fine KPs or none at all

C. INCIDENCE AND PREVALENCE OF UVEITIS (HOW MUCH?)

1. Generally stated at about 15 per 100,000 population

a. $\dfrac{\text{Drawing population}}{100,000} \times 15 =$ Potential number of uveitis cases in your community (a)

b. $\dfrac{\text{Number of active patient files}}{100,000} \times 15 =$ Potential number of active uveitis cases among your patients (b)

c. $\dfrac{\text{Number of active patient files}}{\text{Drawing population}} \times 100 =$ Your practice's (%) of community eye care (c)

d. $((a) \times (c)) + b =$ Potential number of active uveitis presentations to your practice (d)

e. 80% of (d) = Approximate number of active anterior uveitis cases among your patients

2. About 80 percent (12 of 15) are anterior uveitis

3. Calculations for primary eye care practices

D. EPIDEMIOLOGY AND DEMOGRAPHY (WHO, WHEN, AND WHERE?)

1. Age distribution

a. Important clinical diagnostic consideration

b. Most prevalent from ages 20 to 50

c. Highly diagnostic in childhood and adolescence up to ages 15 to 20

d. Uncommon as primary diagnosis beyond age 70

2. Sex distribution

a. Greater in males due to trauma, ankylosing spondylitis and Reiter's syndrome

b. Granulomatous type greater (two times) in females due to sarcoidosis

c. Childhood uveitis greater in females due to Still's disease (chronic juvenile rheumatoid arthritis, greater in young girls)

3. Race

a. Related to uveitis syndromes

b. Caucasians have higher frequency of ankylosing spondylitis, Reiter's and other HLA-B27 diseases

c. Blacks have a significantly higher rate

of sarcoid (10 to 15 times greater) than general population
  i. Especially black females
  ii. Especially in the southeastern United States
  d. Orientals have highest frequency of Vogt–Koyanagi–Harada syndrome and Behçet's disease
  e. Mediterranean races have a higher frequency of Behçet's disease
4. Geography
  a. Again, relative to uveitic-related diseases of a specific region
  b. Always consider sarcoid in the southeastern-American, Swedish, and Norwegian patients
    i. Interestingly, sarcoid is not common (in any race) in South Pacific
    ii. Virtually nonexistent in South African blacks
  c. Vogt–Koyanagi–Harada syndrome and Behçet's disease most prevalent in Orientals

5. Other factors
  a. Increased frequency in "type A" (high strung) personalities
    i. Stress increases risk of uveitis
    ii. Especially pars planitis
  b. Hazardous occupations, sports, avocations increase risk of traumatic uveitis

E. ETIOLOGY

1. Exogenous (external) causes
  a. Unknown (most common)
  b. Trauma
  c. Ocular infection
  d. Allergic reactions
2. Endogenous (internal) causes
  a. Unknown (most common)
  b. Systemic diseases
  c. Immunologic factors
3. More specific and extensive coverage of etiologies covered under "Assessment"

II. Primary Care (by SOAP) of Acute Anterior Uveitis

Subjective

- Presenting symptoms range from none to severe
  1. Range of symptoms is not necessarily directly proportional to severity of uveitis
  2. Many times chronic granulomatous uveitis presents with little to no symptomatology
  3. Conversely, acute iridocyclitis (mild to moderate) may be excruciatingly painful and debilitating
- Pars planitis generally has little or no symptoms and must be diagnosed objectively
- However, anterior uveitis (iritis and iridocyclitis) have such clear-cut predictable symptoms, the diagnosis can almost be made on the basis of subjective symptomatology alone
- Classic symptom pattern
  1. A deep, boring, pressure-type pain
    a. Usually reported as "in or behind" the eyeball
    b. Headache-type pain around the eye
    c. Patient denies or minimizes surface irritation, foreign-body sensation, burning, or itching
    d. Topical anesthetic does not relieve the pain
    e. Lid usually spasms or closes due to the pain
    f. When uveitis is associated with other conditions (e.g., trauma), try to ellicit the "quality" of the pain (as well as quantity) to confirm uveitic component
  2. Photophobia ranges from mild to severe
    a. Patient may flinch slightly to bright light or may require lights be diminished or put out because of pain
    b. Lid(s) may show increased blink rate, winking, or complete spastic closure
    c. More severe photophobia usually produces difficulty in slit-lamp examination especially during anterior chamber evaluation for cells and flare
  3. Vision is usually variable, depending on degree and type of uveitic presentation
    a. Ranges from normal to hazy in acute anterior uveitis (AAU) and pars planitis
    b. Chronic uveitis usually produces more haziness and blurring of vision in spite of minimal discomfort (versus AAU)
    c. Increased discomfort with near (accommodation) vision often reported
  4. Hyperlacrimation ranges from watery sensation to glassy appearance to frank tearing and epiphora
    a. Important to note that no other form of discharge is associated with uveitis (pure inflammation)
    b. Important in differential diagnosis

c. Any mucoid or purulent discharge should be considered a potential associated disease entity

■ Beyond straightforward entering symptoms, the most important part of the uveitic workup is the subjective *history* and *risk factors*

1. Age
   a. The key initial diagnostic milestone
   b. Narrows differential etiologies to highest risk possibilities of greatest frequency (Table 5–1)
2. Sex
   a. Further narrows high-risk possibilities between women and men
   b. Always compare risk factors in history
3. Race
   a. Blacks have a distinct increased risk (10 times greater) for sarcoidosis (especially young females)
   b. Caucasians and Orientals have varying predispositions to certain HLA diseases
4. Habitation
   a. Where does the patient live?
   b. Where was the patient born and raised?
5. Cohabitation
   a. Does patient live with someone?
   b. How long has patient lived with person(s)?
   c. Ocular and general health and well-being of cohabitants?
6. Sexual history
   a. Is patient sexually active?
   b. Any recent changes in sexual partners?
   c. Active or history of venereal disease?
   d. Exposure to any known venereal disease patients?

7. Personal history
   a. Diet
   b. Vocational
   c. Avocational
   d. Travel (risk of exposure to foreign disease)
   e. Medical and family history
   f. Active medications (or habitual drug use)
   g. Allergies or atopias
   h. Pets
8. Ocular history
   a. Disease, injury, or surgery (what and when?)
   b. Family history of ocular disease
9. Systemic disease
   a. Carefully assess direct or indirect possibilities of high-risk uveitic diseases or syndromes (Table 5–2)
   b. Question patient for diagnosed history of such conditions or signs and symptoms of such conditions
10. Onset of current ocular signs and symptoms
    a. As exact a starting point as possible
    b. Consider duration as criteria for diagnosis of acute versus chronic uveitis

■ Significant diagnostic indicators

1. These include the most important differential diagnostic clinical criteria in uveitis (acute versus chronic)
   a. Onset and duration
      i. Conditions lasting less than 6 weeks are usually acute
      ii. Conditions lasting greater than 6 weeks are usually chronic
   b. Response to standard therapies
      i. Acute conditions will respond in 6 weeks or less

TABLE 5–1. RISK FACTORS ASSOCIATED WITH ANTERIOR UVEITIS[a]

Clinical Diagnosis	Less Than 20 Years Old		20 to 50 Years Old		Greater Than 50 Years Old	
	Primary Care[b] (%)	Referral Clinics[c] (%)	Primary Care[b] (%)	Referral Clinics[c] (%)	Primary Care[b] (%)	Referral Clinics[c] (%)
Unknown	~25	>40	>50	>35	>40	>30
Trauma	~50	—	~30	~10	~30	~10
Pars planitis	~20	~15	~10	>10	>1	<5
Sarcoid	<1	~4	~3	~3	—	<3
Adult rheumatoid	—	—	~2	~15	~15	>20
JRA	~1	~30	—	~2	—	—
Other HLA distrophy	—	~2	~2	~3	~1	<2
Fuchs' heterochromic iridocyclitis	~1	~6	~1	>10	~1	~2
Infectious	~1	~2	~1	~10	~10	~18
GI	<1	<1	<1	~2	~2	~10

[a]By age of patient
[b]Catania
[c]Specialists

TABLE 5–2. RANK ORDER OF COMMON ANTERIOR UVEITIS ETIOLOGIES[a]

Age of Patient (yr)	Etiology	Rank Order of Primary Care Risk Factors
Less than 20	Trauma	1
	Unknown	2
	Pars planitis	3
	Infection	4
	JRA	5
	Fuchs'	6
	Sarcoid	7
	GI	8
20 to 50	Unknown	1
	Trauma	2
	Pars planitis	3
	Sarcoid	4
	HLAs	5
	Infection	6
	Fuchs'	7
	GI	8
Greater than 50	Unknown	1
	Trauma	2
	HLAs	3
	Infection	4
	GI	5
	Fuchs'	6
	Pars planitis	7

[a]By age of patient.

ii. Most frequently, acute conditions will respond to topical medications alone
c. Recurrence
   i. Exacerbation upon discontinuation of medication (after appropriate course) is indicative of potential chronicity and possible endogenous (systemic) cause
   ii. History of recurrent episodes separated by variable time intervals is also suspicious
   iii. Clinical guidelines
      • Fewer than three recurrences with negative history and risk factors: assume acute
      • Three or more recurrences with or without postitive history: assume chronic
d. Bilateral presentations
   i. Usually highly suggestive if endogenous and chronic uveitic response
   ii. Granulomatous bilateral uveitis is almost certainly systemically related
e. Alternating eye recurrences
   i. Effectively, a combination of points c and d above
   ii. A history revealing uveitis in one eye followed by a recurrence in the opposite eye can be thought of as a "bilateral" condition

f. Systemic history
   i. The presence of virtually any systemic disease should be considered, confirmed, or ruled out as contributing to an ocular manifestation
   ii. Suspicious signs and symptoms of systemic disease should also be considered relative to an ocular manifestation
   iii. All systemic conditions directly associated with uveitis (with or without other "significant indicators") must be documented and considered in the differential diagnosis of a concommittant (or previous) uveitis (acute or chronic)

Objective*

■ Visual acuity (VA)
   1. May remain as normal 20/20
   2. Moderate reduction: 20/25 to 20/60
   3. Severe reduction: 20/60 to 20/400
   4. Higher-risk reductions: less than 20/200
   5. Accommodation (near VA) usually moderately reduced and painful
   6. General "haziness" usually reported
■ Eyelid signs
   1. Blepharospasms
      a. Secondary to photophobia
      b. Unilateral uveitis can produce a bilateral response
   2. Congestion and edema
      a. Usually mild to moderate
      b. Erythema (redness) absent or mild
      c. Any pain on palpation is result of pressure on globe itself
   3. Pseudoptosis
■ Conjunctiva (Color Plate 80)
   1. Pink or purplish circumcorneal (perilimbal) flush
   2. Circumcorneal hyperemia (flush) usually produces a deep (scleral or episcleral) radiating vessel pattern (versus superficial, irregular conjunctivitis pattern) with injection decreasing further away from the limbus (versus anterior uveitis pattern increasing toward limbus) (Fig. 5–1)
   3. Circumcorneal flush may be 360° or sectional
      a. Usually never much less than 90°
      b. Any amount from 90° to 360° possible
   4. Often cul-de-sacs in uveitis are white and quiet
■ Cornea
   1. Epithelial edema
      a. Frequently present in acute presentations
      b. Microcystic edemas usually present in chronic (or advanced endothelial KP) cases
   2. Band keratopathy may develop in advanced, chronic cases (e.g., Still's triad in JRA of uveitis, cataract, and band keratopathy)
   3. Stromal edema
      a. Present in acute (hot) presentations

*See also Appendix 2.

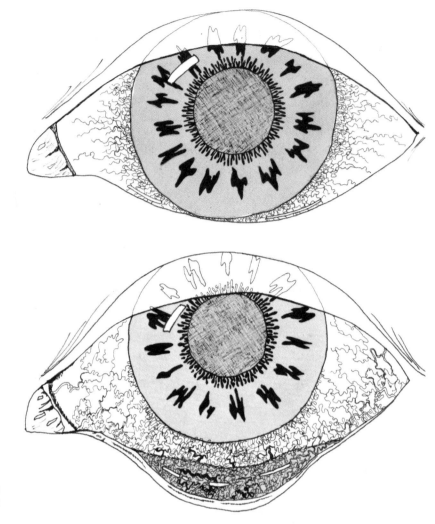

Figure 5–1.
Circumcorneal flush (top) versus
conjunctivitis hyperemic pattern
(bottom)

b. Present with dense KP
c. Present in advanced and chronic cases
4. Striate keratitis
    a. Usually in advanced and chronic conditions
    b. Usually secondary to stromal edema
5. Keratic precipitates
    a. Fine
        i. Whitish-gray fibrin or epithelioid cells adherent to posterior cornea
        ii. Discrete small to medium size dots (always less than 0.5 mm)
        iii. Apparent three-dimensional appearance (as if raised off posterior corneal surface)
        iv. Usually take days to form and weeks or months (or never) to disappear
        v. Old KPs usually flatten first and then disappear
    b. "Mutton fat" KP (Color Plate 82)
        i. Synonymous with chronic granulomatous types
        ii. Large, flat, confluent-looking KP
        iii. Greasy, waxy, grainy-appearing surfaces

        iv. Accummulate pigment with age
        v. Usually do not disappear completely (as fine KP)
    c. Pigmented KP (Color Plate 83)
        i. May be diffuse in AAU
        ii. Most often aqueous convection currents produce vertically oriented configurations called Kruchenburg's spindle or Arlt's triangle (both with base down and apex up) on inferior posterior corneal surface (Figs. 5–2 and 5–3)
6. Other endothelial changes (e.g., guttata) infrequent
■ Anterior chamber (Color Plate 81)
1. Cells in the aqueous (classic uveitic sign)
    a. Usually white blood cells (WBC), abnormal in aqueous, leak from the ciliary body
    b. Red blood cells (RBC) or pigment cells may also be seen (less common than WBC)
    c. Usually move in slow upward direction
    d. Best viewing technique
        i. Good slit lamp is essential

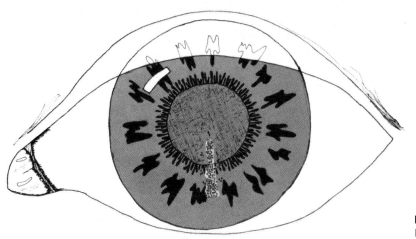

Figure 5–2.
Kruckenburg's spindle

ii. Dark (black) room
iii. Dilated pupil makes ideal backdrop for best viewing
iv. Direct illumination with approximately 45 to 60° viewing angle
v. A 3- to 4-mm vertical beam at inferior

cornea with small portion over iris and balance over pupil
vi. Beam width should be about 1 to 2 mm wide
vii. Focus beam first clearly on corneal surface

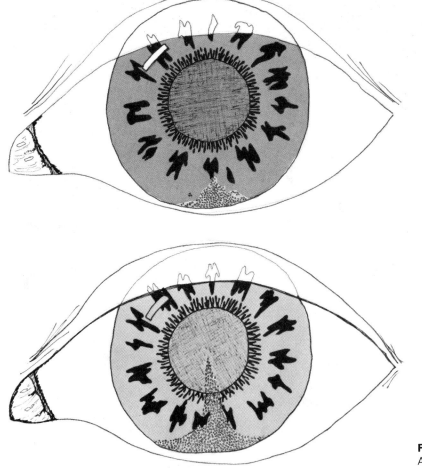

Figure 5–3.
Arlt's triangle

viii. With a "joystick," move back slowly to clear focus on anterior lens capsule

ix. Repeat refocusing from lens to cornea to lens two or three times to get feel of full distance of excursion with joystick

x. After two or three times, move only half-full distance from cornea to lens and hold

xi. Both cornea and lens capsule should be out of focus

xii. Optically "black" space between out of focus cornea and lens images will be clear, focus on aqueous

xiii. Concentrate your view on optically black space and watch for "cells" moving through field of view in a slow, upward (or irregular) motion

xiv. Compare lighter backdrop of iris with darker pupil backdrop for lighter and darker cells

xv. Take at least 30 to 60 seconds or longer in suspect eyes (Table 5–3; Fig. 5–4)

2. Flare in the aqueous
   a. Caused by protein leaking from iris (triggered by prostaglandins)
   b. Produces an optically impure (versus black, clear) aqueous
   c. Slit-lamp examination procedure is same as described for cells

TABLE 5–3. RELATIVE GRADING OF CELLS[a]

Grade	Aqueous Finding
0–1+	1–5 cells in 30–60 sec
1–2+	5–10 cells in beam at once
2–3+	Cells scattered throughout beam
3–4+	Dense cells in beam

[a]In 2-mm-wide × 4-mm-high beam.

d. Flare appears as turbidity or haziness in the aqueous
   i. Tyndall (Brownian movement) effect described in textbooks is difficult to appreciate
   ii. Best approach is to view many optically pure aqueous media first (in normal patients) and then flare will be comparatively obvious
   iii. Also, compare aqueous bilaterally in unilateral uveitis cases (for comparison)
e. Flare is usually greater and more persistent in chronic granulomatous uveitis
   i. Often persists indefinitely
   ii. May also persist as "trace" flare in AAU (Table 5–4; Fig. 5–5)

3. Hypopyon (endophthalmitis)
   a. Dense accumulation of WBC, usually poly-

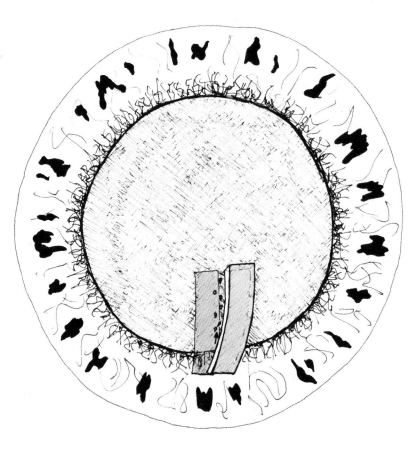

Figure 5–4.
Viewing cells in the anterior chamber

TABLE 5-4. RELATIVE GRADING OF FLARE[a]

Grade	Aqueous Finding
0–1 +	Trace flare (by bilateral comparison)
1–2 +	Obvious presence (by comparison)
2–3 +	Hazy aqueous
3–4 +	Dense haze or plasmoid aqueous

[a]In 2-mm-wide × 4-mm-high beam.

morphonuclear cells (PMN), in severe acute uveitis

   b. Gravity produces inferior pooling and fluid level (straight top) in anterior chamber

   c. Make certain to rule out infectious keratitis (i.e., corneal ulcer synonymous with hypopyon)

4. Plasmoid aqueous (plastic iritis)

   a. Dense accumulation of flare or fibrin cells producing translucent to cloudy or opaque strands and sheets with small to large lumps (coagulates) of proteinous material in the anterior chamber

   b. Usually in severe acute uveitis

   c. Cells move sluggishly (if at all) through thick cloudy aqueous

   d. Often associated with trauma

   e. Easily mistaken for lens material from assumed ruptured lens capsule (especially with history of blunt trauma)

5. Synechiae (Color Plate 84)

   a. Anterior (peripheral)

      i. Fibrous adhesions between peripheral cornea and iris

      ii. Not as common as posterior synechiae

   b. Posterior

      i. Fibrous adhesions between iris (usually at or just behind pupillary border or on posterior surface of iris surface) and anterior lens capsule

      ii. Form readily in heavy flare, chronic and AAU

      iii. May occur in conjunction with iris nodules

      iv. Sometimes mistaken for persistent pupillary membranes

        • Membranes come off collarette

        • Membranes are nonfibrous

      v. Seclusio pupillae (immobile pupil) is 360° posterior synechiae (usually in chronic AU)

■ Iris

1. Atrophy in prolonged chronicity and certain specific forms (e.g., Fuchs' heterochromic iridocyclitis)

   a. Produces transillumination defects

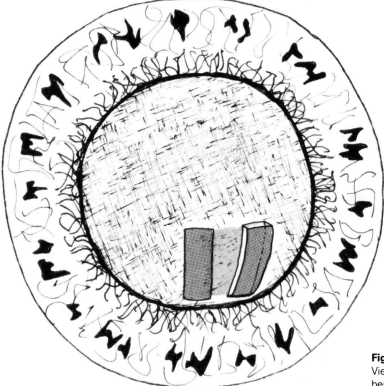

Figure 5-5.
Viewing flare in the anterior chamber

b. May produce decrease in iris pigment (Fuchs')

2. Granuloma

   a. Fleshy, whitish-pink, slightly vascularized mass

   b. Usually larger than other iris nodules

   c. Pupil border, anterior surface of iris or angle locations

   d. Common in sarcoid (especially at angle location)

3. Nodule

   a. Busacca

      i. Whitish-yellow lumps away from pupil border

      ii. Internal iris stroma

      iii. Always associated with granulomatous uveitis

   b. Koeppe

      i. Most common nodule in uveitis

      ii. Round or oval solid tissue (cellular aggregates) masses

      iii. Located at pupil border in varying sizes

      iv. May accumulate pigmentation over time

4. Swelling (or "boggy") iris

   a. Loss of iris crypt definition

   b. Smooth velvety surface appearance

   c. Usually associated with dense flare

- Pupil (Color Plate 85)

1. Reactions range from normal to sluggish

2. Usually but not always miotic in acute presentations

3. Frequent corectopia (undilated or upon dilation) secondary to posterior synechiae

4. Fixed pupils may occur with advancing complications or chronicity

   a. Seclusio pupillae

   b. Iris bombe (seclusio with iris bowing anteriorly)

   c. Secondary glaucomas

- Intraocular pressure (IOP)

1. Usually reduced by 3 to 6 mm (as compared with contralateral eye) in early stages of acute presentations due to ciliary body hypotony (reduced aqueous production)

   a. Prolonged hypotony in chronic conditions could potentiate phthisis bulbi

   b. Chronic IOP below 5 mm Hg are at risk

2. IOP may increase in untreated acute or chronic forms because of angle (trabecular) congestion reducing outflow

   a. Also consider iatrogenic, steroid-related increase in IOP

   b. Monitor IOP frequently

3. Acute glaucoma (Posner–Schlossman syndrome or glaucomatocyclitic crisis)

   a. IOP increases to greater than 30 mm Hg

   b. Total congestion of trabecular meshwork due to inflammatory debri

4. Chronic glaucoma

   a. High risk in prolonged uveitis

b. Multiple-angle etiologies

c. Seclusio pupillae

- Crystalline lens

1. Epicapsular stars or pigment debri may occur in acute or chronic cases

   a. Frequently associated with posterior synechiae

   b. Clumps of pigment may persist

2. Posterior subcapsular cataracts most common in chronic endogenous forms

   a. May be associated with long-term steroids (oral or topical) in treatment

   b. Also associated with Fuchs' heterochromic iridocyclitis

3. Mature cataracts usually limited to advanced rheumatoid cases (e.g., Still's disease)

- Vitreous

1. Anterior and retrolental (Berger's) space

   a. Observable with direct slit-lamp illumination

   b. Cells appear adherent to vitreous strands (usually greater inferiorly)

   c. Strands may be broad and dense

2. Posterior

   a. Must be viewed with Hruby, Goldmann, or Volk 90D lens

   b. Involvement called vitritis and associated with posterior, chronic, endogenous uveitic syndromes

- Posterior globe (retina, choroid, optic nerve)

1. Peripheral retinal involvements associated with pars planitis ("snowballing" on pars plana)

2. Posterior involvements are always diagnostic of advanced peripheral uveitis (pars planitis) or a chronic uveitic syndrome (Tables 5–5 and 5–8)

Assessment*

- Carefully examine subjective and objective presentations

- Rule out primary anterior segment ocular diseases and masquarade syndromes that mimic anterior uveitis (Table 5–6)

- Try "Henkind" test (easy, but not always accurate, i.e., beware of false-negative results)[3]

1. Occlude involved eye while shining light in contralateral (opposite) pupil

2. Indirect (consensual) pupillary reflex should produce pain in occluded (involved) eye if uveitis present

- Consider significant indicators for acute versus chronic anterior uveitis

1. Onset and duration (6 weeks or less = acute)

2. Response to standard therapies (within 6 weeks)

3. Recurrences (2 = acute; 3 = chronic potential)

4. Bilateral (= chronic potential)

5. Alternating eye recurrences (= bilateral = chronic)

---

*See also Appendix 3.

TABLE 5–5. OBJECTIVE (PHYSICAL) FINDINGS IN ANTERIOR UVEITIS[a]

Clinical Classification	Objective (Physical) Findings	Acute	Chronic	Pars Planitis	Nongranulomatous	Granulomatous
Vision	20/20 (normal)	X		X	X	
	20/25 to 20/60	X		X	X	
	20/60 to 20/200		X			X
	High risk (<20/400)		X			X
	Painful accommodation	X			X	
Lids and conjunctiva	Blepharospasm	X			X	
	Lid congestion/edema	X			X	
	Circumcorneal flush	X	X		X	X
Cornea	Epithelial edema	X	X		X	X
	Band keratopathy		X			X
	Stromal edema/striae		X			X
	Fine KP	X			X	
	Pigmented KP	X	X			X
	Mutton fat KP		X			X
Anterior chamber	Cells and flare	X	X		X	X
	Hypopyon		X		X	X
	Plasmoid aqueous	X			X	
Iris	Posterior synechiae	X	X		X	X
	Iris atrophy		X		X	X
	Granulomas		X		X	X
	Busacca nodule		X			X
	Koeppe nodule		X		X	X
	Swelling		X			X
Pupil	Sluggish	X	X	X	X	X
	Miosis	X			X	
	Corectopia	X	X		X	X
	Fixed (nonreactive)		X		X	X
Intraocular pressure	Reduced	X			X	
	Chronic hypotony		X		X	X
	Increasing	X	X		X	X
	Acute glaucoma	X	X		X	X
	Chronic glaucoma		X		X	X
Lens	Capsule pigment	X	X		X	X
	Posterior subcapsular		X		X	X
	Mature cataract		X			X
Vitreous posterior chamber	Anterior vitreous cells			X		
	Posterior vitreous cells		X			X
	Peripheral retinal exudation			X		
	Posterior retinal involvement		X	X		X

[a]By clinical classification.

6. Systemic history (positive = chronic potential) (Tables 5–7 and 5–8)

- Consider major risk factors
  1. Age
  2. Race
  3. Sex
  4. Geographic considerations
  5. Other factors
- Consider risk factors by age of presenting patient (Tables 5–1 and 5–2)
- Attempt to differentiate exogenous from endogenous causes

1. Exogenous causes
  a. Unknown
  b. Trauma
  c. Infection
  d. Drug induced (toxic)
  e. Allergic response
  f. Keratitis (prostaglandins)
  g. Surgery
2. Endogenous causes
  a. Unknown
  b. HLA antigens
  c. Sarcoid

TABLE 5–6. DIFFERENTIATING PRIMARY ANTERIOR SEGMENT DISEASES FROM ANTERIOR UVEITIS[a]

Condition	Findings	Compared with Anterior Uveitis
Conjunctivitis		
Subjective	No pain	Pain and photophobia
Objective	Discharge	No discharge
	Hyperemia greater farther from limbus	Circumcorneal (perilimbal) flush
Episcleritis		
Subjective	No photophobia	Photophobia
Objective	Hyperemic sector decreasing toward limbus	Hyperemia greatest at limbus
	Clear chamber	Cells and flare
Keratitis		
Subjective	Superficial pain	Deep pain
	Pain relieved with topical anesthetic	No relief with topical anesthetic
Objective	Corneal staining	No direct corneal involvement
Scleritis		
Subjective	General malaise	No systemic symptoms
Objective	Deep injection all the way to fornices	Injection (circumcorneal) decreasing toward fornices
Acute glaucoma		
Subjective	Sudden VA decrease	Insidious VA reduction
Objective	Increased IOP with corneal edema	Decreased (acute) IOP with clear cornea
Masquerade syndrome		
Retinoblastoma	Posterior lesion	No posterior
Leukemia	Systemic	No systemic
Intraocular FB	Contributory history	Secondary
Malignant melanoma	Posterior lesion	No posterior
Retinal detachment	Fundus finding	Secondary
Retinitis pigmentosa	Fundus finding	Secondary
Lymphoma	Systemic	Secondary
Multiple sclerosis	Neurological signs	No neurological signs

[a]By selected subjective and objective findings.

TABLE 5–7. SUMMARY OF SUBJECTIVE AND OBJECTIVE SYMPTOMS IN ACUTE AND CHRONIC ANTERIOR UVEITIS

Acute	Chronic
Subjective	
Usually moderate to severe	Usually mild to moderate
Rapid onset	Slow, insidious development
Mild to moderate haziness or VA reduction	Moderate to severe "haziness" or VA reduction
Moderate to severe dull, aching pain, usually reported in or behind eye	Mild to moderate pain response (sometimes no pain at all)
Distinctly photophobic	Mild photophobia
Presentations <2 times	Recurrent (>2 times)
Responsive to therapy in <6 weeks	Poor response to therapy, usually >6 weeks
No systemic history	Frequent systemic history
Objective	
Usually unilateral	Bilateral or changing eyes
Lid congestion	No lid involvement
Moderate circumcorneal flush	Mild circumcorneal flush
Fine KPs	Mutton fat KPs
Cells and flare	Cells and flare
Posterior synechiae (fresh)	Dense synechiae (fibrous)
Occasional boggy iris	Iris nodules and granulomas
Occasional miotic pupil	Occasional fixed pupil
IOP reduced	Frequent secondary glaucoma
No vitreoretinal complications	Frequent vitreoretinal involvement
Minimal potential for complications	Greater potential for complications

   d. Granulomatous disease
   e. Infections
   f. Phacoantigenic
   g. Sympathetic ophthalmia
■ Consider and compare all clinical signs and symptoms (subjective and objective), risk factors, epidemiology, and (most important) significant indicators, and assess the following
   1. Anterior versus posterior (or disseminated)
   2. Acute versus chronic
     a. More or less than 6 weeks
     b. First, second, third (or greater) presentation(s)
   3. Granulomatous versus nongranulomatous
   4. Exogenous versus endogenous etiology
   5. Mild, moderate, or severe degree
   6. Risk of complications
     a. Low
     b. High
   7. Prognosis
     a. Good
     b. Guarded
     c. Poor

Plan*

■ Goals in treating anterior uveitis
   1. Protect vision
   2. Reduce tissue changes (e.g., KPs, cells, and flare)
   3. Reduce scarring potential (e.g., synechiae)
   4. Reduce pain
   5. And above all, "Do no harm" (Hippocrates)
■ Always make sure that any known cause of a uveitic response is treated and managed in conjunction with the uveitis (the eye) itself
■ Therapeutic agents used for anterior uveitis
   1. Topical agents (Table 5–9)
     a. Mydriatic and cycloplegic agents
       i. Avoid atropine due to pupil immobilization effect for prolonged period increasing risk of synechiae
       ii. Conversely, atropine, may be useful in some situations
         • Intensely severe presentations
         • Prolonged therapies
         • Noncompliant patients
       iii. Scopolamine may have a more positive effect on darkly pigmented and black patients
     b. Anti-inflammatory agents and steroids
     c. Antibiotics (when indicated)
   2. Oral agents
     a. Steroids (usually prednisone)
     b. Nonsteroidal anti-inflammatory drugs (NSAIDs)

       i. Aspirin
       ii. Ibuprofen[4]
   3. Other agents
     a. Injectable (depot) steroids
     b. Cytotoxic agents
     c. Anticancer (immunosuppressive agents)
     d. Investigational substances
■ Nontherapeutic therapies
   1. Hot packs (for ciliary muscle spasm pain)
   2. Dark glasses (for photophobia and dilation)
   3. Temporary plus for near work (due to cycloplegia)
■ Mild presentations (cells and flare: trace to 1+; no KP)
   1. Therapy is optional (depending on symptoms)
   2. Mydriacyl or homatropine bid to tid
   3. Oral ibuprofen (1200 to 1600 mg/day)
   4. Hot packs q3–4h
   5. RTC 48 hours, or PRN if worsening
   6. Reassure patient
■ Moderate presentations (cells and flare: 1 to 3+ and KPs)
   1. Five percent homatropine qid
   2. One percent prednisolone q3–4h
     a. Use FML (fluorometholone) if there is a direct or family history of glaucoma
     b. Always shake steroid suspensions thoroughly before use (and instruct patient on such)
   3. Oral ibuprofen (1600 mg/day)
   4. Hot packs q3–4h
   5. Dark glasses
   6. Temporary plus for near work (optional for needs)
   7. Counsel and advise patient carefully
     a. Especially on nature, severity, and probable duration of pain
     b. Explain medications
       i. Their use
       ii. Their side effects (i.e., near blur, dilation)
     c. Discuss disease and its clinical course
   8. RTC 48 hours
     a. PRN (or phone) after 24 hours, if symptoms worsen
     b. May get worse before getting better
     c. Should stabilize with meds in within 48 hours
■ Severe presentations (cells and flare >3+ with KPs)
   1. Five percent homatropine q4h
   2. One percent prednisolone q2h (see "moderate presentations" regarding FML)
   3. Oral ibuprofen (1600 to 2000 mg/day)
   4. Hot packs q2–3h
   5. Dark glasses
   6. Temporary plus for near (if needed)
   7. Counsel and advise (see "moderate presentations")
   8. RTC 24 hours (Tables 5–10 and 5–11)
■ Pars planitis presentations
   1. Mild to moderate presentations should be

---

*See also Appendix 4.

TABLE 5–8. SUMMARY OF ANTERIOR UVEITIS

Cause of Anterior Uveitis	Age <20	Age 20–50	Age >50	Acute	Chronic	Nongranulomatous	Granulomatous	Anterior	Posterior	Exogenous	Endogenous	Male	Female	Unilateral	Bilateral	Degree Mild	Degree Moderate	Degree Severe	Compl. Potential Low	Compl. Potential High	Prognosis Good	Prognosis Guarded	Prognosis Poor
Adult rheumatoid disease		X	X	X		X		X			X			X			X		X		X		
Ankylosing spondylitis		X		X		X		X			X	X			X		X	X	X		X		
Behçet's disease		X			X	X	X	X			X	X	(X)		X			X		X		X	
Crohn's disease		X			X	X		X			X	X		X			X		X		X		
Fuchs' heterochromic	X	X			X	X		X			X			X			X		X		X		
Glaucomatocyclitic		X	X	X		X		X		X	X			X			X	X	X		X		
Infectious disease		X		X	X	X		X		X	X			X	X	X	X		X		X		
Juvenile rheumatoid arthritis (JRA)	X	X		X	X	X	X	X			X		X		X		X	X	X				
Juvenile xanthogranuloma (JXG)	X			X			X	X			X		X		X		X	X	X				X
Keratouveitis		X	X	X		X		X		X				X			X	X	X		X		
Lens induced		X	X	X			X	X		X				X			X	X		X			X
Mononucleosis		X		X		X		X			X				X	X	X		X		X		
Pars planitis		X			X	X		X	X		X				X	X	X		X		X		
Reiter's syndrome	X	X		X		X		X	X	X		X			X		X		X		X		
Sarcoidosis		X		X		X	X	X	X		X				X		X	X		X		X	
Sclerouveitis		X		X	X	X		X	X	X	X			X			X	X		X		X	
Subacute sclerosing panencephalitis	X			X	X		X	X	X		X				X			X		X		X	
Sympathetic ophthalmia		X			X	X	X	X	X		X			X	X		X	X		X		X	
Syphilis		X		X	X		X	X	X	X	X				X		X	X		X		X	
Trauma				X		X		X			X			X			X		X		X		
Tuberculosis		X	X		X	X	X	X	X		X				X		X	X	X			X	
Ulcerative colitis		X	X		X	X		X		X	X	X			X		X	X	X		X		
Unknown		X		X		X	X	X		X	X				X				X		X		
Vogt-Koyanagi-Harada		X			X	X	X	X	X		X				X	X	X		X		X		

TABLE 5–9. COMMON TOPICAL AGENTS USED IN ANTERIOR UVEITIS THERAPY

Generic Name	Sample Brand(s)	Concentration (%)	Duration	Potential Risks
Mydriatic/cycloplegics				Angle closure (remote)
Atropine	Isopto Atropine	0.5, 1, 2	7–14 days	Atropine toxicity
Cyclopentolate	Cyclogyl	0.5, 1, 2	6–12 hr	Atropine (remote)
Homatropine	Isopto Homatropine	2, 5	18–24 hr	Atropine (remote)
Phenylephrine	Neo-Synephrine	2.5, 10	4–8 hr	Cardiovascular (remote)
Scopolamine		0.25	5–7 days	Atropine (remote)
Tropicamide	Mydriacyl	0.5, 1	3–6 hr	Angle closure (remote)
Steroids				↑IOP, PSC, HSV
Dexamethasone	Decadron	0.1	Greatest with epithelial defect	↑IOP, HSV, PSC (remote)
Fluorometholone	FML	0.1	Fluorinated	HSV
Hydrocortisone	Hydrocort	2.5	Very mild	↑IOP, HSV
Medrysone	HMS	1.0	Very mild	↑IOP, HSV
Prednisolone	Pred Mild/Forte	0.125, 1.0	Best with intact epithelium (e.g., anterior uveitis)	↑IOP, HSV PSC (remote)
	Econopred	1.0		
	Inflamase	1.0		

treated with oral aspirin (2 tabs q4h or minimum 10 tabs/day) or ibuprofen (1600 mg/day) and hot packs q3–4h

2. Moderate to severe presentations usually produce posterior or disseminated uveitis requiring advanced therapies by skilled specialist and medical co-management
3. No topical therapies are indicated in pars planitis
4. RTC 3 to 5 days for re-evaluation
5. Often require long-term low-grade chronic management care

Follow-up (Table 5–12)

■ Mild presentations
1. RTC 48 hours (or PRN) is usually valuable
   a. 48 hours RTC if medications provided
   b. PRN if mild or no medications prescribed
2. If appointment scheduled, do not be surprised on "no show" (owing to complete resolution)

   a. Especially very mild cases
   b. Phone call follow-up is always appreciated
3. If condition worsens, initiate or increase therapy to "moderate presentation" level
■ Moderate presentations
1. Upon 48 hour return compare subjective and objective signs and check IOP for steroid responders
   a. If positive, discontinue (D/C) steroids
   b. Treat glaucoma, if no IOP reduction in 48 to 72 hours or if IOP greater than 30 mm Hg
2. Uveitis should be no worse or better
   a. Sometimes it is difficult to assess changes on the basis of cells and flare alone
   b. Try quantifying (counting) KPs in given area on first visit and recount same area in follow-up (Fig. 5–6)
      i. Increased count: uncontrolled condition
      ii. Stable count: controlled condition
3. If condition is worsening
   a. Question compliance

TABLE 5–10. CLINICAL DEGREE OF ACUTE ANTERIOR UVEITIS

Mild	Moderate	Severe
Mild to moderate symptoms	Moderate to severe symptoms	Moderate to severe symptoms
VA 20/20 to 20/30	VA from 20/30 to 20/100	VA ≤20/100
Superficial circumcorneal flush	Deep circumcorneal flush	Deep circumcorneal flush
No KPs	Scattered KPs	Dense KPs
Trace to 1+ cells and flare	1–3+ cells and flare	3–4+ cells and flare
IOP reduced <4 mm Hg	Miotic, sluggish pupil	Sluggish or fixed pupil
	Mild posterior synechiae	Posterior synechiae (fibrous)
	IOP reduced from 3–6 mm Hg	Boggy iris (no crypts)
	Mild iris swelling	Raised IOP
	Anterior vitreous cells	Moderate to heavy anterior cells

TABLE 5–11. ACUTE ANTERIOR UVEITIS: TREATMENT AND FOLLOW-UP[a]

A. Mild uveitic therapy
1. Optional (depending on symptoms)
2. Mydriacyl or homatropine (bid–tid)
3. Oral aspirin or ibuprofen (Motrin)
4. Warm compresses
5. RTC 48 hours (or PRN if worsening)

B. Refer to nonophthalmological physician for systemic evaluation (with significant indicators)

C. Moderate uveitic therapy
1. 5% homatropine qid
2. 1% prednisolone q3–4h
   a. Use FML if direct or family history of glaucoma
   b. Shake steroid suspensions well before using
3. Oral aspirin or ibuprofen, 2 tabs q4h
4. Warm compresses
5. Dark glasses
6. Plus for near (optional)
7. Advise patient carefully (e.g., pain, course, compliance)
8. RTC 48 hours (or PRN if necessary)

D. Heavy uveitic therapy
1. 5% homatropine q4h
2. 1% prednisolone q2h (see C.2.a, b)
3. Oral aspirin or ibuprofen, 2 tabs q3–4h
4. Warm compresses (q2–3h)
5. Dark glasses
6. Plus for near (optional)
7. Advise patient carefully
8. RTC 24 hours

E. Refer to ophthalmologist for possible depot or oral steroid therapy

F. Counsel, education, advise patient regarding potential chronic uveitis syndromes and dismiss (PRN)

[a]Giving letter code to be used with Table 5–14.

b. Check dilation
   i. May want to increase potency of dilator from shorter-acting to longer-acting drug (e.g., 1 percent tropicamide to 5 percent homatropine)
   ii. Also increase dosage (to q2–3h)
c. Increase steroid dosage to q2h
d. RTC 24 hours
4. If condition is stable (usually the case)
   a. Continue all medications
      i. Never D/C steroids sooner than 7 to 10 days
      ii. Maintain dilation for 5 to 7 days (minimum)
   b. RTC 3 to 4 days (check IOP)
      i. Dilation can be discontinued (tapering optional)
      ii. Always taper steroids
         • Use any gradual decrease, taking about 4 to 6 days

• Suggest decreasing existing dose by one per day to zero
• Whatever, keep instructions simple
5. See patient once again about 3 to 5 days after all medications have been discontinued
6. Trace cells and flare may persist (sometimes indefinitely)

■ Severe presentations
1. Upon 24-hour return, compare findings from initial visit (check IOP)
2. Flare and cells may often appear worse
3. Count KP for baseline (see "moderate presentations")
4. If plasmoid aqueous developing (or more likely still present from initial visit) increase steroids to every hour
5. Otherwise, reassure patient (regarding pain and likely improvement), continue all medications and RTC 24 hours
6. On return visit, look for signs of stabilization
   a. Cells and flare holding
   b. KP count stable
   c. Any plasmoid aqueous dissolving
   d. Subjective pain diminishing
7. Attempt to break any posterior synechiae with strong pupil dilators

TABLE 5–12. ACUTE ANTERIOR UVEITIS: FOLLOW-UP PROTOCOL[a]

Mild presentations
48 hr or PRN
PRN if no medication provided
Phone call valuable in PRN or RTC no show
If worsening, initiate or upgrade therapy
Moderate
Compare subjective and objective findings at 48 hr
Check IOP (for steroid responders)
Should be no worse or better (count KPs)
If worsening
   Question compliance
   Check dilation
   Increase dosages
   RTC 24 hr
If stabilizing
   Continue medication for ≈1 week, then taper steroids
   RTC 3–5 days
   RTC 3–5 days after medication discontinued
Severe
Compare subjective and objective findings at 24 hr
Check IOP (for steroid responders and secondary glaucomas)
May be worse than initial presentation (count KPs)
Hold all medication or increase steroids to q1h
Reassure and reinstruct
RTC 24 hr
If stabilizing RTC 48 hr
If worsening after 3–5 days, depot or oral steroids may be indicated

[a]By degree of presentation.

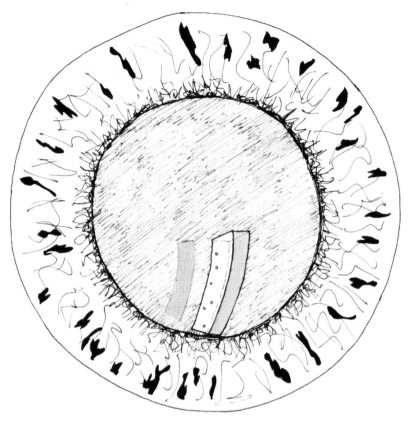

Figure 5–6.
Counting keratic precipitates

a. If synechiae unresponsive to dilation efforts (multiple dilators every 15 minutes for 1 to 2 hours), monitor patient closely during 6- to 12-week follow-up period

b. Chronic synechiae increase the risk of follow-up complications (i.e., increased IOP, recurrences)

8. RTC 48 hours upon stabilization

9. If condition is still progressive beyond 3 to 5 days, depot or oral steroids may be indicated

a. Also, reassess your diagnosis at this point (e.g., acute versus chronic, exogenous versus endogenous)

b. Consider co-management of oral steroid therapies with patient's primary physician

■ Potential complications (Table 5–13)

1. Steroid induced (iatrogenic)

a. Increased IOP (steroid responders)

b. Infectious reactions (especially HSV epithelial keratitis)

c. Posterior subcapsular cataracts (with extended or oral steroids)

2. Band keratopathy

3. Intractable synechiae (e.g., seclusio pupillae: 360°)

4. Secondary glaucomas

a. Acute (Posner–Schlossman syndrome)

b. Chronic

TABLE 5–13. ANTERIOR UVEITIS: COMPLICATIONS

Steroid induced (iatrogenic)
   Increased IOP (steroid responder)
   Infectious reactions (especially HSV epithelial keratitis)
   Posterior subcapsular cataracts
Band keratopathy
Intractable synechiae (e.g., seclusio pupillae)
Secondary glaucomas (e.g., Posner–Schlossman)
Cataracts
Chronic corneal edema
Chronic KP formations
Bullous keratopathy
Chronic cells and flare (anterior chamber and vitreous)
Posterior involvements
Optic nerve damage
Phthisis bulbi

5. Cataracts

6. Chronic corneal edema

7. Chronic KP formations

8. Bullous keratopathy

9. Chronic cells and flare (anterior chamber or vitreous)

10. Posterior changes

a. Macula edema

b. Retinal detachment

TABLE 5 – 14. ANTERIOR UVEITIS MANAGEMENT (BY AGE OF PRESENTATION)

Age at Presentation (yr)	Rate of Recurrence	Degree of Disease	Initial Therapy[a]	Follow-up Care[a] Response in Less Than 6 Weeks	Follow-up Care[a] Response in Greater Than 6 Weeks
Less than 20	First occurence	Mild	A	B	B[b]
		Moderate	C	F	B[b]
		Severe	D,B[b]	—	—
	Second occurrence	Mild	A	F	B[b]
		Moderate	C, B[b]	—	—
		Severe	D, B[b]	—	—
	Third occurrence or significant indicators	Mild	A, B[b]	—	—
		Moderate	C, B[b]	—	—
		Severe	D, B, E	—	—
From 20 to 50	First occurrence	Mild	A	F	B[b]
		Moderate	C	F	B[b]
		Severe	D	F	B, E
	Second occurrence	Mild	A	F	E
		Moderate	C	F	E
		Severe	D	F	B, E
	Third occurrence or significant indicators	Mild	A, B	F[b]	E
		Moderate	C, B[b]	—	—
		Severe	C, B, E	—	—
Greater than 50	First occurrence	Mild	A	F	B[b]
		Moderate	C	F	B[b]
		Severe	D	F	B, E
	Second occurrence	Mild	A	F	B[b]
		Moderate	C, B	F[b]	B[b]
		Severe	D, B, E	—	—
	Third occurrence or significant indicators	Mild	A, B	F[b]	B, E
		Moderate	C, B	F[b]	B, E
		Severe	D, B, E	—	—

[a]Refer to Table 5–11 for letter code.
[b]Occurrence of any progressive ocular complications at this point indicates treatment E.

11. Optic nerve damage
12. Phthisis bulbi
■ Prognosis
   1. Evaluation should be based on presentation and diagnosis (Tables 5–8 and 5–14)

   a. Degree of presentation
   b. Acute versus chronic
   c. Nature of etiologic cause (if determined)
  2. Advise, educate, and counsel patient carefully

III. Chronic Anterior Uveitis

A. GENERAL CONSIDERATIONS

  1. Terminology
    a. Granulomatous
      i. Refers to small collections of modified macrophages or histiocytes surrounded by lymphocytes (giant cells)
      ii. Associated systemic granulomatous diseases

      • Tuberculosis
      • Sarcoidosis
      • Syphilis
      • Cat scratch fever
      • Fungal infections
    b. Autoimmune
      i. Tissue injury associated with humeral or cell-mediated responses to body constituents
      ii. Hypersensitivity reactions are im-

mune responses that injure the host by four types (Table 5–15)

c. HLA

　i. On the surface of nucleated cells

　ii. Important in tissue transplantation and diagnosis of certain diseases

　iii. More than 50 diseases are directly associated with a particular HLA antigen[5]

　　• HLA-B27
　　　Ankylosing spondylitis
　　　Reiter's syndrome
　　　Crohn's disease
　　　Ulcerative colitis

　　• HLA-B5
　　　Behçet's syndrome

　　• HLA-Dw4
　　　Rheumatoid arthritis

2. Specific diagnosis of cause

　a. Made in about 10 to 12 percent of all cases

　b. Therefore, therapy is specific for only 10 to 12 percent of cases

　c. Remaining (90 percent) therapy is empiric and general

3. Diagnostic workup for cause

　a. Expensive, with literally hundreds of tests available and payoff on most limited

　b. The more common causes of anterior uveitis make up most of the 10 to 12 percent definitive diagnosed cases

　c. Most anterior uveitis looks alike, irrespective of cause

4. Pathophysiology

　a. Prostaglandins

　b. Hypersensitivity reaction (immune response)

　c. Human leukocytic antigens (HLA) related

B. CLINICAL MEDICINE

1. Preliminary systemic evaluation by primary eye practitioner before referral for complete medical workup

Subjective

- History most important part of evaluation
- Careful review of systems to illicit specific associated symptoms (including but not limited to)
  1. Joint problems
  2. Stiffness
  3. Lower back pain
  4. Past medical illnesses
  5. Family medical history
  6. Infectious conditions
  7. Urinary tract problems (e.g., infection)
  8. Trauma

Objective

- Slit-lamp examination and dilated fundus examination
- Blood tests
  1. Venereal disease, Reagan Laboratory (VDRL)
  2. Fluorescein treponema absorption (FTA-ABS)
  3. Complete blood count (CBC)
  4. WBC
  5. Electrolytes (increased calcium)
- Radiological studies
  1. Chest radiograph (x-ray)
  2. Tuberculosis
  3. Sarcoid
  4. Sacroiliac (S-I) joint film (for men)
- Skin tests: Purified protein derivative (PPD)
- Other tests
  1. Angiotensin-converting enzyme (ACE)
  2. Antinuclear antigens (ANA)
  3. Biopsy of conjunctiva
  4. Enzyme-linked immunosorbent assay (ELISA)
  5. Fixation reaction
  6. Histoplasmin complement
  7. HLA typing
  8. Rheumatoid factor
  9. Sedimentation rate
  10. Toxoplasmin dye test
  11. Kviem test

Assessment*

- Chronic nongranulomatous
  1. Exogenous
     a. Trauma
        i. Sterile inflammation following penetrat-

---

*See also Appendix 3.

TABLE 5–15. THE FOUR TYPES OF HYPERSENSITIVITY REACTIONS

Type	Manifestation	Immune Mechanism	Ocular Example
I	Immediate	IgI	Atopic iritis from allergy to shellfish
II	Cytotoxicity	IgG, IgM, ± complement	Microbial iritis involved in pathogenesis of uveitis
III	Immune complex	IgG, IgM, + complement	Autoimmune lens induced sympathetic ophthalmitis
IV	Cell mediated	Sensitized T lymphocytes	Possible chronic uveitic relationship

ing injury from small FB with resultant decomposing tissue
  ii. Secondary to viral introduction at time of intraocular injury
  b. Postsurgical
2. Endogenous
  a. Unknown (most frequent)
  b. Ocular
    i. Pars planitis
    ii. Fuch's heterochromic iridocyclitis
    iii. Posner–Schlossman glaucomatocyclitic crisis
  c. Infection
    i. Herpes simplex
    ii. Herpes zoster
    iii. Rubeola
    iv. Subacute sclerosing panencephalitis (SSPE)
  d. Systemic
    i. Reiter's syndrome
    ii. Behçet's syndrome
    iii. Arthritides
    iv. Ankylosing spondylitis
    v. JRA
    vi. Regional enteritis (Crohn's disease)
    vii. Ulcerative colitis
    viii. Whipple's disease (extremely rare)
■ Chronic granulomatous
  1. Infectious
    a. Tuberculosis (TB)
    b. Syphilis
    c. Leprosy
    d. Mycotic
    e. Parasitic
  2. Noninfectious
    a. Sarcoidosis
    b. Juvenile xanthogranuloma (JXG)
    c. Vogt–Koyanagi–Harada disease
    d. Sympathetic ophthalmitis
    e. Phacoanaphylactic

  2. Referral to physician for uveitic workup should be as specific as reasonably possible based on ocular impressions, suspicions, and preliminary systemic evaluation
    a. Consider patient's primary physician as potential coordinator of medical and laboratory workup
    b. Specialist may be consulted if no primary or family physician indicated by patient and preliminary systemic evaluation produces high index of suspicion in specific organ system or pathophysiological area (e.g., gastrointestinal, rheumatoid, infectious)
      i. Internist (internal medicine)
      ii. Rheumatologist

C. SPECIFIC DISEASES

1. Ankylosing Spondylitis
  a. Pathophysiology
    i. Chronic proliferative inflammation of joint capsules and intervertebral ligaments
    ii. Arthritic syndrome
  b. Physical
    i. Limitation of motion of lumbar spine
    ii. Lower back pain with morning stiffness
    iii. Limitation of chest expansion (late in disease)
  c. Radiology
    i. Calcification of sacroiliac joint
    ii. "Bamboo spine"
  d. Diagnosis
    i. History
    ii. Clinical examination
    iii. Males four times females in severe forms
    iv. Eighty percent HLA-B27 positive (10 percent in normal population)
  e. Treatment
    i. Steroids
    ii. Nonsteroidals
      • Indomethacin
      • Phenylbutazone
      • Sulindac
  f. Ocular
    i. Related to duration of disease: 50 percent occur after 15 years of disease
    ii. Anterior uveitis usually unilateral
  g. Course
    i. Mild cases often undiagnosed
    ii. Disease progressive in severe forms

2. Behçet's Disease
  a. Etiology
    i. Proposed viral etiology with many immunological features
    ii. Associated with HLA-B5, 70 percent of the time
  b. Epidemiology
    i. Young adults
    ii. Greater in Oriental race
    iii. Women two times more frequent than men
  c. Clinical
    i. Recurrent oral ulcerations (aphthous type)
    ii. Genital ulcerations

iii. Uveitis and cutaneous vasculitis

iv. Phlebitis

v. Aneurysms

vi. Meningoencephalitis

vii. Synovitis

d. Diagnosis

   i. Recurrent oral aphthous ulcers plus any two additional associated (above) signs

e. Treatment

   i. Steroids

   ii. Antimetabolites (e.g., chlorambucil)

   iii. No treatment is curative

f. Course

   i. Often unrelenting

   ii. Visual prognosis is poor

3. Crohn's Disease (Regional Enteritis)

a. Epidemiology

   i. Usually 20- to 30-year range

   ii. Males greater than females

b. Clinical

   i. Symptoms similar to ulcerative colitis

   ii. Relapsing granulomatous inflammatory disorder affecting any portion of GI tract

   iii. Most common site is terminal ileum or colon

c. Diagnosis

   i. History

   ii. "String sign" on barium enema

   iii. Intestinal biopsy

   iv. Must rule out ulcerative colitis

d. Treatment

   i. Medical

   • Azothriopine

   • Steroids

   ii. Surgical

   • Resection of diseased section of tract

   • Seventy percent of patients require surgery

e. Ocular

   i. Symptomatic anterior uveitis in 5 percent of cases

   ii. Symptomatic forms rare

f. Course

   i. Classically recurs and remits

   ii. Occasionally it remits permanently

   iii. Usually chronic and progressive

   iv. Complications

   • Metabolic disturbances

   • Hemorrhage

   • Perforation of tract

   • Adhesions

   • Peritonitis

   • Fistulas

   v. Unlike ulcerative colitis, Crohn's presents no increased risk for cancer

4. Fuchs' Heterochromic Iridocyclitis

a. Etiology: unknown

b. Incidence: 2 to 3 percent of all uveitis

c. Clinical

   i. Ninety percent unilateral

   ii. Syndrome

   • Recurrent chronic anterior uveitis

   • Heterochromia (loss of iris pigment)

   • Cataract

   • Glaucoma (occasionally)

d. Treatment

   i. Standard anterior uveitic therapy

   ii. Treat complications appropriately

   iii. Associated glaucomas are difficult to control

5. Glaucomatocyclitic Crisis (Posner–Schlossman Syndrome)

a. Clinical

   i. Chronic unilateral anterior uveitis with pain in young adults with marked dissociation between degree of uveitis and high IOP

b. Diagnosis

   i. Acute glaucoma

   ii. Open angles

   iii. Anterior chamber reaction

c. Treatment

   i. Topical treatment for uveitis

   ii. IOP control

d. Course

   i. Intermittent attacks of 3- to 10-day duration

   ii. Condition resolves during middle age

6. Juvenile Rheumatoid Arthritis (JRA)

a. Epidemiology

   i. Children

   ii. Females four times greater than males

b. Pathophysiology

   i. Chronic synovial inflammation

ii. Erosion of articular cartilage
c. Clinical
   i. Ocular involvement most common (30 percent) in mono- and oligoarticular types
   ii. Joints
      • Swollen, stiff, warm, and tender
      • Limited range of motion
   iii. Still's ocular triad
      • Iridocyclitis
         Seventy percent of patients reduce to 20/200 over 10 to 20 years with disease
         Eyes often remain white
      • Band keratopathy
      • Cataract
d. Diagnosis
   i. No specific test available
   ii. Some nonspecific tests
      • Rheumatoid factor
      • ANA
      • HLA typing
   iii. Rule out joint infection, malignancy, trauma, and avascular necrosis
   iv. Should have minimum of 6 weeks of chronic observed synovitis
e. Treatment
   i. Standard therapy for uveitis
   ii. Nonsteroidal anti-inflammatory agents for arthritis
f. Course
   i. Arthritis prognosis is guarded
   ii. Ocular prognosis is poor

7. Juvenile Xanthogranuloma (JXG)
a. Etiology: unknown
b. Clinical: dermatological disease in children
c. Diagnosis: biopsy
d. Ocular
   i. Anterior uveitis
   ii. Epibulbar mass
   iii. Spontaneous hyphema
e. Treatment
   i. Standard and supportive uveitic therapies
   ii. Monitor for secondary glaucoma

8. Pars Planitis[6]
a. Etiology: unknown
b. Incidence
   i. Ten percent of all uveitis
   ii. Seventy percent bilateral
c. Clinical

   i. Anterior uveitis with organization of the vitreous base
   ii. Vitreous cells and opacities (anteriorly)
   iii. Possibly cystoid macula edema
   iv. "Snowbanking"
   v. Vision may reduce to 20/40 or less
d. Treatment
   i. Standard topical therapy rarely useful
   ii. May need periocular depo injections of 40 to 80 mg Depo-Medrol steroids in more advanced cases
   iii. Sometimes oral nonsteroidal and steroids
e. Course
   i. Can remit and exacerbate
   ii. Severe cases can be unrelenting

9. Reiter's Syndrome[7]
a. Etiology
   i. Postvenereal exposure usually chlamydial
   ii. Postdysentery cause is *Shigella*
b. Clinical
   i. Triad (syndrome)
      • Arthritis (usually monoarticulate, especially knee)
      • Nongonococcal urethritis
      • Conjunctivitis
   ii. Other findings
      • Anterior uveitis
      • Circinate balanitis
      • Keratodermic blenorrhygicum
c. Diagnosis
   i. Any two of the triad warrant presumptive diagnosis for syndrome
   ii. Anterior uveitis usually present
d. Ocular
   i. Conjunctivitis or uveitis present in at least 30 percent of syndrome
   ii. Conjunctivitis may be mild and self-limiting or severe with secondary inflammatory iridocyclitis
e. Treatment
   i. Tetracycline with chlamydial urethritis
   ii. Nonsteroidal anti-inflammatory agents
f. Course
   i. Usually prolonged course of remissions and exacerbations
   ii. Occasionally resolves spontaneously

10. Rheumatoid Arthritis
a. Incidence of anterior uveitis in patients with rheumatoid arthritis (RA) parallels that of the general population
b. Uveitis not considered a specific part of disease

11. Sarcoidosis[8]
a. Etiology: unknown
b. Clinical
   i. Multisystem disorder
   ii. Granulomatous disease
   iii. Noncaseating epithelioid tubercles
   iv. Pulmonary node(s) most common
c. Diagnosis
   i. Diagnosis of exclusion
   ii. Lymph node (or tissue) biopsy (e.g., conjunctiva)
   iii. Kviem test
   iv. Hilar adenopathy on chest radiograph
d. Ocular
   i. Any part of eye or adnexa may be involved
   ii. Ocular involvement from 25 to 50 percent of cases
e. Treatment
   i. Nonsteroidals
   ii. Steroids
   iii. Antimalarial (alkylating) agents
f. Course
   i. Highly variable
   ii. If only benign hilar adenopathy, 80 percent remission rate

12. Syphilis
a. Etiology
   i. *Treponema pallidum* infection
   ii. Congenital or acquired
b. Clinical
   i. "Great mimicker" (i.e., highly variable signs and symptoms imitating many different disease conditions)
   ii. Acquired and congenital
   iii. Primary, secondary, and tertiary involvement
c. Diagnosis
   i. Clinical suspicion
   ii. FTA ABS (for inactive conditions)
   iii. FTA ABS and VDRL in active conditions
   iv. Hutchinson's triad

- Leuitic interstitial keratitis (90 percent of all interstitial keratitis)
- Notched incisor teeth
- Eighth nerve deafness
   v. May have flattened nasal bridge
d. Ocular
   i. Anterior or posterior uveitis
   ii. Interstitial keratitis
   iii. Argyll–Robertson pupil
   iv. Chorioretinitis
e. Treatment
   i. Penicillin
   ii. Steroids (oral and topical) for uveitis and interstitial keratitis
f. Course
   i. Progressive, if it is not medically treated
   ii. Often produces permanent damage and (if not treated) death

13. Tuberculosis
a. Etiology
   i. *Mycobacterium* tuberculosis
   ii. Granulomatous disease
b. Clinical
   i. Variable presentation
   ii. Pulmonary form most common
c. Diagnosis
   i. Chest radiography
   ii. PPD
   iii. Tissue biopsy characteristic of tuberculosis
d. Ocular
   i. Any portion of eye may be involved
   ii. Anterior uveitis
   iii. Phlyctenular keratoconjunctivitis
e. Treatment
   i. Systemic isoniazid
   ii. Ethambutol
   iii. Rifampin
   iv. Streptomycin

14. Ulcerative Colitis
a. Epidemiology
   i. Greater in females
   ii. Greater in whites than blacks
   iii. Familial incidence is 15 percent
b. Clinical
   i. Abdominal pain, cramping, and diarrhea
   ii. Inflammatory disease of mucosa and submucosa of the colon
   iii. Frequent relapses
   iv. Recurrence risk always present

c. Diagnosis
   i. History
   ii. Sigmoidoscopy
   iii. Barium enema
   iv. Differential considerations
      • Dysentery
      • Crohn's disease
      • Diverticulitis
      • Cancer of the colon
d. Ocular
   i. Bilateral anterior uveitis in 5 percent of cases
   ii. Colon resection cures uveitis in 20 percent of cases
   iii. Patients with accompanying arthritis have much higher incidence of anterior uveitis
e. Treatment
   i. Steroids for symptomatic relief
   ii. Colon resection for cure
f. Complications
   i. Chronic exacerbations
   ii. Colon cancer expected in 10 percent of patients with disease for 10 years or more

D. SYSTEMIC MANAGEMENT CONSIDERATIONS

1. Immediate considerations in chronic anterior uveitis
   a. Ongoing suspicion of recurrences
   b. Early recognition of recurrences
   c. Management and co-management
      i. Reinstitution of uveitic therapies
      ii. Preliminary systemic evaluation
      iii. Referral to appropriate ophthalmic or medical specialist for more extensive diagnostic evaluation
2. Long-term management considerations for the primary eye practitioner in management of chronic anterior uveitis
   a. Continued monitoring and recognition of exacerbation
   b. Prevention and maintenance of controllable and treatable complications
   c. Close monitoring and maintenance of visual needs
   d. Continued coordination of care with specialists
3. Management responsibilities of co-managing ophthalmic or medical specialist(s)
   a. Ongoing monitoring of systemic condition and any potential complications
   b. Management of immunosuppressive therapies and associated risks and complications
   c. Continued communication with patient's primary eye care practitioner

IV. Hyphema (Color Plate 86)

Background Information [9,10]

A. Accumulation of whole red blood in the anterior chamber
   1. Usually less than one third of chamber involved
   2. Most common involvement is inferior (owing to gravitational effect)

B. Contusive injury most common cause

C. Microhyphema: diffuse RBC in anterior chamber

D. "Eight-ball" hemorrhage: anterior chamber completely filled with whole red blood

E. Important clinical statistics regarding risk of hyphema (excluding microhyphema, which has low risks for glaucoma or rebleed) [11]
   1. Approximately 5 percent develop secondary glaucoma
   2. Approximately 25 percent rebleed (increasing risk of secondary glaucoma)
   3. Approximately 30 percent have temporary IOP increase during acute phase (first 5 to 7 days)
   4. Approximately 75 percent demonstrate some degree of recession or rupture of iris root (increasing risk of secondary glaucoma)

Subjective

■ Usually history of blunt trauma associated
   1. Racket sport injuries (ball or racket)
   2. Hockey injuries (puck or stick)
   3. Fists
■ More common in children (through teenage years)
■ Vision widely variable based on degree of blood
   1. May be normal (in microhyphema)
   2. May be hazy (in aqueous clouded with blood)

3. Variable degrees of reduction, depending on blood level

4. Light perception (LP) to no light perception (NLP) in "eight-ball" hemorrhage

■ Pain varies from mild to severe

   1. Relative to uveitic reaction

   2. Relative to acute IOP increases

■ Frequently an unexplainable drowsiness (somnolence) is reported or demonstrated during acute phase

   1. Especially in children

   2. Not necessarily proportional to degree of blood

   3. Produces suspicion of neurological complications, especially when hyphema is associated with head trauma

Objective*

■ Injured eyes usually have all findings associated with blunt trauma to the lids, conjunctiva, and cornea

■ Anterior chamber appearance varies with amount, position, and degree of accumulated blood

   1. Least degree is microhyphema with discrete RBC seen with slit lamp in anterior chamber

   2. Blood may produce a red haze to the aqueous with increasing amounts (but not enough for a level)

   3. Free blood clots may be seen fixed or floating in the aqueous

     a. May be seen floating anywhere in chamber, but usually greatest in inferior chamber

     b. May be fixed anywhere

       i. Iris stromal surface

       ii. Chamber angle

       iii. Corneal endothelial surface

   4. Most typically, blood accumulates inferiorly with a distinct blood level visible without instrumentation

     a. This is the superior level of the inferior blood accumulated pool (from gravitational effects on the loose RBC in the aqueous)

     b. Occasionally coagulates may produce an irregular (versus straight) line

   5. Anterior chamber completely filled with blood is called an "eight-ball" hemorrhage

     a. Ominous appearance of blackish–purplish–red anterior chamber

     b. Iris, pupil aperture, angle, and red reflex (with ophthalmoscope) are not visible

       i. Slit-lamp examination demonstrates clear or edematous cornea anterior to dense blood mass

       ii. Fundus examination (even with pupil dilation) is impossible and must be postponed

         • If posterior damage is feared (with blunt trauma), B-scan ultrasonography may be indicated

         • Foreign-body concerns may indicate ultrasonography or radiographs

     c. "Eight-ball" hemorrhages often produce small to extensive peripheral anterior synechiae after reabsorption

■ Upon resorption of major portion of blood, gonioscopy may reveal varying degrees of angle recession or rupture of the iris root

   1. Usually appears as black strip or elongated whole at base of iris (between ciliary body and trabeculum)

   2. Recession may be small (<10°) or large (up to 360°)

   3. Degree of hyphema need not be proportional to amount of recession or rupture

   4. The greater amount of recession, the greater the risk of secondary glaucoma

     a. Recessions greater than 180° pose an extremely high risk (about 75 percent) for secondary glaucoma

     b. May occur as long as 10 to 15 years after injury

     c. Thus, unilateral contusive injury (with angle recession, diagnosed or undiagnosed) should be considered the leading cause of any unilateral glaucoma at any time in life

■ IOP varies during acute phase

   1. Often (30 percent) raised dramatically (>35mm Hg) because of acute congestion from anterior chamber blood

   2. Infrequently reduced because of ciliary body hypotony

■ Pupil size, shape, and reactions may vary during acute phase

   1. Normal

   2. Corectopia (irregular shape)

   3. Sluggish or no reactions

   4. Miosis (due to accompanying uveitis)

■ Rebleeds usually occur during the first 2- to 5-day period following initial bleed (or rebleed)[12]

   1. Rebleeds are usually worse than original presenting hyphema

   2. Almost always occur before seventh day after first bleed

Assessment

■ Rule out other associated tissue damage in cases of contusion injury

■ Rule out neurological complications in cases associated with unexplained somnolence

■ In children, rule out underlying risks

   1. Juvenile xanthogranuloma (recurrent spontaneous hyphema)

   2. Retinoblastoma (microhyphema)

■ Rule out herpes simplex uveitis (usually microhyphema)

Plan

■ Reduce all ambulatory activity to a minimum

   1. Noncompliant patients should be hospitalized for 5- to 7-day period during resolution

---

*See also Appendix 2.

2. Rate of rebleeds no greater with minimal activity versus strict bed rest
3. Sedation not indicated in ambulatory patient
- Apply unilateral shield over involved eye
  1. Bilateral shielding proven to be of no value
  2. Rate of rebleeds same with unilateral or bilateral
- Have patient sleep with head raised 30° to 45°
  1. Lowers venous pressure to reduce IOP
  2. Promotes more rapid blood resorption
- Topical or oral steroids not indicated unless required for treatment of associated anterior uveitis
- Pupil dilation is optional
  1. Varied opinions on value in reducing rebleeds or enhancing resorption
  2. Atropine (0.5 percent bid) has shown some value in reducing rebleeds
- If IOP raised, use topical and oral antiglaucoma agents
  1. Anticoagulants also valuable with increased IOP
  2. Need for rapid reabsorption (to reduce angle congestion) essential
- Antifibrinolytic agents have proved useful in reducing rate of rebleeds[12] (controversial)
  1. Oral aminocaproic acid, 100 mg/kg body weight (not to exceed 30 g/day) qid for 5 days
  2. Contraindicated in renal disease
  3. May cause nausea and vomiting
- Surgical intervention should be avoided in patients with less than 50 percent hyphema or complicated cases
  1. Corneal blood staining
  2. "Eight-ball" (total) hyphema lasting longer than 7 days with normal IOP, or
     a. After 6 days if IOP exceeds 25 mm Hg or
     b. After 5 days if IOP exceeds 50 mm Hg

Follow-up

- Patient must be seen daily for close monitoring during first 5 to 7 days
  1. Visual acuities
2. Slit-lamp examination
3. IOP by applanation tonometry
4. Monitoring of corneal clarity (regarding blood staining)
5. Size of hyphema
6. Compliance with instructions (regarding activities)
- Rebleeds will almost always occur before seventh day
  1. Upon rebleed, all management steps must be reinstituted as from day number 1
  2. Prognosis with rebleeds worsens (e.g., regarding risk of secondary glaucoma, corneal blood staining)
- Corneal blood staining is produced by entrance of hemoglobin and hemosiderin into corneal stroma
  1. Primary causes
     a. Duration of blood exposure 6 to 7 days or more
     b. Greater than 50 percent hyphema (of anterior chamber)
     c. Corneal endothelial defect(s)
     d. Increased IOP (drives blood into stroma)
  2. Staining may (or may not) clear within months to years
     a. Often a residual posterior corneal line results (at site of blood level)
     b. Most resultants corneal stains are mild
     c. Greater at periphery
- Optic atrophy may result from severe acute or uncontrolled secondary glaucomas
- Generally, most mild hyphemas run a 5- to 7-day course and resolve without complications
  1. More severe involvements (e.g., >50 percent, rebleeds) may produce permanent damage and ongoing glaucoma problems
  2. All (mild through severe) hyphemas should be managed as lifelong risk factors for glaucoma
     a. IOP in involved eye may rise any time in life
     b. Advise patient and recheck annually

V. Iris and Ciliary Body Abnormalities*†

A. ANGLE RECESSION

Refer to "Hyphema" in this chapter, under "Objective, part C" of the SOAP section

B. ANIRIDIA

1. Congenital absence of iris or small 360° stump of iris base
2. Usually associated with other congenital anomalies

   a. Sensory nystagmus
   b. Lens opacities and dislocations
   c. Retinopathies
   d. Mental retardation
   e. Neurological disorders
3. Visual prognosis usually poor
4. Best diagnosed by slit lamp and gonioscopy
5. Increased risks
   a. Corneal pannus
   b. Secondary glaucoma
6. May be associated with Wilms' tumor (Miller's syndrome)

---

*In alphabetical order.
†See also Appendix 2.

7. Condition generally produces difficult management problems

C. ATROPHIES (Color Plate 87)

1. Aging
a. Thinning of iris stroma with flattening of architecture
   i. Disappearance of crypts (especially at pupillary zone)
   ii. Sphincter becomes more visible (brownish)
   iii. Pupillary ruff appears eroded
b. Miosis and pupillary immobility often present

2. Essential Iris Atrophy
a. Usually white females at 30 to 40 years of age
b. Unilateral condition
c. Development of through-and-through iris holes (pseudopolycoria)
d. Progresses over a 1- to 3-year period
e. Pupil distortion and displacement caused by peripheral anterior synechiae
f. Complications
   i. Secondary glaucoma
   ii. Corneal edema
   iii. Pain
   iv. Reduced vision
g. Mimics Chandler's syndrome
   i. Corneal endothelial changes
   ii. Iris atrophy
   iii. Milder glaucoma

3. Iridoschisis
a. Bilateral in patients over 65 years of age

b. Anterior iris stroma splits into fibers (with associated blood vessels versus persistent pupillary membranes), with one end remaining attached to iris and other floating freely in anterior chamber ("shredded wheat" appearance)
c. Significant (50 percent) risk of primary angle closure glaucoma
d. Monitor closely

4. Secondary Atrophies
a. Glaucomatous
b. Ischemic
c. Neurogenic (syphilitic)
d. Postinflammatory
e. Posttraumatic

D. COLOBOMA

1. Autosomal-dominant hereditary trait
2. Unilateral or bilateral incomplete closure (cleft)
3. Keyhole pupil (down to ciliary body) at inferior 6 o'clock position (slightly medialward)
4. May be associated with other colobomas
   a. Choroid
   b. Retina
   c. Optic nerve

E. CONFIGURATIONS OF THE IRIS

1. Iris Bombé (Fig. 5–7)
a. Iris bowed anteriorward from posterior 360° synechiae at pupillary border
b. Usually secondary to anterior segment inflammation
c. Results in secondary glaucoma

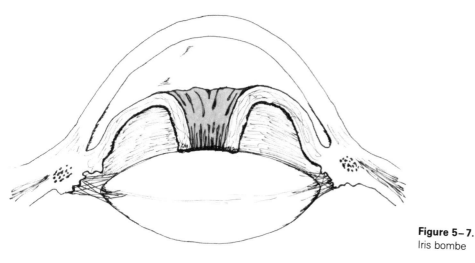

Figure 5–7.
Iris bombe

2. **Corectopia**
   a. Irregularly shaped pupil(s)
   b. Variable causes

3. **Plateau Iris (Fig. 5–8)**
   a. Anterior insertion of iris on ciliary body with deep anterior chamber
   b. Slight increased risk of angle closure

4. **Polycoria**
   a. Multiple pupillary apertures within single iris
   b. Variable causes

F. CYSTS[13]

1. Uncommon, multiple cysts of iris or ciliary body
2. Produce "bumpy," irregular peripheral iris surface or abrupt, localized bulge(s)
3. May block trabeculum and raise IOP
4. Pupil dilates normally (versus masses)
5. Best viewed through gonioscopy
6. Treatable with laser therapy and iridectomy
7. Cysts may be secondary
   a. Intraocular surgery
   b. Pharmaceutical agents (e.g., phospholine iodide)

G. IRIDOCYCLITIS

Refer to Anterior Uveitis (Chapter 5, section II)

H. IRIDODIALYSIS

1. Disinsertion of iris base from ciliary body
2. Produces irregular iris configurations and pseudopolycoria
3. Common in large hyphemas
4. Increased risk of glaucoma
5. No treatment indicated in absence of symptoms (e.g., diplopia)

I. IRIDODONESIS

1. Tremulous (quivering or shakey) iris
2. Multiple causes
   a. Rupture of zonules
   b. Dislocation of crystalline lens
   c. Marfan's syndrome
   d. Megalocornea

J. IRIDOSCHISIS

Refer to Atrophies

K. IRITIS

Refer to Anterior Uveitis (Chapter 5, section II)

L. MASSES AND NEOPLASIAS (Color Plate 88)

1. Amyloidosis
2. Brushfeld's spots (e.g., Downs' syndrome)[14]
3. Granulomas
4. Hemangiomas
5. Iris nevus (Cogan–Reese) syndrome
6. Juvenile xanthogranuloma (nevoxanthoendothelioma)
7. Leiomyoma (neoplastic)
8. Leukemia (neoplastic)[15]
9. Lymphoma (neoplastic)
10. Medulloepitheliomas
11. Melanomas (neoplastic)
12. Metastatic tumors (neoplastic)
13. Neurilemmomas

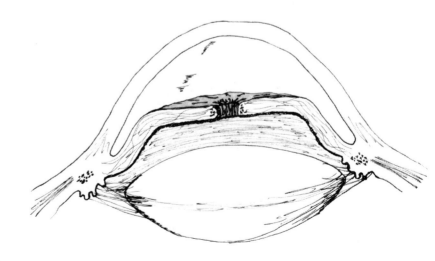

Figure 5–8.
Plateau iris

14. Neurofibromas
15. Nevi (iris freckles)[16]
16. Reactive lymphoid hyperplasia
17. Reticulum cell sarcoma (neoplastic)
18. Retinoblastoma (neoplastic)

M. PERSISTENT PUPILLARY MEMBRANE(S) OR REMNANT(S) (Color Plate 89)

1. Fine avascular threads, often pigmented (less than iris stroma)
2. May be single threads, branched, or meshwork
3. One end attached to iris collarette and other end loose or attached to pupil, iris stroma (elsewhere), or anterior lens capsule
4. Rather common (especially in children)
5. May break with pupil dilation (pharmaceutically induced or natural), trauma, spontaneously, and so forth; disappear or persist
6. No treatment indicated
7. No increased risks

N. PIGMENTATION VARIATIONS*

1. **Albinism**
   a. Oculocutaneous albinism
      i. Sex-linked recessive trait (female carrier, males affected)
      ii. Normal skin and hair pigmentation
      iii. Deficient ocular pigmentations with iris transillumination defects
      iv. Poor visual acuity
   b. Tyrosinase-negative oculocutaneous albinism
      i. Complete pigment deficiency (skin, hair, and eyes)
      ii. Marked iris transillumination defects
      iii. Poor visual prognosis
         • Serious visual reduction
         • Nystagmus
         • High myopia
         • Severe photophobia
   c. Tyrosinase-positive oculocutaneous albinism
      i. Milder form of complete albinism
      ii. Skin, hair, and eyes have mild pigmentation that may increase with age

   iii. Visual prognosis is better than negative form

2. **Heterochromia (Variations in Pigmentation)**
   a. Irregular unilateral or bilateral distribution
   b. Occasional wedge-shaped sectors of hyper- or hypopigmentation
   c. "Heterochromia iridum": condition in which the pigment of one iris is completely different from that of the opposite iris
   d. Pathological causes
      i. Fuch's heterochromic iridocyclitis
      ii. Intraocular foreign-body hemosiderosis
      iii. Intraocular neoplasias

3. **Nevus (Iris Freckle)**
   a. Hyperpigmented spot on iris stroma
   b. May be flat or raised
   c. Creates no distortions to iris architecture, pupil or upon pupil dilation (versus melanoma)
   d. Slight increased risk of melanoma (iris or choroid)
   e. Monitor for changes and photodocument (if possible)
   f. No treatment indicated

O. RUBEOSIS IRIDIS[17,18] (Color Plate 90)

1. Proliferation of neovascular network on anterior surface of iris and anterior chamber angle
2. Circumferential pattern with greatest concentration of vessels at pupillary zone and angle
3. Leads to fibrovascular peripheral anterior synechiae secondary glaucoma (resistant to treatment)
4. Multiple causes
   a. Diabetes mellitus
   b. Ocular inflammation
   c. Intraocular tumors (with necrosis)
   d. Neovascular glaucoma
   e. Vascular occlusive disease

P. TRAUMA†

1. Produced by direct, contrecoup, or contusive injuries

---

*Little to no iris pigmentation = "blue eyes." Increasing iris pigmentation = "green" to "hazel" to "brown" eyes.

†See specific clinical entities.

2. Clinical results of trauma to iris and ciliary body
   a. Angle recession
   b. Cyclodialysis
   c. Hyphema
   d. Iridodialysis
   e. Iridoschisis

f. Iritis
g. Pigmentary disturbances
h. Sphincter pupillae rupture (miosis or mydriasis)
i. Vossius ring (pigment on anterior lens capsule)

VI. Self-assessment Questions

1. The leading cause of uveitis according to most authorities is:
   a. Infection
   b. HLA diseases
   c. Unknown
   d. Sarcoid

2. Acute anterior uveitis should respond to standard nonspecific therapies in:
   a. Less than 6 weeks
   b. Greater than 6 weeks
   c. From 6 to 12 weeks
   d. Greater than 12 weeks

3. Which of the following considerations is *not* a significant diagnostic indicator in chronic uveitis?
   a. Recurrence
   b. Vision
   c. Bilaterality
   d. Systemic disease

4. The most prominent subjective symptoms associated with acute anterior uveitis include all of the following, *except*:
   a. Deep, aching pain
   b. Photophobia
   c. "Hazy" vision
   d. Foreign-body sensation

5. The most prominent objective findings associated with acute anterior uveitis include all of the following, *except*:
   a. Mucoid discharge
   b. Circumcorneal flush
   c. Cells and flare
   d. Fine keratic precipitates

You have diagnosed a second recurrence of a 2 to 3+ acute anterior uveitis in a 30-year-old man:

6. Immediate care should include all of the following steps, *except*:
   a. Detailed patient interview

   b. Complete medical and laboratory evaluation
   c. Topical therapies
   d. Palliative (symptomatic) care

7. Topical therapies might include all of the following, *except*:
   a. Homatropine
   b. Predisolone
   c. Fluorometholone (FML)
   d. Atropine

8. Palliative care might include any of the following, *except*:
   a. Decongestants (topical and oral)
   b. Oral aspirin or ibuprofen
   c. Warm compresses
   d. Dark glasses

9. Recommended dosage for topical medications should be
   a. hs (at bedtime)
   b. tid
   c. bid
   d. q2–4h

10. Your patient should be rechecked:
    a. In 1 week
    b. In 3 to 5 days
    c. In 24 to 48 hours
    d. By a specialist

Select the systemic manifestation in column B most closely associated with the uveitic related disease in column A

Column A	Column B
11. Ankylosing spondylitis	a. Glaucoma
12. Juvenile rheumatoid arthritis (JRA)	b. Nongonococcal urethritis
13. Reiter's syndrome	c. Positive FTA-ABS
14. Crohn's disease	d. Fever, sore throat, and lymphadenopathy
15. Sarcoidosis	e. Lower back pain
16. Behçet's disease	f. Cramping and diarrhea
	g. Vitiligo

Column A
17. Posner–Schlossman syndrome
18. Syphilis
19. Vogt–Koyanagi–Harada syndrome
20. Mononucleosis

Column B
h. Aphthous mouth ulcers
i. Positive chest radiograph
j. Still's triad

For answers, refer to Appendix 6

REFERENCES

1. Henderly DE, Genstler AJ, Smith RE, et al: Changing patterns of uveitis. Am J Ophthalmol 103:131, 1987
2. Rothova A, van Veenendaal WG, Linssen A, et al: Clinical features of acute anterior uveitis. Am J Ophthalmol 103:13, 1987
3. An Y-K, Henkind P: Pain elicited by consensual pupillary reflex: A diagnostic test for acute iritis. Lancet 2:1254, 1981
4. March WF, Coniglione TC: Ibuprofen in the treatment of uveitis. Am J Ophthalmol 17:103, 1985
5. Wakefield D, Easter J, Robinson P, et al: Immunological features of HLA-B27 anterior uveitis. Inst J Ophthalmol 11:15, 1983
6. Henderly DE: Par planitis. Trans Ophthalmol Soc UK 105:227, 1986
7. Lee DA, Barker SM, Su WP, et al: The clinical diagnosis of Reiter's syndrome. Ophthalmol 93:350, 1986
8. Jabs DA, Johns CJ: Ocular involvement in chronic sarcoidosis. Am J Ophthalmol 102:297, 1986
9. Trouch ERJ: Traumatic hyphema. J Pediatr Ophthalmol 23:95, 1986
10. Canavan YM, Archer DB: Anterior segment consequences of blunt ocular trauma. Br J Ophthalmol 66:549, 1982
11. Witteman GJ, Brubaker SJ, Johnson M, et al: The incidence of rebleeding in traumatic hyphema. An Ophthalmol 17:525, 1985
12. Trouch ERJ: Traumatic hyphema. J Pediatr Ophthalmol 23:95, 1986
13. Waeltermann JM, Mettinger ME, Cibis GW: Congenital cysts of the iris stroma. Am J Ophthalmol 100:549, 1985
14. Shapiro MB, France TD: Ocular features of Down's syndrome. Am J Ophthamol 99:659, 1985
15. Kincaid MC, Green WH: Ocular and orbital involvement in leukemia. Surv Ophthalmol 27:4:211, 1983
16. Kliman GJ, Augsburger JJ, Shields JA: Association between iris color and iris melanocytic lesions. Am J Ophthalmol 100:547, 1985
17. Gartner S, Henkind P: Neovascularization of the iris (rubeosis iridis). Surv Ophthalmol 22:291, 1978
18. Tauber J, Lahau M, Erzurum SA: New clinical classification for iris neovascularization. Ophthalmol 94:542, 1987

ANNOTATED REFERENCES

Duane DD, Jaeger EA (eds): Clinical Ophthalmology, Vol IV: External Disease. Philadelphia, Harper & Row, 1987
Chapters by most prominent uveitic experts on standard approaches and new methods of care regarding diseases of the uvea, including anterior uveitis and hyphema.

Duke-Elder WS: Diseases of the Uveal Tract. Systems of Ophthalmology, Vol IX, part II. St. Louis, CV Mosby, 1975
Most comprehensive work on all congenital developmental, anomalous and disease entities of the uveal tract. Essential for understanding of uveitis and other anterior chamber, iris and ciliary body abnormalities.

Kraus-Mackiw E, O'Connor GR: Uveitis, Pathophysiology and Therapy. New York, Thieme–Stratton, 1983
Limited clinical applications, but comprehensive approach to basis and understanding of uveitic involvements.

Schlaegal TF (ed): Current aspects of uveitis, in International Ophthalmology Clinics. Boston, Little, Brown, 1977
Classical work by the pre-eminent authority on uveitis. Comprehensive in most areas and valuable for understanding of the disease process and care.

Smith RE, Nozik RA: Uveitis: A Clinical Approach to Diagnosis and Management. Baltimore, Williams & Wilkins, 1984
Totally clinical approach to uveitic disease. Covers all aspects of workup, differential diagnosis, and care in the most comprehensive and clinical manner of any other text.

6

Systemic Considerations in Anterior Segment Care: Diagnostic Entities by Medical Specialties and Classifications

Chapter Outline

I. **Cardiology**
   A. Marfan's syndrome
   B. Subacute bacterial endocarditis
II. **Dermatology**
   A. Acne rosacea
   B. Allergic contact dermatitis
   C. Basal cell epithelioma
   D. Herpes zoster (varicella virus)
   E. Molluscum contagiosum
   F. Nevus of Ota
   G. Psoriasis
   H. Stevens–Johnson syndrome
III. **Endocrinology**
   A. Diabetes mellitus
   B. Hyperparathyroidism
   C. Hyperthyroidism (Graves' disease)
   D. Hypoparathyroidism
   E. Hypothyroidism
IV. **Gastroenterology**
   A. Crohn's disease (regional enteritis)
   B. Ulcerative colitis
   C. Wilson's disease
V. **Hematology**
   A. Anemias
   B. Polycythemia
   C. Sickle cell anemia
VI. **Infectious disease**
   A. Cat-scratch disease
   B. Sexually transmitted diseases
   C. Sinusitis
VII. **Nephrology**
   A. Cystinosis
   B. Nephrotic syndrome
   C. Uremia
   D. Post-transplant

   E. Wilms' tumor
VIII. **Neurology**
   A. Myasthenia gravis
   B. Temporal arteritis (cranial or giant cell arteritis)
IX. **Oncology**
   A. Breast cancer
   B. Bronchogenic (lung) cancer
   C. Metastatic neoplasm
   D. Multiple myeloma
   E. Primary neoplasm
X. **Pediatrics**
   A. Chickenpox
   B. Galactosemia
   C. Kawasaki's disease
   D. Mumps
XI. **Rheumatology**
   A. Ankylosing spondylitis
   B. Gout
   C. Reiter's syndrome
   D. Rheumatoid arthritis
   E. Sarcoidosis
   F. Sjögren's syndrome
XII. **Trauma**
   A. Head injury
XIII. **"Top 100" Systemic Diagnoses Related to Anterior Segment Care**
   A. "Top 100" specific diagnoses
   B. "Top 100" diagnoses by pathological classification
   C. "Top 100" diagnoses by ocular anatomical classification
XIV. **Self-assessment Questions**
References

I. Cardiology

A. MARFAN'S SYNDROME (Color Plate 91)

1. Etiology and pathogenesis
   a. Autosomal-dominant with variable expression
   b. Defective formation of collagen and elastic fibers
   c. May occur sporadically as mutation
2. Physical findings
   a. Skeletal
      i. Slender, elongated habitus
      ii. Long arms, legs, fingers
      iii. High arched palate
      iv. Hyperextensible joints
   b. Cardiac
      i. Floppy heart valves
      ii. Aneurysmal dilation
      iii. Dissecting aneurysm
   c. Ocular
      i. Ectopic lentis superotemporally
      ii. Segmental hypoplasia of iris
      iii. Fetal anterior chamber angle
      iv. Zonular lysis
      v. Blue sclera
3. Laboratory test
   a. Urinary excretion of hydroxyproline
   b. Differentiate from homocystinuria
4. Clinical course
   a. May survive to age 70
   b. Average age of death 30 to 40, attributable to aortic rupture

B. SUBACUTE BACTERIAL ENDOCARDITIS

1. Epidemiology
   a. Occurs on damaged heart valves, as in rheumatic heart disease or congenital heart disease
   b. Artificial valves
   c. Intravenous (IV) drug abusers
2. Etiology and pathogenesis
   a. *Streptococcus viridens* infection of a previously damaged heart valve in presence of turublent blood flow
3. Symptomatology
   a. Fever, night sweats, malaise, fatigue, backache, myalgia, arthralgia
   b. Symptoms for weeks or months
   c. Often responsible for fevers of unknown origin (FUO)
4. Physical findings
   a. Roth spot hemorrhage of retina or conjunctiva
   b. Osler's nodes: raised tender lesions on pads of fingers
   c. Janeway lesions: hemorrhagic lesions of palms or soles
   d. New or changing cardiac murmur
   e. Pale skin, splenomegaly
5. Diagnostic tests
   a. Blood cultures, echocardiogram
   b. Increased erythrocyte sedimentation rate (ESR), leukocytosis, anemia
   c. Cardiac ultrasound
6. Treatment
   a. Antibiotics: prolonged IV therapy 4 to 6 weeks
   b. Prophylaxis: patients with acquired valve disorder or artificial valves should take antibiotics prior to any surgical manipulation (i.e., dental work)
7. Clinical course
   a. Untreated, it is usually fatal
   b. Usual cause of death in treated cases is congestive heart failure
   c. Cardiac valve destruction
   d. Renal damage
   e. Hemiplegia or other embolic phenomena 25 percent

II. Dermatology

A. ACNE ROSACEA[1] (Color Plates 68 and 92)

1. Epidemiology
   a. Approximately 60 percent female 30 to 60 years old
   b. More common with alcoholics, high carbohydrate intake, and hyperchlorhydria
   c. Approximately 20 percent of patients have ocular findings
   d. Approximately 4 percent keratitis

2. Symtomatology
   a. Transient attacks of flushing of the nose and cheeks occur initially
   b. Variable ocular (lids and eye) involvement
3. Physical findings
   a. Mid-face: chronic congestion of capillaries, telangiectasis, sebaceous gland hypertrophy, rhinophyma of nose
   b. Red areas of malar region with blepharitis, keratitis, conjunctivitis
4. Treatment
   a. Tetracycline (TCN) orally to decrease propionibacteria and free fatty acid (FFA)
   b. Balanced nutrition
   c. Cleansing and drying preparations
   d. Penetrating keratoplasty, if severe keratitis
5. Clinical course
   a. Approximately 25 percent recur soon after TCN stopped
   b. Approximately 50 percent recur within 6 months of stopping TCN
   c. Approximately 20 percent long-term remission
6. Anterior segment manifestations
   a. Blepharoconjunctivitis: thickened vascularized lids
   b. Keratitis: marginal vascular infiltration followed by subepi-infiltrates that ulcerate and progress centrally
   c. Recurrent chalazia secondary to superimposed staphylococcal infection

B. ALLERGIC CONTACT DERMATITIS

1. Etiology
   a. Local allergic reaction to a caustic agent
   b. Frequent lid involvement secondary to makeup or rubbing the eyes with contaminated fingers
2. Physical findings: Classic signs of inflammation (redness, swelling, warmth)
3. Diagnosis
   a. Inspection
   b. History
4. Treatment
   a. Removal of caustic agent
   b. Topical steroid
   c. Benadryl for itching

C. BASAL CELL EPITHELIOMA[2]

1. Epidemiology
   a. Most common malignancy of eyelid, 20 to 40 times more common than squamous cell
   b. Sun-exposed skin
   c. Lower lid more frequently than upper
   d. Light-skinned patients most often affected
   e. Usually over 40 years of age
2. Etiology and pathogenesis
   a. Excessive exposure to ultraviolet (UV) irradiation from sunlight
   b. Cumulative throughout life
3. Physical findings
   a. Painless, indurated, firm, pearly nodule, with heaped-up telangiectatic border
   b. Ulceration may or may not be present
   c. Less than 2 cm in diameter
   d. Multiple sites
   e. Individual lesions may vary greatly from classic lesions
4. Diagnostic tests
   a. Inspection
   b. Excisional biopsy, confirmation by microscopy
5. Treatment
   a. Excision most frequently
   b. Chemosurgery and lasers
   c. Topical fluorouracil
6. Clinical course
   a. Incapable of metastasis but recurs if incompletely excised
   b. Morpheoform rare but aggressive

D. HERPES ZOSTER (VARICELLA VIRUS)[3] (Color Plate 93)

1. Etiology
   a. Herpesvirus
   b. Curetting core usually a benign self-limited disease
   c. However may be debilitating, even fatal
2. Underlying causes
   a. Immunosuppression secondary to steroids, chemotherapy
   b. Patient with a malignancy (e.g., lymphoma)
3. Physical findings
   a. Rash of vesicles on an erythematous base in a dermatomic distribution
   b. Thoracic: 70 percent
   c. Trigeminal: 25 percent
   d. Rash is characteristic, but hallmark is pain
4. Clinical course
   a. Ocular (globe) involvement >50 per-

cent or variable when tip of nose involved (Hutchinson's sign)
   b. Postherpetic neuralgia: subsides in 6 months but may last years
      i. Painful
      ii. Has caused patients to commit suicide
   c. Vesicles, conjunctivitis, keritis, uveitis, secondary glaucoma, anything!
5. Treatment
   a. Isolation from immunosuppressed patients
   b. Prednisone: 100 mg PO, for 1 week
   c. Acyclovir: 400 mg 5×/day for 10 days (controversial)

E. MOLLUSCUM CONTAGIOSUM

1. Etiology
   a. Viral infection that causes a skin growth
   b. Sometimes confused with basal cell carcinoma or papilloma
   c. Can lead to chronic unilateral conjunctivitis
2. Diagnosis
   a. Inspection
   b. Biopsy
3. Treatment
   a. Surgical removal
   b. Curette out central core during active phase

F. NEVUS OF OTA

1. Epidemiology
   a. Common in Orientals, no risk of malignancy
   b. Rare in Caucasians; malignancy reported only with whites: uveal melanoma
   c. Melanosis oculi: when only eye is involved
2. Etiology/pathogenesis
   a. Hyperpigmentation
   b. A type of blue nevus
3. Symptomatology
   a. Asymptomatic
   b. Cosmetic concern
4. Physical findings
   a. Usually unilateral
   b. Blue hyperpigmentation of sclera, conjunctiva, and skin in the distribution of the ophthalmic and maxillary divisions of the trigeminal nerve
5. Course: benign

G. PSORIASIS (Color Plate 94)

1. Epidemiology
   a. Two percent of adult white population, uncommon in blacks
   b. Hereditary in 30 percent of cases
   c. Onset 10 to 50 years of age
   d. Thirty percent have positive family history
2. Symptomatology
   a. Twenty percent of patients symptomatic
   b. Painful at times, most lesions asymptomatic
   c. Mono- and polyarticular pain, tenderness, and morning stiffness
3. Physical findings
   a. Sharply demarcated red plaques covered with silvery scales
   b. Location: scalp, elbows, knees, back, buttocks
   c. Removal of scales; multiple punctate bleeding points: Auspitz sign
   d. Pitting of nail surface
   e. Ocular psoriatic blepharitis produces yellowish red plaques on conjunctiva with neovascularized marginal keratitis
4. Diagnostic tests
   a. Clinical appearance
   b. Biopsy of confusing cases
   c. Increased ESR
   d. Hyperuricemia, +rheumatoid factor (RF)
5. Treatment
   a. Topical steroids, coal tar
   b. Systemic steroids in severe cases
   c. Methotrexate in severest forms
   d. Phototherapy PUVA*
      i. Dermatologist may refer for eye consultation prior to treatment for baseline lens evaluation
      ii. Periodic monitoring during treatment course (months) also advisable
6. Clinical course
   a. Exacerbation and remissions
   b. Can be disabling (with arthritis)
   c. Koebner reaction: lesions appear in areas of epidermal injury, beltline typical

---

*Psoralen plus ultraviolet light of "A" wavelength.

H. STEVENS–JOHNSON SYNDROME

1. Epidemiology
   a. Most frequent in young adult men, recurrences yearly in spring or fall for 2 to 3 weeks duration
   b. Fifty percent have ocular involvement
2. Etiology and pathogenesis
   a. Reactive to drugs, infections, visceral malignancy, keralytic gel, or food allergic reactions
   b. Autoimmune, infectious, and allergic mechanisms have been implicated
   c. Associated with sulfa drugs frequently; beware of glaucoma patients on Diamox (sulfa derivative)
3. Symptomatology
   a. Prodromal symptoms: fever, malaise, headache, upper respiratory infection (URI) symptoms
   b. Bullous eruptions of skin and mucous membranes
4. Physical findings
   a. Target lesion: red with clear center: characteristic lesion
   b. Macules, papules, vesicles, and bullae on extremities
   c. Mucous membrane lesions: oral, pharynx, larynx, esophagus, trachea, bronchi
   d. Ocular
      i. Conjunctivitis: pseudo- or membranous
      ii. Corneal ulceration
      iii. Symblepharon
      iv. Entropia
      v. Destruction of goblet cells and lacrimal punctae
      vi. Keratitis sicca syndrome
      vii. Necrosis and purulent inflammatory reactions
5. Diagnostic tests
   a. Clinical appearance
   b. Keratitis sicca testing
6. Treatment
   a. Supportive
      i. Compresses
      ii. Colloid baths
      iii. Ointments
      iv. Vitamin A (topical)
   b. Systemic steroids
   c. Correction of electrolyte imbalances
7. Clinical course
   a. Mortality 20 percent without steroid treatment
   b. Erythema multiforme is minor form, only involving skin

III. Endocrinology

A. DIABETES MELLITUS[4]

1. Epidemiology
   a. Five million diabetics in United States (second leading cause of blindness in U.S.)
   b. Appears at any age
   c. Prevalence increases with each decade; 10 percent of population by age 70
   d. Rapidly increasing in gene pool
2. Etiology and pathogenesis
   a. Disease of insufficient insulin action secondary to either not enough insulin or peripheral resistance to insulin
   b. Genetics
      i. Type 1: Insulin-dependent diabetes mellitus (IDDM), or juvenile-onset diabetes, is not hereditary; persons have their disease much longer before development of diabetic retinopathy but, when it comes, it is severe
      ii. Type 2: Non-insulin-dependent diabetes mellitus (NIDDM), or adult-onset diabetes, has more hereditary pattern; persons have their disease over a shorter time period before development of retinopathy, usually not as severe
3. Symptomatology
   a. Polyuria, polydipsia, polyphagia
   b. Blurred vision, weight loss, fatigue
   c. Slow healing
   d. Women: *Monilia* vaginitis
   e. Refractive fluctuation
      i. Increased minus
      ii. Decreased plus
4. Physical findings
   a. Affects all organs and systems, sec-

ondary to metabolic or vascular involvement
  b. Basement membrane thickening
  c. Microangiopathy
5. Diagnostic tests
  a. Elevated serum glucose (hyperglycemia)
  b. Glycosuria
  c. Glucose tolerance test (GTT), fasting blood sugar (FBS), 2 hour postprandial
6. Treatment
  a. Diet control, weight reduction
  b. Oral therapy with sulfonylureas (i.e., tolbutamide)
  c. Insulin injections, NPH or regular
    i. Primarily for type I
    ii. Sometimes in type II
7. Clinical course
  a. Atherosclerosis: 50 percent of adult onset die from coronary disease
  b. Renal failure: leading cause of death in juvenile diabetes
  c. Neuropathy
    i. Most common
    ii. Bilateral symmetric sensory impairment in lower extremities
  d. Retinopathy, at same time as glomerulonecrosis of kidneys
  e. Cerebrovascular accident (CVA), myocardial ischemia (MI), gangrene
  f. Ketoacidosis (always a threat)
  g. Shortens life expectancy by 8 to 10 years

B. HYPERPARATHYROIDISM

1. Etiology and pathogenesis
  a. Excessive production of parathormone usually due to parathyroid adenoma
  b. Sometimes by ectopic production from cancer of lung or kidney
2. Symptomatology
  a. Nonspecific due to hypercalcemia
    i. Malaise
    ii. Fatigue
    iii. Headache
    iv. Diffuse aches and pains
  b. Polyuria and obstructive uropathy from nephrolithiasis
  c. Nausea, anorexia, vomiting
3. Diagnostic tests
  a. Elevated blood levels of calcium, uric acid, and parathormone
  b. Decreased serum phosphate

  c. Increased urine calcium and phosphate
  d. Radiographic findings of bone cortex reabsorption
4. Treatment
  a. Surgical exploration
  b. Removal of parathyroid adenoma
5. Clinical course
  a. The disease of "bones, stones, abdominal groans, and psychic moans"
  b. Peptic ulcer disease, gout, hypertension, osteitis fibrosa cystica, renal stones
6. Anterior segment manifestations
  a. Band keratopathy of Bowman's layer
  b. Limited to intrapalpebral area

C. HYPERTHYROIDISM (GRAVES' DISEASE)[5]

1. Epidemiology
  a. Female to male ratio: 7:1
  b. Young to middle age
  c. Marked familial pattern
  d. Approximately 50 percent of Graves' patients have ophthalmic signs
  e. Approximately 10 percent have infiltrative ocular signs
  f. Approximately 20 percent with infiltrative ophthalmopathy are euthyroid
2. Etiology/pathogenesis
  a. Thyroid-stimulating immunoglobulins (TSI) in the blood
    i. LATS (long-acting thyroid stimulator)
    ii. LATS protector
  b. Exophthalmos-producing substance
3. Symptomatology
  a. Nervousness, restless overactivity, tremor, palpitation
  b. Sensitivity to heat, sweating, weight loss
  c. Occasionally headache, nausea, diarrhea
4. Physical findings
  a. Diffuse goiter
  b. Infiltrative ophthalmopathy
  c. Infiltrative dermopathy (pretibial myxedema, reddish nodules on anterior surface of lower legs)
  d. Thyroid acropachy (a form of clubbing of the digits)
  e. Smooth skin, tachycardia
5. Diagnostic tests
  a. Radioimmunoassay (RIA) tests
    i. Triiodothyronine (T3), thyroxine

(T4), free T3, free T4, thyroid-stimulating hormone (TSH)

    ii. Usually T3 and T4 increased, TSH decreased

  b. Ninety percent of euthyroid Graves' patients positive to T3-suppression test

6. Treatment

  a. Hyperthyroidism

    i. Thyroidectomy

    ii. Radioactive iodine

    iii. Antithyroid drug therapy: propylthiouracil

  b. Ocular complications, treated as warranted

  c. In general, treatment palliative

7. Clinical course

  a. Highly variable

  b. Continuously present

  c. Intermittent flareup or even spontaneous hypothyroidism

  d. Ocular proptosis not affected by thyroid treatment

  e. Heart failure may develop

8. Anterior segment manifestations

  a. Most common cause of unilateral and bilateral proptosis

  b. Thickened extraocular muscles

  c. Exposure keratitis

D. HYPOPARATHYROIDISM

1. Etiology and pathogenesis

  a. Iatrogenic: when parathyroids are removed during thyroid surgery

  b. Congenital: DiGeorge's syndrome

  c. Caused by severe magnesium deficiency

2. Symptomatology

  a. Relates to hypocalcemia: tingling in lips, fingers

  b. Cramps, spasm, tonic contraction of any muscle

3. Physical findings

  a. Chovstek's sign: tap facial nerve at zygomatic arch; watch involuntary contractions of orbicularis oris muscle

  b. Trousseau's sign: tetany of hand following 2 minutes of upper arm constriction with sphygmomanometer (above systolic pressure)

4. Diagnostic tests

  a. Serum tests: low Ca, high P, normal alkaline phosphatase

  b. No urine Ca

  c. Radiographs show increased bone density

5. Treatment

  a. Supplemental calcium salts

  b. Vitamin D analogues: 50,000 to 150,000 IU/day

6. Anterior segment manifestations

  a. Cataracts: tetanic (lamellar) in children, subcapsular in adults

  b. Progressive superficial keratitis with opacification and superficial vascularization, in idiopathic type

E. HYPOTHYROIDISM

1. Epidemiology

  a. Most common cause: Hashimoto's thyroiditis, in women aged 20 to 50 years

  b. Secondary to thyroid surgery or radioiodine (^{131}I) therapy

2. Etiology/pathogenesis

  a. Congenital: cretinism

  b. Adult

    i. Pituitary origin

    ii. Primary thyroid disorder (atrophy)

3. Symptomatology[6]

  a. Gradual onset of lethargy, intolerance to cold, weight gain, constipation

  b. Mental confusion, slowing of mentation, forgetfulness

  c. Voice changes: deep, harsh, thick tongue

  d. Bizarre sense of humor, frank psychosis—often inappropriately committed to mental institutions

4. Physical findings

  a. Skin cool, coarse, dry, yellow-orange (carotene), puffy face

  b. Hair: brittle, alopecia

  c. Deep tendon reflexes, relaxation phase delayed

  d. Bradycardia, hypothermia

  e. Myxedema, nonpitting edema

5. Diagnostic tests

  a. Same tests as for hyperthyroidism

  b. TSH increased; T4 decreased, T3 resin uptake decreased

  c. Serum Na depressed, elevated CPK, CSF protein elevated

6. Treatment

  a. Oral T4

  b. Lifelong replacement of levo-thyroxine (L-T4) 100 to 200 mg/day PO

7. Clinical course

  a. Ability to handle stress is diminished

b. Mild illnesses may cause coma
c. Drug metabolism is decreased
d. Associated risks
 i. Anemia 20 percent
 ii. Increased risk for arteriosclerotic heart disease

8. Anterior segment manifestations
 a. Ptosis, edema, cataract, KCS, extraocular muscle myotonia
 b. Loss of lateral one third of eyebrows

IV. Gastroenterology

A. CROHN'S DISEASE (REGIONAL ENTERITIS)

Refer to Chapter 5 for a complete discussion.

B. ULCERATIVE COLITIS

Refer to Chapter 5 for a complete discussion.

C. WILSON'S DISEASE (HEPATICOLENTICULAR DISEASE)

1. Epidemiology
 a. Autosomal recessive
 b. Under age 30, can present as chronic active hepatitis without mental or corneal changes
2. Etiology and pathogenesis
 a. Unknown metabolic defect
 b. Copper deposits in brain, kidney, liver, cornea
3. Symptomatology
 a. Neuropsychiatric signs present later with a loss of coordination
 b. Neuroses, dementia, psychosis

4. Physical findings
 a. All patients with neuropsychiatric signs have Kayser–Fleisher ring
 b. Tremors
 c. Masked facies
 d. Hypersalivation
5. Diagnostic tests
 a. Low serum ceruloplasmin level
 b. Low serum copper
 c. Urine copper level increased
6. Treatment
 a. Penicillamine: chelates copper
 b. One of few treatable cause of dementia and liver disease
7. Clinical course
 a. Can be reversible with treatment
 b. Cirrhosis of liver begins by age 6, often fatal
 c. Cavitations develop in lenticular nucleus in the brain
8. Anterior segment manifestations[7]
 a. Copper deposits in peripheral Descemet's membrane (Kayser–Fleischer ring)
 b. Sunflower cataract (copper under anterior lens capsule)

V. Hematology

A. ANEMIAS

1. Etiology and pathogenesis
 a. Excessive blood loss
 b. Deficient red blood cell (RBC) production (nutritional, suppression)
 c. Excessive RBC destruction (hemolytic)
 d. Disorders with both deficient RBC production and excessive RBC destruction (hemoglobinopathies, infection, thalassemia)
2. Symptomatology
 a. Weakness, vertigo, headache, tinnitus, spots before eyes, fatigue
 b. Drowsiness, irritability, euphoria, psychotic behavior
 c. Amenorrhea, loss of libido, gastrointestinal (GI) complaints, jaundice
3. Physical findings: Pale skin and mucous membranes
4. Diagnostic tests
 a. Hemoglobin and hematocrit are decreased
 b. Reticulocyte count: increased or normal, depending on type of anemia

c. RBC indices: microcytic, macrocytic hypochromic, hyperchromic

5. Treatment
   a. Symptomatic: rest
   b. Diet: high protein
   c. Iron supplements
   d. Transfusion when necessary: packed red blood cells (PRBC)

B. POLYCYTHEMIA

1. Etiology and pathogenesis
   a. Preleukemic disorder of bone marrow causing an excess of circulating RBC
   b. Can be secondary to chronic lung disease
2. Symptomatology
   a. Headache, tinnitus, pruritis, dyspnea, weakness, GI complaints
   b. Amaurosis fugax, hemianopia, blurring (secondary to impaired cerebral circulation)
3. Physical findings
   a. Ruddy facial cyanosis, with ecchymoses
   b. Hepatosplenomegaly, hypertension
4. Diagnostic tests
   a. Increased hematocrit, hypouricemia, hyperuricosuria
   b. Bone marrow hyperplasia
   c. CBC shows leukocytosis with basophils and eosinophils
5. Treatment: Phlebotomy (to reduce RBC mass)
6. Clinical course
   a. Variable, depending on occurrence of serious cerebrovascular vascular hemorrhage (CVA) and thrombosis, from which 30 percent of patients die
   b. Survival 15 years
   c. Fifteen percent of patients will develop leukemia
7. Ocular manifestations
   a. Vascular congestion of conjunctiva
   b. Vascular engorgement of iris
   c. Fundus appears like impending central retinal vein occlusion

C. SICKLE CELL ANEMIA

1. Epidemiology
   a. 1:600 blacks in the United States
   b. Eight percent blacks heterozygous for HbS (trait)
2. Etiology and pathogenesis
   a. Genetic: substitution of a valine for a glutamine in the sixth position of the β-hemoglobin (Hb) chain
   b. The altered hemoglobin forms crystalline aggregates, leading to sickled shape of RBC
3. Symptomatology
   a. Episodes of arthralgia, abdominal pain, fever, other symptoms of anemia (crisis)
   b. Deep bone pain secondary to microvascular necrosis
4. Physical findings
   a. Comma-shaped capillary segments on bulbar conjunctiva
   b. "Sun-ray" finding on radiographs of the skull
   c. Recurrent leg ulcers
   d. Poorly developed, short trunk with long extremities, tower skull
5. Diagnostic tests: Electrophoresis demonstrating HbS
6. Treatment
   a. Symptomatic
   b. Transfusion when necessary
   c. Pain relief (narcotics)
7. Clinical course
   a. Disease apparent by age 2 to 3 years
   b. Chronic course of exacerbations of the anemia accompanied by pain of abdomen or skeleton secondary to microvascular occlusions
   c. Many patients still die before age 30 as a result of intercurrent infection, pulmonary emboli, or thrombosis
8. Other ocular manifestations
   a. Angioid streaks in 6 percent of cases
   b. Salmon-patch retinal findings
   c. Seafan neovascular tuft
   d. Occlusive retinal pattern

VI. Infectious Disease

A. CAT-SCRATCH DISEASE

1. Etiology and pathogenesis
   a. Cat scratch or bite 2 to 4 weeks prior to symptoms
   b. Granulomatous abscess formation
   c. Virus has been implicated
2. Symptomatology
   a. Fever

b. Headache

c. Malaise

3. Physical findings

   a. Regional lymphadenitis with enlargement, tenderness, and occasional suppuration in 50 percent of patients

   b. Inflamed scratch or papular lesion with central necrosis

   c. Unilateral conjunctivitis and adenitis of preauricular node

4. Diagnostic tests

   a. Skin test: injection into the skin of the suppurative exudate from a known case

      i. Positive if induration and erythema 48 hours after intradermal injection

5. Treatment

   a. Supportive

   b. Antibiotics?

6. Clinical course

   a. Relatively benign disease with spontaneous remissions in weeks to months

B. SEXUALLY TRANSMITTED DISEASES

1. Epidemiology

   a. Most common infectious diseases

   b. Rising incidence because of availability of multiple sexual partners, asymptomatic infection, increasing affluence, leisure time, and mobility of patients

2. Etiology and pathogenesis

   a. *Chlamydia, Gonorrhea,* pediculosis, venereal warts, genital herpes, trichomoniasis, syphilis, and acquired immune deficiency syndrome (AIDS)

   b. Acquired through sexual contact with infected partner

3. Symptomatology

   a. Male heterosexuals: infections of pharynx, urethra, anorectal region

   b. Male heterosexuals: urethral, pharyngeal less common

   c. Female heterosexuals: pharyngeal, vaginal, cervical, anorectal infection

   d. Female homosexuals: very monogamous, hence rare infection

4. Physical findings

   a. Urethral discharge, vaginal discharge, genital sore, rash, scabies, proctitis

   b. Skin lesion: condylomata

   c. Mucosal sore

   d. Corneal infiltrates in chlamydial

5. Diagnostic tests

   a. Cultures of infected areas

b. FTA–ABS, VDRL for syphilis

c. HIV-III test for AIDS

6. Treatment

   a. Antibiotics (for bacterial causes) to infected patients and sexual contacts

   b. Education: to prevent infection

7. Clinical course

   a. Homosexual male: leads to intestinal pathology because of fecal–oral contact, hepatitis, Kaposi's sarcoma, AIDS

   b. AIDS: suppression of cell-mediated immunity with life threatening opportunistic infections

      i. Risk group: homosexual males, intravenous drug abusers, hemophiliacs, blood transfusion recipients

      ii. Kaposi's sarcoma: red placque-like growth on lid or conjunctiva

      iii. Up to 5-year incubation period

      iv. One hundred percent mortality, infections

C. SINUSITIS (SUPPURATIVE)

1. Predisposing conditions

   a. Ciliary injury secondary to dryness, chemical irritants, inhalation of dust, exposure or change in temperature

   b. Most common in children

2. Etiology and pathogenesis

   a. Inflammation obstructing the drainage orifices leads to secondary infection in the nasal sinuses

   b. *Streptococcus pneumonia, Staphylococcus aureus, Hemophilus influenzae,* group A *Streptococcus*

3. Symptomatology

   a. Fever, chills, headache with changes in intensity with position

   b. Dull aching around eyes

4. Physical findings

   a. Pain over infected sinuses

   b. Erythema or edema of turbinates

   c. Visualization of mucopus in the nose or nasopharynx

5. Diagnostic tests

   a. Anterior–posterior (Caldwell) radiographs; Waters and lateral views for air–fluid levels and thickening of sinus membranes

   b. Stain and culture of sinus exudate

   c. Transillumination

6. Treatment

   a. Medical: appropriate antibiotics

      i. Amoxicillin

ii. Ampicillin
iii. Erythromycin
iv. Penicillin
  b. Medical: decongestants, vasoconstrictors
  c. Surgical: drainage
7. Clinical course[8]
  a. May lead to orbital cellulitis and osteomyelitis
  b. Orbital abscess

c. Meningitis: death
d. Cavernous sinus thrombosis with clinical hallmarks
  i. Proptosis
  ii. Chemosis
  iii. Ophthalmoplagia
  iv. Blindness in contralateral eye
  v. Fifty percent fatal, even with today's antibiotics

VII. Nephrology

A. CYSTINOSIS (ADULT FORM)

1. Epidemiology
  a. 1:600
  b. Autosomal-recessive trait
  c. Eye involvement only significant factor in adult form
2. Etiology and pathogenesis: suspected enzyme deficiency but not identified
3. Symptomatology: photophobia, headache, burning, itching of eyes
4. Physical findings
  a. Hexagonal cystine crystals in anterior stroma centrally and all layers peripherally
  b. Clusters around vessels in conjunctiva
5. Diagnostic tests: quantified determination of cystine in blood leukocytes (approximately 30 times normal)
6. Treatment
  a. Adult form benign, no treatment necessary
  b. Differential is multiple myeloma, similar corneal crystals
7. Clinical course
  a. Infantile type: Fanconi syndrome, renal insufficiency during first decade of life
  b. Juvenile type: renal disease during second decade of life
  c. Adult type: benign with no renal disease

B. NEPHROTIC SYNDROME

1. Definition: the clinical expression of any glomerular disease that produces massive proteinuria
2. Etiology and pathogenesis: the decreased plasma oncotic pressure results in consequent edema and serosal effusion
3. Causative renal pathology

a. Renal vein thrombosis, sickle cell anemia, diabetes, multiple myeloma
b. Secondary to drugs, infection, neoplasia, toxemia, myxedema
4. Physical findings
  a. Weight gain
  b. Generalized edema
  c. Edema of eyelids
  d. Increased melanin "allergic shiner" in recurrent periorbital edema
5. Diagnostic tests
  a. Urine protein loss exceeding 3 to 4 g/day (hallmark finding)
  b. Albuminuria, hypoalbuminemia, hyperlipidemia
6. Treatment
  a. Treat underlying cause
  b. Diet high in protein
  c. Gradual reduction of edema
  d. Treat complications when appropriate

C. UREMIA

1. Widespread systemic disorder associated with chronic renal failure
2. Pathogenesis: unknown, but accumulation of metabolic by-products may be cause
3. Symptoms: pruritis, polydipsia, nausea, vomiting
4. Physical findings
  a. Wasting, sallow complexion, mouth ulcers, hypertension
  b. Band keratopathy, pericarditis, neuropathies, pleural effusions
5. Laboratory findings
  a. Elevated BUN and creatinine, anemia
  b. Urine specific gravity 1.010, isothenuria, proteinuria, tubular casts
6. Treatment
  a. Protein restriction
  b. Dialysis
  c. Transplantation

D. POST-TRANSPLANT

1. One hundred percent of patients develop posterior subcapsular cataracts

E. WILMS' TUMOR

1. Kidney tumor
2. Third most common organ cancer in children under age 10
3. Mesodermal in origin, hence association with aniridia
4. Symptoms caused by tumor's large size, abdominal
5. Treatment: radiotherapy, chemotherapy, nephrectomy
6. Two-year survival rate implies cure

VIII. Neurology

A. MYASTHENIA GRAVIS

1. Epidemiology
   a. Any age
   b. One in 20,000 patients
   c. Thymoma: 10 percent
   d. Two peaks: 20 years (female to male, 3:1) and middle age (male greater than female)
2. Etiology and pathogenesis
   a. Defective neuromuscular transmission across motor end plates of skeletal muscles
   b. Autoimmune reaction against acetylcholine receptors (AChR)
3. Symptomatology
   a. Ocular complaint: 75 percent of initial complaints; 95 percent of patients
   b. Five percent have thyrotoxicosis
4. Physical findings
   a. Weakness without other signs of neurological deficit
   b. Variability of muscle function within minutes, hours, or weeks
   c. Predilection for extraocular, facial, and oropharyngeal muscles
5. Diagnostic tests
   a. Tensilon test 10 mg (IV effects immediate)
   b. Chest radiographs, to rule out thymoma
   c. Must be considered in any extraocular muscle problem
6. Treatment
   a. The domain of the neurologist
   b. Neostigmine, pyridostigmine PO
   c. Thymectomy: beneficial in more than 50 percent of patients
7. Clinical course
   a. Long, chronic course with periods of remission
   b. Highly variable and not predictable in any one patient

c. Can be fatal if respiratory muscles involved
d. Remission achieved in 25 percent of patients
e. One third remain ocular after 3 years duration
f. If only ocular after 2 years, low chance of progression

B. TEMPORAL ARTERITIS (CRANIAL OR GIANT CELL ARTERITIS)

1. Epidemiology
   a. Rare under 60 years of age (80 percent are over 70 years of age)
   b. Females incidence greater than males
   c. Ophthalmic artery involved in more than 50 percent of cases
   d. Rare among blacks
2. Etiology and pathogenesis
   a. Autoimmune reaction to elastin fibers
   b. An inflammatory disorder affecting medium-size arteries
3. Symptomatology
   a. Headache, scalp tenderness, intermittent jaw claudication
   b. Polymyalgia rheumatica: stiffness, aching, and pain in the muscles of the neck, shoulders, lower back, hips, and thighs
   c. Loss of vision
   d. Pain on combing hair
4. Physical findings
   a. Palpable nodular enlargement of temporal artery
   b. Overlying skin: edematous, erythematous
   c. Skip lesions: long segments of involved arteries unaffected
5. Diagnostic tests
   a. ESR elevated, usually over 100
   b. Biopsy of temporal artery, loss of internal elastic lamina
   c. Anemia, leukocytosis

6. Treatment
   a. Systemic corticosteroids to reduce ESR (prednisone 60 mg/day)
   b. Continued for several months
   c. Pain relief with aspirin, indomethacin (Indocin)
7. Clinical course
   a. Once blindness occurs, return of vision rare

b. Chronic course, eventually leading to remission
c. Blindness in other eye 25 percent if untreated
d. Aorta often involved with aneurysm, dissection
e. Mesenteric arteritis, MI, claudication of legs (if iliacs involved)

IX. Oncology

A. BREAST CANCER

1. Currently the most common form of cancer in women in the United States
2. May soon be overtaken by lung cancer because of increase in smoking in women during the past 40 years
3. 1:7 to 1:12 in women
4. Prognosis depends on type of tumor, lymph node, involvement, age, and size of tumor
   a. Best prognosis: <2 cm
5. Treatment
   a. Lumpectomy
   b. Radiation
   c. Chemotherapy
   d. Hormonal treatment (estrogen)
   e. Surgery (radical or modified mastectomy)

B. BRONCHOGENIC (LUNG) CANCER

1. Symptoms
   a. Twenty-five percent asymptomatic: found incidentally on chest radiograph
   b. Seventy-five percent symptomatic: cough, weight loss, chest pain, dyspnea, hemoptysis
2. May present with ipsilateral Horner's syndrome (ptosis, miosis, anhidrosis) and ulnar nerve pain
   a. Pancoast tumor
   b. In apical field, it impinges on cervical sympathetic plexus
3. Overall 5-year survival, 10 percent

C. METASTATIC NEOPLASM

1. General
   a. Malignant neoplasms disseminate by one of three pathways

i. Direct seeding within body cavity (basal cell rare)
ii. Lymphatic spread (breast cancer)
iii. Hematogenous spread (colon cancer)
2. Ocular involvement
   a. No predilection for right or left eye
   b. Bilateral 20 percent
   c. Commonly carcinomas, not melanoma or sarcoma
   d. Women: breast cancer, history of breast cancer of 2 years duration
   e. Men: lung cancer, ocular metastasis before primary is found, also typical of kidney cancer
   f. Forty percent of metastatic tumors to anterior segments have iridocyclitis
3. Rare for primary ocular malignancy to metastasize

D. MULTIPLE MYELOMA

1. Epidemiology
   a. 3:100,000
   b. 50 to 70 years of age
2. Etiology and pathogenesis: Proliferation of abnormal plasma cells in the bone marrow
3. Symptomatology
   a. Severe bone pain, initial symptom in two thirds of patients
   b. Symptoms of anemia: fatigue, malaise, anorexia
4. Physical findings
   a. Pathological fractures
   b. Recurrent infections
5. Diagnostic tests
   a. Test for serum protein electrophoresis (SPEP), characteristic M spike
   b. Imunoelectrophoresis
   c. Osteolytic bone lesions on radiographs
   d. Bone marrow biopsy: plasma cells

6. Treatment: chemotherapy (alkylating agents and steroids)
7. Clinical course
   a. Infection is most common cause of death, secondary to patients depressed immunological defenses
   b. Bone pain can be exceptionally disabling
   c. Five-year survival rate low
   d. Uremia and hypercalcemia are worst prognostic signs
8. Anterior segment manifestations
   a. Crystals in cornea and conjunctiva
   b. Sludging in conjunctiva vessels
   c. Ciliary body cysts
   d. Lid edema, if kidneys are damaged

E. PRIMARY NEOPLASM

1. Hodgkin's disease
   a. One third of systemic lymphomas
   b. Diagnosis: microscopic presence of Reed–Sternberg cells
   c. Prognosis: depends on staging
   d. Ocular: extremely rare involvement
2. Non-Hodgkin's lymphoma
   a. Majority of systemic lymphomas
   b. Majority of lymphomas affecting ocular adnexa
   c. Symptom: lymphadenopathy
   d. Diagnosis: biopsy
   e. Prognosis: nodular better than diffuse
   f. Most common: Nodular, poorly differentiated, lymphocyctic tumors
      i. Conjunctival lymphoid tumors
         • Fifty to 60 years of age
         • Ninety percent not associated with systemic disease
         • Predilection for inferior conjunctiva
         • Biopsy is the only way to tell benign from malignant
         • Eighty percent of lymphoid tumors represent reactive hyperplasia
      ii. Orbital lymphoid tumors
         • Orbital pseudomotor: explosive onset, pain, proptosis, EOM disturbance
         • Orbital lymphoid tumors:
            Insidious onset, painless, usually anterior superior location
            Fifty percent have systemic disease
            Diagnosis based on biopsy, computed tomography (CT) scans
            Treatment: excision, radiation
3. Malignant melanoma
   a. Skin cancer
      i. Any age, peak incidence 50 to 60 years
      ii. Incidence increasing annually secondary to changing dress modes
      iii. Most arise from pre-existing nevi or moles
      iv. Thirty percent of population have nevi, 1:25,000 have melanoma
         • Nevi: rounded, regular, distinct borders, tan to brown
         • Melanomas: irregular margins, brown to black background with foci
      v. Metastasis based on depth of skin penetration
      vi. Death by visceral involvement
   b. Malignant melanoma of iris
      i. Arise from iris nevi
      ii. Six percent of all uveal melanoma
      iii. Presents at mass, heterochromia, glaucoma, uveitis
      iv. Rarely metastasize
      v. Mortality rate 4 percent
   c. Malignant melanoma of conjunctiva
      i. Arise from nevi, acquired melanosis, and de novo
      ii. Rare from congenital ocular melanocytosis
      iii. Exceedingly rare in blacks
      iv. Mortality
         • Nevi: 20 percent in those acquired from nevi
         • 40 percent in those that are de novo

X. Pediatrics

A. CHICKENPOX

1. Varicella virus
   a. Chickenpox in nonimmune host (usually child)
   b. Shingles (zoster) in the immune host (always adult)
2. Droplet infection communicable from 1 day prior to 6 days after appearance of physical findings

3. Discrete erythematous macules and papules over thorax, scalp, and mucous membranes
   a. Crust forms in 2 to 4 days
   b. Duration of 2 to 3 weeks
4. Pruritis: most annoying feature
5. Treatment symptomatic

B. GALACTOSEMIA

1. Epidemiology
   a. Autosomal-recessive trait
   b. One percent of population is heterozygous for galactosemia gene
   c. Incidence 1:50,000
2. Etiology and pathogenesis
   a. Deficiency of galactose 1-phosphate uridyltransferase
      i. Cataract
      ii. Cirrhosis
      iii. Mental retardation
   b. Deficiency of galactokinase—cataract formation
3. Symptomatology
   a. Days to weeks after birth, failure to thrive
   b. Reluctant to ingest breast milk or formula
4. Physical findings
   a. Oil droplet cataracts develop over weeks to months secondary to galacticol
   b. Jaundice, hepatomegaly, liver disease
5. Diagnostic tests
   a. Non-glucose-reducing substance in urine, high galactose in blood

b. Definitive: demonstrating the enzyme deficiency in RBC
   c. Can be diagnosed by amniocentesis
6. Treatment
   a. Galactose-free diet: usually leads to dramatic improvement
   b. All clinical features (except mental retardation) may improve
   c. Lenses clear or regress if treated early

C. KAWASAKI'S DISEASE

1. Mucocutaneous lymph node syndrome
2. Fever of 1 to 2 weeks
3. Injection of conjunctiva
4. Acute nonsuppurative swelling of cervical nodes
5. Polymorphous exanthem of trunk without crusts, vesicles
6. Reddening of palms, soles, and oral and pharyngeal mucosa
7. One to 2 percent die from coronary artery thrombosis, aneurysm, myocarditis, or pericarditis
8. Treatment: aspirin

D. MUMPS

1. Paramyxovirus
2. Humans: only natural host for mumps
3. Peak ages 6 to 10
4. Rapidly declining in incidence
5. Sudden onset of parotitis
6. Lacrimal gland may become involved
7. Orchitis in 30 percent of postpubertal males
8. Supportive treatment
9. Live attenuated vaccine for prevention

XI. Rheumatology

A. ANKYLOSING SPONDYLITIS

Refer to Chapter 5 for a complete discussion.

B. GOUT

1. Epidemiology
   a. Disease of middle-aged or elderly men (85 to 90 percent of patients)
   b. Associated with overeating, alcohol, and periods of stress
   c. Ten percent preceded by nephrolithiasis

2. Etiology
   a. Release of microcrystals of monosodium urate monohydrate into joint cavities
   b. Disorder of purine metabolism
3. Symptomatology
   a. Acute monoarticular pain often of nocturnal onset
   b. Symptoms of acute inflammation: erythema, heat, swelling, pain
4. Physical findings
   a. Initial presentation: first metatarsophalangeal joint (big toe)

b. Recurrent attacks may also involve ankles, knees, fingers, wrist, olecranon bursa
5. Diagnostic tests
   a. Elevated serum uric acid level
   b. Synovial fluid analysis: urate crystals
6. Treatment
   a. Acute: high dose, tapering regimen of nonsteroidal agents
   b. Chronic: allopurinol, colchicine
7. Clinical course
   a. Can lead to bony erosion, joint deformity, and renal insufficiency
   b. Variable beginning; many months to years between attacks; later attacks are more frequent and more severe and affect more and more joints
8. Anterior segment manifestations
   a. Cornea: scintillating crystals scattered in Bowman's membrane
   b. Chronic conjunctivitis with congested vessels and subconjunctival hemorrhages (SCH)
   c. Uveitis, scleritis, episcleritis

C. REITER'S SYNDROME

Refer to Chapter 5 for a complete discussion.

D. RHEUMATOID ARTHRITIS

1. Epidemiology
   a. Affects four percent of women and 1.5 percent men
   b. Onset: young adulthood
   c. All races and ethnic groups
   d. Typical case: women 30 to 50 years of age
2. Etiology and pathogenesis
   a. Autoimmune
   b. Nonsuppurative, proliferative synovitis
   c. Anti-IgG antibodies
3. Symptomatology
   a. Joint pain, stiffness, limited motion, morning stiffness greater than 30 minutes
   b. Constitutional symptoms precede arthritis: fatigue, fever, neuroasthenia
4. Physical findings
   a. Ulnar deviation of wrist
   b. Swan neck deformity of fingers
   c. Rheumatoid nodules: asymptomatic, subcutaneous, 25 percent of patients
   d. Carpel tunnel syndrome
5. Diagnostic tests

a. Rheumatoid factor (RF) in serum
b. Synovial fluid analysis: polymorphonuclear cells (PMN) and decreased complement level
6. Treatment
   a. Nonsteroidal anti-inflammatory drugs (NSAID)
      i. ASA 3 to 6 g/day
      ii. Indomethacin
      iii. Phenylbutazone
      iv. Ibuprofen
   b. Physical therapy
   c. Arthritic surgery
7. Clinical course
   a. Leads to destruction of articular cartilage and progressive disabling arthritis in 10 percent of patients after 20 years duration
   b. Extra-articular involvement of skin, heart vessels, muscles, lungs (amyloidosis in 5 to 10 percent)
   c. After 10 years, disease stabilizes in 50 percent of patients
   d. Not predictable, but men do slightly better than women

E. SARCOIDOSIS

Refer to Chapter 5 for a complete discussion.

F. SJÖGREN'S SYNDROME

1. Epidemiology
   a. Ninety percent are women
   b. Average age 50
   c. All races involved
2. Etiology and pathogenesis
   a. Immunological attack on exocrine organs
   b. B-cell dysfunction
3. Symptomatology
   a. Dry eye
   b. Difficulty chewing, swallowing, phonation
4. Physical findings
   a. Filamentary keratitis
   b. Fissures and ulcers of tongue, buccal mucosa, and lips
   c. Rampant dental caries
   d. Fifty percent have parotid or submandibular gland enlargement
5. Diagnostic tests
   a. Diagnosis: made if two of the following findings are present:
      i. Lymphocytic infiltrate in salivary gland
      ii. Definite KCS

iii. Any connective tissue or lymphoproliferative disorder presenting RA, SLE, systemic sclerosis, polymyositis
   b. Differential: local glandular disorder, depression, parasympathomimetic drugs
6. Treatment
   a. Symptomatic
      i. Artificial tears
      ii. Sugar-free lozenges
   b. Corticosteroids and immunosuppressive drugs for
      i. Severe functional disability
      ii. Life-threatening complications

7. Clinical course
   a. One third only have KCS and xerostomia (dry mouth)
   b. Raynaud's in 20 percent
   c. One third have interstitial nephritis
   d. Lymphomas occur more frequently than in general population
   e. Esophageal webs may develop
8. Anterior segment manifestations
   a. Ocular complications: corneal ulceration, vascularization, opacification, and rarely perforation
   b. All secondary to dry eye–keratitis sicca problems

XII. Trauma

A. HEAD INJURY

1. General
   a. Leading cause of death under 40 years of age
   b. Severity of head injury may not become manifest for days to weeks
2. Special entity
   a. Carotid cavernous fistulas
      i. Traumatic three times more common than spontaneous type
      ii. Usually in men 20 to 30 years of age, following severe head trauma
      iii. Symptoms: bothersome orbital bruit
      iv. Signs: pulsating exophthalmos, chemosis, exposure keratitis
      v. Diagnosis: cerebral angiography
      vi. Surgery: indicated for intolerable bruit, progressive vascular loss, or hemorrhage
   b. Epidural hematoma
      i. One to 3 percent of major head injuries
      ii. Male to female, 4:1 Auto accidents—common, also with trivial falls and sports injuries
      iii. Fracture of temporal skull in 80 percent of cases
      iv. Clinical picture: "talk and die picture"
         • Unconscious, then regains relatively normal function
         • As hematoma enlarges, it causes herniation of the uncus compressing cranial nerve III ipsilateral pupil dilation or ptosis
         • Contralateral hemiparesis develops
   c. Basal skull fracture
      i. If anterior basilar fracture is present, damaging the anterior venous sinuses, blood leaks into periorbital tissue, producing raccoon or panda sign (dark discoloration of lids with no subconjunctival involvement)

XIII. "Top 100" Systemic Diagnoses Related to Anterior Segment Care

A. "TOP 100" SPECIFIC DIAGNOSES (Table 6–1)

Use Table 6–1 when patient provides a specific systemic diagnosis during history (subjective)

TABLE 6–1. "TOP 100" CHART: ALPHABETICAL LISTING OF 100 SYSTEMIC DISORDERS WITH ANTERIOR SEGMENT MANIFESTATIONS

Systemic Disorder	Pathological Classification	Anterior Segment Manifestation	Primary Eyecare Management	Co-management or Referral
1. Acne rosacea	Dermatological	Blepharitis Recurrent chalazia Keratitis	Antibiotics Steroids	Dermatologist
2. Addison's disease	Endocrine	Lid pigmentation Conjunctiva pigmentation	Counsel	Internist
3. Albinism	Metabolic	Depigmentation	Palliative	Vision rehabilitation
4. Alcoholism	Nutritional	Meibomianitis Conjunctivitis	Antibiotics Steroids (limited)	Primary physician
5. Alkaptonuria	Metabolic	Pigmentation	Counsel	Internist
6. Allergies	Allergic	Edema Hyperemia	Cold compresses Antihistamine–decongestants Steroids (limited)	Primary physician Allergist
7. Alport's syndrome	Renal	Anterior lenticonus Anterior polar cataract	Counsel	Internist
8. Amyloidosis	Metabolic	Lid nodules Conjunctival nodules Corneal deposits	Counsel	Internist
9. Anemia(s)	Hematologic	Pallor Subconjunctival hemorrhage	Counsel	Primary physician
10. Ankylosing spondylitis	Collagen vascular	Anterior uveitis	Cycloplege and dilate Steroids	Rheumatologist
11. Asthma	Pulmonary	Conjunctivitis	Decongestants Steroids (limited)	Internist
12. Behçet's disease	Dermatological (?) Ophthalmologic (?)	Anterior uveitis Keratitis	Cycloplege and dilate Steroids	Gynecologist Primary physician
13. Breast cancer (carcinoma)	Neoplastic	Metastasis	Counsel	Surgeon Ophthalmologist
14. Cardiovascular disease	Cardiovascular	Arcus senilis Lipid keratopathy	Counsel	Cardiologist Primary physician
15. Cat-scratch fever	Infectious (?)	Follicular conjunctivitis	Supportive	Primary physician
16. Chlamydial disease	Infectious	Conjunctivitis Keratitis	Topical tetracycline Steroids (limited)	Primary physician
17. Cogan's syndrome	Neurological (?)	Interstitial keratitis	Counsel	Neurologist Cardiologist
18. Crohn's disease (regional enteritis)	Gastrointestinal	Anterior uveitis	Cycloplege and dilate Steroids	Gastroenterologist
19. Dermatitis	Dermatological	Blepharitis Conjunctivitis	Antibiotics (limited) Steroids	Dermatologist
20. Dermatomyositis (polymyositis)	Collagen vascular	Lid edema Lid erythema	Cold compresses	Dermatologist Internist
21. Diabetes mellitus	Endocrine	Recurrent erosion Rubeosis irides	Supportive	Internist
22. Downs' syndrome	Chromosomal	Epicanthal folds Keratoconus Brushfield's spots	Monitor closely	Pediatrician
23. Eczema	Dermatological	Blepharoconjunctivitis Dry-eye syndrome	Supportive	Dermatologist

Subjective Systemic Highlight	Objective Systemic Highlight	Standard Medical Management	Complications (Ocular and Systemic)	Prognosis (Ocular and Systemic)
Recurrent Middle age	Skin flush Papillae Telangiectasia	Tetracycline	O: Scarring S: Recurring	O/S: 10–15-yr course
Weakness	Skin pigmentation in body creases	Steroids	O: Papilledema S: Diabetes	O/S: Good
Genetic	Depigmentation	Counsel	O: Numerous S: Sunlight	O: Guarded S: Good
Addiction	Gastrointestinal Dermatological	Rehabilitation	O: Neurological S: Liver disease	O: Good S: Guarded
Genetic	Skin pigmentation	Vitamin C	O: Posterior uvea S: Arthritis	O/S: Good
Long history Seasonal	Congestion Asthmatic	Antihistamines Decongestants Steroids	O: Recurrent S: Steroids	O: Guarded S: Good
Genetic	Nerve deafness Hypertension	Antihypertensive	O: Posterior S: Cardiovascular	O/S: Guarded
Genetic	Serum protein Amyloid deposits	Surgery	O: Posterior glaucoma	O: Guarded S: Poor
General weakness	Laboratory blood workup	Vitamins and minerals	O: Posterior S: Numerous	O: Good S: Guarded
Lower back pain	HLA–B27 +	Steroids	S: Rheumatoid arthritis, steroids	O: Good S: Guarded
Family history	Breathing problems	Steroids Cromolyn sodium	O: Steroids S: Steroids	O: Good S: Guarded
Greater in Orientals	Mouth ulcers Genital lesions	Steroids	O: Hyphema S: Vascular	O: Poor S: Guarded
Cancer history	Biopsy +	Surgery	O: Posterior S: Metastasis	O/S: Poor
Risk factors	Angina Arteriosclerosis	Reduce risk factors	O: Posterior S: Renal	O: Guarded S: Poor
Cat history	Lymphadenopathy Fever	Palliative	O: Keratitis	O/S: Good
Veneral	Genitourinary	Tetracycline Counsel	O: Adult scarring	O/S: Good
Tinnitus Vertigo	Vestibular deafness	Rehabilitation	O: Photophobia S: Cardiovascular	O/S: Guarded
Recurrent cramping	Bloody diarrhea	Steroids Surgery	S: Arthritis	O: Good S: Guarded
Atopic history Contact history	Skin rash Erythema	Steroids	O: Keratitis S: Steroids	O: Good S: Guarded
	Dermatological Systemic	Steroids	O: Posterior S: Steroids	O: Good S: Guarded
Polyuria	Hyperglycemia	Insulin	O: Posterior S: Numerous	O/S: Guarded
Congenital Trisomy 21	Stigmata of syndrome (FLK)	Counsel	O: Cataracts numerous S: Cardiac	O: Good S: Guarded
Atopia	Skin cracking Rhinitis	Steroids (limited)	O: Cataract S: Asthma	O: Good S: Guarded

continued

TABLE 6-1. (Cont.)

Systemic Disorder	Pathological Classification	Anterior Segment Manifestation	Primary Eyecare Management	Co-management or Referral
24. Ehlers–Danlos syndrome	Dermatological	Blue sclera Microcornea	Counsel	Primary physician
25. Fabry's disease	Metabolic	Conjunctival tortuosity Corneal swirls	Monitor closely	Pediatrician Internist
26. Facial deformity syndromes	Musculoskeletal	Lower lid colobomas Epibulbar dermoids	Counsel	Pediatrician
27. Galactosemia	Metabolic	Cataract	Counsel	Pediatrician
28. Gaucher's disease	Metabolic	Conjunctival infiltrates Corneal opacity	Counsel	Pediatrician Corneal surgeon
29. Gonorrhea	Infectious	Hyperacute purulent conjunctiva	Antibiotic	Primary physician
30. Gout	Metabolic	Corneal crystals Sclerouveitis	Steroids	Internist
31. Hay fever	Allergic	Conjunctivitis	Antihistamine–decongestants Steroids (limited)	Primary physician Allergist
32. Hemophilia	Hematological	Ecchymosis Subconjunctival hemorrhage	Cold compresses Monitor closely	Hematologist Primary physician
33. Herpes simplex	Infectious	Blepharitis Dendritic keratitis	Trifluridine Acyclovir	Primary physician
34. Herpes zoster	Infectious	Dermatoblepharitis Keratitis Anterior uveitis	Supportive Steroids (limited)	Dermatologist
35. Histiocytosis	Metabolic	Unilateral exophthalmos	Monitor exophthalmometry	Pediatrician
36. Histoplasmosis	Infectious	Palpebral conjunctivitis	Palliative	Primary physician
37. Hives (urticaria)	Allergic	Lid edema Lid erythema Conjunctivitis	Cold compresses Supportive Steroids (limited)	Primary physician
38. Homocystinuria	Metabolic	Dislocated lens (downward)	Monitor closely	Pediatrician
39. Hyperparathyroidism	Endocrine	Band keratopathy Conjunctival calcifications	Monitor closely	Internist
40. Hypertension	Cardiovascular	Arcus senilis Subconjunctival hemorrhage	Counsel	Primary physician
41. Hyperthyroidism (Grave's disease)	Endocrine	Lid signs Exophthalmos Exposure keratitis SLK	Monitor closely	Internist
42. Hypervitaminosis	Nutritional	Band keratopathy Conjunctival deposits	Monitor closely	Primary physician
43. Hypoparathyroidism	Endocrine	Blepharospasm Photophobia	Monitor closely	Internist
44. Hypothyroidism	Endocrine	Lid edema Loss of lateral one third of eyebrows	Monitor closely	Internist
45. Impetigo	Infectious	Lid pustules Conjunctivitis	Antibiotics Hygiene	Pediatrician Primary physician
46. Influenza	Infectious	Mild keratitis "Itchy-burnies"	Palliative	Primary physician

Subjective Systemic Highlight	Objective Systemic Highlight	Standard Medical Management	Complications (Ocular and Systemic)	Prognosis (Ocular and Systemic)
Skin fragility	Hyperelasticity	Counsel	O: Angioid streaks S: Hematomas	O: Guarded S: Good
Genetic	Serum lipids	Counsel	O: Posterior S: Cardiovascular	O/S: Guarded
FLK syndromes	Goldenhar Hallerman–Streiff	Counsel	O: Numerous S: Retardation	O: Guarded S: Good
Congenital	Galactose intolerance	D/C galactose	O: Amblyopia	O/S: Good
Congenital	Lipoidoses	Supportive	O: Posterior	O: Guarded S: Poor
Venereal	Genitourinary	Penicillin	O: Corneal ulcer Uveitis	O: Guarded S: Good
Pain	Arthritis	Steroids	O: Blepharitis S: Nephritis	O/S: Guarded
Seasonal	Rhinitis	Antihistamine– decongestants Steroids	S: Steroids	O/S: Guarded
Genetic	Hemorrhaging	Precaution	S: Blood loss	O: Good S: Guarded
Venereal	Genitourinary	Acyclovir	O: Scarring S: Recurrence	O/S: Guarded
Severe pain	Dermatitis (shingles)	Pain medications Steroids	O: Numerous S: Scarring	O: Guarded S: Poor
Childhood	Granulomas	Steroids	O: Granulomas S: Musculoskeletal	O/S: Guarded
Regional	Laboratory workup	Counsel	O: Posterior S: Respiratory	O: Guarded S: Good
Atopic history Allergen	Dermatitis Edema	Remove allergen Steroids (limited)	S: Anaphylaxis	O: Good S: Guarded
Congenital	Fair complexion Urinanalysis	Counsel	O: Cataract S: Vascular disease	O/S: Guarded
Pain	Hypercalcemia	Anticalcemic Surgery	O: Conjunctival S: Renal	O/S: Guarded
Risk factors	Increased pulse	Antihypertensives	O: Posterior S: Cardiovascular	O: Good S: Guarded
Aggitation	Laboratory workup Enlarged thyroid	Euthyroid	O: Neurological S: Numerous	O: Good S: Guarded
Headache	Intracranial pressure	Dietary	O: Cataract	O/S: Good
Personality changes	Tetany	Calcium	O: Cataract S: Cardiac	O/S: Good
Cretinism	Dry skin, hair	Thyroid substitute	O: Cataract S: Myxedema	O: Good S: Guarded
Hygiene problems	Maculopapule rash	Antibiotics Hygiene	O/S: Secondary infection	O/S: Good
General malaise	Myalgia	Palliative	O/S: Rare neurological	O/S: Good

continued

TABLE 6–1. (Cont.)

Systemic Disorder	Pathological Classification	Anterior Segment Manifestation	Primary Eyecare Management	Co-management or Referral
47. Kaposi's sarcoma	Neoplastic	Lid tumor Conjunctival tumor	Counsel	Internist Ophthalmologist
48. Leukemia(s)	Neoplastic	Proptosis Subconjunctival hemorrhages	Counsel	Internist
49. Lipidoses	Metabolic	Arcus senilis Xanthelasma	Monitor closely Counsel	Primary physician
50. Liver disease	Nutritional	Icteric sclera Keratitis sicca	Monitor closely	Internist
51. Louis–Barr syndrome (ataxia telangectasia)	Phakomatoses	Conjunctival telangectasia	Monitor	Gynecologist Neurologist
52. Lowe's syndrome	Renal	Cataracts Posterior lenticonus	Monitor closely	Nephrologist
53. Lung cancer (carcinoma)	Neoplastic	Metastasis	Counsel	Surgeon Ophthalmologist
54. Lymphoma(s)	Neoplastic	Uveitis Proptosis	Cycloplege and dilate Steroids	Internist
55. Malnutrition	Nutritional	Edema Keratopathy	Supportive	Primary physician
56. Marfan's syndrome	Metabolic	Blue sclera Persistent pupillary membranes	Monitor closely	Internist
57. Measles (rubeola)	Infectious	Conjunctivitis Koplik's spots	Supportive	Pediatrician
58. Melanoma (skin cancer)	Neoplastic	Conjunctival lid nevus	Monitor closely	Dermatologist
59. Mononucleosis	Infectious	Conjunctivitis Uveitis	Palliative Steroids (limited)	Primary physician
60. Mucopolysac-charidosis	Metabolic	Corneal opacities	Counsel	Pediatrician
61. Multiple myeloma	Hematological	Corneal crystals Iris cysts	Monitor closely	Internist
62. Multiple sclerosis	Neurological	Ptosis	Counsel	Neurologist
63. Mumps	Infectious	Keratoconjunctivitis	Warm compresses Steroids (limited)	Pediatrician
64. Muscular dystrophy	Musculoskeletal	Ptosis	Counsel	Pediatrician
65. Myasthenia gravis	Neurological	Ptosis	Monitor	Neurologist
66. Nevus of Ota	Dermatological	Lid pigmentation Scleral pigmentation	Counsel	Primary physician
67. Occlusive arterial disease	Cardiovascular	Hypoxia Hemorrhages	Counsel	Primary physician Cardiologist
68. Occlusive venous disease	Cardiovascular	Edema Rubeosis iridis	Counsel Cold compresses	Primary physician Cardiologist
69. Osteogenesis imperfecta	Musculoskeletal	Blue sclera	Monitor	Primary physician
70. Pemphigoid (benign, ocular)	Dermatological	Conjunctivitis Keratitis sicca	Supportive	Ophthalmologist Dermatologist

Subjective Systemic Highlight	Objective Systemic Highlight	Standard Medical Management	Complications (Ocular and Systemic)	Prognosis (Ocular and Systemic)
Predominant male	AIDS victim	Radiation	S: Metastasis	O: Guarded S: Poor
Weakness	Hematologic	Chemotherapy	O: Posterior Anterior uveitis	O/S: Guarded
Diet Risk factors	Laboratory workup	Diet control	S: ˙Cardiovascular	O: Good S: Guarded
Malaise Weakness	Jaundice	Steroids	O: Night and color vision S: Hetatitis	O: Good S: Guarded
Familial (rare)	Spasms	Counsel	O: Motility S: Cerebellar	O/S: Poor
Congenital Males	Mental retardation	Counsel	O: Glaucoma S: Dwarfism	O/S: Guarded
Cancer history	Biopsy +	Surgery	O/S: High-risk metastasis	O/S: Poor
Weakness	Hematologic	Chemotherapy	O: Posterior S: Recurrence	O: Good S: Guarded
History of weakness	Weight loss	Nutrition	O: Xerophthalmia Nightblindness	O: Guarded S: Good
Tall, slender stature	Arachnodactylae (long fingers) Cardiovascular	Counsel Monitor	O: Myopia, lens dislocation Retinal detachment	O: Guarded S: Good
Childhood	Koplik's spots	Palliative	S: Subacute sclerosing panencephalitis	O/S: Good
Metastasis	Pigmented lesions	Surgery	O: Hyphema	O: Guarded S: Poor
General weakness	Laboratory workup	Rest	O: Posterior vitritis	O/S: Good
Congenital	FLKs Laboratory workup	Counsel Supportive	O: Pigmentary retinopathy	O/S: Guarded
Weakness	Laboratory workup	Transfusion	O: Posterior S: Paraplegia	O: Guarded S: Poor
Uthoff's sign La Hermit sign	Neurological workup	Supportive	O: Optic neuritis S: Recurrences	O: Good S: Guarded
Malaise	Swollen glands	Isolation	O: Optic neuritis	O/S: Good
Congenital	Muscular	Supportive	O: Ophthalmoplegia	O/S: Guarded
Weakness	Tensilon test	Prostigmine	O: Pupil defects	O/S: Good
Orientals	Hyperpigment spots	Counsel	S: Malignant in Caucasians	O/S: Good
Risk factors	Vascular disease	Anticoagulants	O: Posterior S: MI or stroke	O: Good S: Guarded
Risk factors	Vascular disease	Specific to disease	O: Posterior S: Phlebitis	O: Good S: Guarded
Congenital	Fragile long bones	Supportive	O: Glaucoma S: Deafness	O: Good S: Guarded
Pain	Skin bullae	Steroids	O: Scarring Corneal perforation	O/S: Guarded

continued

TABLE 6–1. (Cont.)

	Systemic Disorder	Pathological Classification	Anterior Segment Manifestation	Primary Eyecare Management	Co-management or Referral
71.	Periarteritis nodosa	Collagen vascular	Episcleritis Uveitis	Supportive Steroids	Internist
72.	Pneumonia	Infectious	Hemorrhagic blepharoconjunctivitis	Antibiotics Supportive	Primary physician
73.	Polycythemia vera	Hematological	Conjunctival hyperemia	Cold compresses Palliative	Internist
74.	Psoriasis	Dermatological	Conjunctivitis Corneal infiltrates	Supportive	Dermatologist
75.	Reiter's syndrome	Collagen vascular	Conjunctivitis Uveitis	Cycloplege and dilate Steroids	Internist
76.	Rheumatoid arthritis (and JRA)	Collagen vascular	Uveitis Sclerouveitis	Cycloplege and dilate Steroids	Rheumatologist
77.	Rubella (German measles) congenital form	Infectious	Corneal clouding Iris atrophy Cataract	Monitor	Pediatrician Low vision
78.	Sarcoidosis	Collagen vascular	Uveitis	Cycloplege and dilate Steroids	Internist
79.	Scleroderma	Collagen vascular	Keratitis	Lubricants Supportive	Dermatologist
80.	Septicemia (bacteremia)	Infectious	Subconjunctival hemorrhage Uveitis	Cycloplege and dilate Supportive	Internist
81.	Sickle cell disease	Hematological	Comma-shaped conjunctival vessels	Counsel	Internist
82.	Sjögren's syndrome	Collagen vascular	Keratitis sicca	Lubricants Supportive	Internist
83.	Stevens–Johnson disease (erythema multiforme)	Dermatological	Conjunctivitis Dry-eye syndrome	Lubricants Supportive	Dermatologist
84.	Sturge–Weber syndrome (encephalotrigeminal angiomatosis)	Phakomatoses	Dilated episcleral veins Port wine stain	Counsel Monitor IOP	Primary physician
85.	Syphilis	Infectious	Interstitial keratitis Uveitis	Cycloplege and dilate Steroids	Internist
86.	Systemic lupus erythematosus	Collagen vascular	Conjunctival hyperemia Episcleritis (?)	Supportive	Internist
87.	Temporal (cranial) arteritis	Collagen vascular	Uveitis	Cycloplege and dilate Steroids	Internist
88.	Toxemia of pregnancy	Cardiovascular	Periorbital edema	Cold compresses Palliative	Obstetrician
89.	Toxoplasmosis	Infectious	Conjunctivitis Uveitis	Cycloplege and dilate Steroids	Internist
90.	Trichinosis (trichinella)	Infectious	Lid edema Chemosis	Cold compresses Palliative	Internist
91.	Tuberculosis	Infectious	Phlyctenular keratoconjunctivitis	Steroids	Internist

Subjective Systemic Highlight	Objective Systemic Highlight	Standard Medical Management	Complications (Ocular and Systemic)	Prognosis (Ocular and Systemic)
Sick male	Fever High ESR	Steroids	O: Hemorrhages S: Vasculitis	O/S: Guarded
Malaise	Laboratory workup	Antibiotics Supportive	O: Corneal S: Vascular	O: Good S: Guarded
Fatigue	Blood workup	Radiophosphorus Phlebotomy	O: Retinal S: Hemorrhage	O: Good S: Guarded
History	Skin scaling	Ultraviolet therapy	O: Lid involvement	O: Good S: Guarded
Arthritic history	Urethritis (nongonococcal)	Tetracycline	O: Keratitis S: Vasculitis	O: Guarded S: Poor
Joint pain	High ESA HLA +	Anti-inflammatories (steroidal and nonsteroidal)	O: Band keratopathy S: Musculoskeletal	O: Guarded S: Poor
Maternal history	Congenital findings	Supportive	O: Posterior S: Numerous	O/S: Guarded
Disseminated	Granulomas Chest radiograph	Steroids Supportive	O: Posterior S: Numerous	O: Guarded S: Good
Skin irritation	Leathery skin	Steroids	O: Lid scarring S: SLE	O/S: Guarded
Gravely ill	Blood workup	Antibiotics	O: Endophthalmitis	O: Guarded S: Poor
Blacks	Hemoglobinopathy	Supportive	O: Posterior S: Numerous	O: Guarded S: Poor
Malaise Fever	Dry mouth Arthritis	Steroids	O: Corneal S: Polymyalgia rheumatism	O: Good S: Guarded
History Sulfa drugs	Erythematous reactions	Steroids	O: Uveitis S: Respiratory	O/S: Guarded
Congenital	Radiological (intracranial calcifications)	Counsel	O: Choroidal hemangiomas	O/S: Good
Acquired Congenital	FTA–ABS	Penicillin	O/S: "Anything"	O/S: Guarded
Females	Butterfly rash	Steroids	O: Keratouveitis S: Numerous	O: Good S: Guarded
Headache Jaw pain Hemianopsia	Prominent, tender temporal artery High ESR	Steroids	O: Posterior Ophthalmoplegia Blindness	O: Poor S: Guarded
Second to third trimester	Edema High BP	Antihypertensives Diuretics	O: Posterior Papilledema	O: Good S: Guarded
Acquired Congenital	Laboratory workup	Pyrimethamine	O: Vitritis Chorioretinitis	O: Guarded S: Good
Diet history	Laboratory workup	Supportive	O: Motility S: Hypersensitivity	O: Good S: Guarded
Hygienic history	Skin test Chest radiograph	Isoniazid	O: Posterior S: Pulmonary	O: Good S: Guarded

continued

TABLE 6–1. (Cont.)

Systemic Disorder	Pathological Classification	Anterior Segment Manifestation	Primary Eyecare Management	Co-management or Referral
92. Turner's syndrome	Chromosomal	Epicanthal folds Oval corneas Corneal opacities	Counsel	Pediatrician
93. Ulcer (peptic)	Gastrointestinal	Uveitis	Cycloplege and dilate Steroids (limited)	Primary physician
94. Ulcerative colitis	Gastrointestinal	Uveitis	Cycloplege and dilate Steroids	Internist
95. Varicella (chickenpox)	Infectious	Lid vescicles Conjunctivitis	Supportive	Pediatrician
96. Vitamin deficiencies	Nutritional	Xerosis	Lubricants	Nutritionist
97. Von Recklinghausen's (neurofibromatosis)	Phakomatoses	Thickened lids Prominent corneal nerves	Counsel	Dermatologist Neurologist Internist
98. Wegener's granulomatosis	Collagen vascular	Corneal margin ulceration	Steroids	Internist
99. Wilms' tumor (nephroblastoma)	Renal	Aniridia	Counsel	Nephrologist Pediatrician
100. Wilson's disease (hepaticolenticular)	Metabolic	Kayser–Fleischer ring (copper on posterior cornea)	Counsel	Neurologist

B. "TOP 100" DIAGNOSES BY PATHOLOGICAL CLASSIFICATION (Table 6–2)

Use Table 6–2 when patient presents symptoms in history (subjective) suggesting a specific pathological category or classification of systemic disease

TABLE 6–2. "TOP 100" SYSTEMIC DISORDERS WITH ANTERIOR SEGMENT MANIFESTATIONS (BY PATHOLOGICAL CLASSIFICATION)

Pathological Classification	Specific Systemic Disorder	No. on Top 100 Chart (Table 6–1)	Lids Adnexa	Conjunctiva	Sclera Episclera	Cornea	Anterior Chamber	Lens
Allergic	Allergies	6	X	X				
	Hay fever	31		X				
	Hives (urticaria)	37	X	X				
Cardiovascular	Arteriosclerosis	14				X		
	Hypertension	40		X		X		
	Occlusive arterial	67		X				
	Occlusive venous	68	X				X	
	Toxemia of pregnancy	88	X					
Chromosomal	Downs' syndrome	22	X			X	X	X
	Turner's syndrome	92	X			X		X
Collagen vascular	Ankylosing spondylitis	10				X		
	Dermatomyositis	20	X			X		
	Periarteritis nodosa	70			X		X	

Subjective Systemic Highlight	Objective Systemic Highlight	Standard Medical Management	Complications (Ocular and Systemic)	Prognosis (Ocular and Systemic)
Congenital Females	FLK Dwarfism	Counsel Estrogens	O: Cataracts Retinal S: Cardiovascular	O: Guarded S: Guarded
GI pain Stressful males	Aggravated by diet	Diet control Tagamet	S: Numerous	O: Good S: Guarded
GI pain	Blood in stool	Steroids	S: Carcinoma	O: Good S: Poor
Childhood	Vesicular patterns	Palliative	S: Adult Shingles (herpes zoster)	O/S: Good
Diet	Serum levels	Dietary	O: Visual S: Numerous	O/S: Good
Disseminated findings	Cafe-au-lait spots Neurofibromas	Supportive	O: Glaucoma nodules S: Numerous	O/S: Guarded
Painful lesions	Necrotizing granulomas	Steroids	O: Orbital S: Numerous	O: Guarded S: Poor
Childhood Congenital	Abdominal	Surgery	O: Orbital mass S: Cardiovascular	O: Poor S: Guarded
Personality changes	Peripheral tremors	Penicillamine	O: Cataract S: Neurologic Cirrhosis	O: Good S: Guarded

TABLE 6–2. (Cont.)

Pathological Classification	Specific Systemic Disorder	No. on Top 100 Chart (Table 6–1)	Lids Adnexa	Conjunctiva	Sclera Episclera	Cornea	Anterior Chamber	Lens
Collagen vascular (cont.)	Reiter's syndrome	75		X		X	X	
	Rheumatoid arthritis	76			X	X	X	
	Sarcoidosis	78				X	X	X
	Scleroderma	79	X			X		X
	Sjögren's syndrome	82		X		X	X	
	Systemic lupus erythematosus	86		X	X	X	X	
	Temporal arteritis	87					X	
	Wegener's granulomatosis	98	X			X		
Dermatologic	Acne rosacea	1	X	X		X	X	
	Behçet's disease	12				X	X	
	Dermatitis	19	X	X		X		
	Eczema	23	X	X		X		X
	Ehlers–Danlos syndrome	24	X		X	X		

continued

TABLE 6–2. (Cont.)

Pathological Classification	Specific Systemic Disorder	No. on Top 100 Chart (Table 6–1)	Lids Adnexa	Conjunctiva	Sclera Episclera	Cornea	Anterior Chamber	Lens
Dermatologic (cont.)	Nevus of Ota	66	X		X			
	Pemphigoid	70		X		X		
	Psoriasis	74	X	X		X	X	
	Stevens–Johnson disease	83		X		X	X	
Endocrine	Addison's disease	2	X	X				
	Diabetes mellitus	21				X	X	
	Hyperparathyroidism	39		X		X		
	Hyperthyroidism	41	X			X		
	Hypoparathyroidism	43	X	X				X
	Hypothyroidism	44	X					X
Gastrointestinal	Crohn's disease	18				X		
	Ulcer (peptic)	93				X		
	Ulcerative colitis	94		X		X		
Hematologic	Anemia(s)	9		X				
	Hemophilia	32	X	X				
	Multiple myeloma	61		X		X	X	
	Polyerythemia vera	73		X				
	Sickle cell disease	81		X				
Infectious	Cat-scratch fever	15		X		X		
	Chlamydial disease	16		X		X		
	Gonorrhea	29		X		X	X	
	Herpes simplex	33	X	X		X	X	
	Herpes zoster	34	X	X		X	X	
	Histoplasmosis	36		X				
	Impetigo	45	X	X				
	Influenza	46		X		X		
	Measles	57		X				
	Mononucleosis	59		X		X		
	Mumps	63		X		X		
	Pneumonia	72	X	X		X		
	Rubella (congenital)	77				X	X	X
	Septicemia	80	X	X			X	
	Syphilis	85				X	X	
	Toxoplasmosis	89		X			X	
	Trichinosis	90	X	X				
	Tuberculosis	91				X	X	
	Varicella (chickenpox)	95	X	X				
Metabolic	Albinism	3	X			X		
	Alkaptonuria	5		X	X	X		
	Amyloidosis	8	X	X		X		
	Fabry's disease	25		X		X		
	Galactosemia	27						X
	Gaucher's disease	28		X		X		
	Gout	30				X	X	
	Histioytosis	35	X					
	Homocystinuria	38						X
	Lipidoses	49	X			X		
	Marfan's syndrome	56			X		X	X
	Mucopolysaccharidosis	60				X		
	Wilson's disease	100				X		X
Musculoskeletal	Facial deformity syndrome	26	X					X
	Muscular dystrophy	64	X					
	Osteogenesis imperfect	69			X		X	
Neoplastic	Breast cancer	13	X	X			X	
	Kaposi's sarcoma	47	X	X				
	Leukemia(s)	48	X	X				
	Lung cancer	53	X	X			X	

TABLE 6–2. (Cont.)

Pathological Classification	Specific Systemic Disorder	No. on Top 100 Chart (Table 6–1)	Anterior Segment Manifestation					
			Lids Adnexa	Conjunctiva	Sclera Episclera	Cornea	Anterior Chamber	Lens
Neoplastic (cont.)	Lymphoma(s)	54	X				X	
	Melanoma	58	X	X			X	
Neurological	Cogan's syndrome	17				X		
	Multiple sclerosis	62	X					
	Mysasthenia gravis	65	X				X	
Nutritional	Alcoholism	4	X	X			X	
	Hypervitaminosis	42		X		X		X
	Liver disease	50			X	X		
	Malnutrition	55	X	X		X		
	Vitamin deficiencies	96		X		X		
Phakomatoses	Louis-Barr syndrome	51		X				
	Sturge-Weber syndrome	84	X		X			
	Van Rechlinghausen's	97	X			X	X	
Pulmonary	Asthma	11		X				
Renal	Alport's syndrome	7						X
	Lowe's syndrome	52					X	X
	Wilms' tumor	99	X				X	

C. "TOP 100" DIAGNOSES BY OCULAR ANATOMICAL CLASSIFICATION (Table 6–3)

Use Table 6–3 when your objective examination of the anterior segment reveals physical signs suggestive of systemic origin

TABLE 6–3. "TOP 100" SYSTEMIC DISORDERS WITH ANTERIOR SEGMENT MANIFESTATIONS (BY OCULAR ANATOMICAL CLASSIFICATION)

Anterior Segment Manifestation	Specific Systemic Disorder(s)	Number on Top 100 Chart (Table 6–1)
Lids and adnexa		
Blepharitis	Acne rosacea	1
	Alcoholism	4
	Dermatitis	19
	Eczema	23
	Herpes simplex	33
	Herpes zoster	34
	Impetigo	45
	Pneumonia	72
	Wegener's granulomatosis	98
Blepharoptosis	Hyperthyroidism	41
	Multiple sclerosis	62
	Muscular dystrophy	64
	Myasthenia gravis	65
Blepharospasm	Hypoparathyroidism	43
Changes in eyebrows	Albinism	3
	Hypothyroidism	44
Colobomas	Facial deformity syndrome	26
Edema	Allergies	6
	Dermatomyositis	20
	Hives (urticaria)	37
	Hypothyroidism	44

continued

TABLE 6–3. (Cont.)

Anterior Segment Manifestation	Specific Systemic Disorder(s)	Number on Top 100 Chart (Table 6–1)
Edema (cont.)	Malnutrition	55
	Occlusive venous disease	68
	Toxemia of pregnancy	88
	Trichinosis	90
Epicanthal folds	Downs' syndrome	22
	Turner's syndrome	92
Erythema	Dermatomyositis	20
	Hives (urticaria)	37
Exophthalmos	Histiocytosis	35
	Hyperthyroidism	41
	Leukemia(s)	48
	Lymphoma	54
Hemorrhage	Hemophilia	32
	Pneumonia	72
Lumps and bumps	Acne rosacea	1
	Amyloidosis	8
	Facial deformity syndrome	26
	Kaposi's sarcoma	47
	Melanoma	58
	Neurofibromatosis	97
Pigmentary changes	Addison's disease	2
	Albinism	3
	Alkaptonuria	5
	Melanoma	58
	Nevus of Ota	66
	Sturge–Weber syndrome	84
Vescicles	Herpes simplex	33
	Herpes zoster	34
	Impetigo	45
	Varicella (chickenpox)	95
Xanthalasma	Lipidoses	49
Conjunctiva		
Chemosis (edema)	Allergies	6
	Asthma	11
	Hives (urticaria)	37
	Occlusive venous disease	68
	Trichinosis	90
Conjunctivitis	Alcoholism	4
	Asthma	11
	Cat-scratch fever	15
	Chlamydial disease	16
	Dermatitis	19
	Eczema	23
	Gonorrhea	29
	Hay fever	31
	Herpes zoster	34
	Histoplasmosis	36
	Hives (urticaria)	37
	Impetigo	45
	Influenza	46
	Measles (rubeola)	57
	Mononucleosis	59
	Pemphigoid	70
	Pneumonia	72
	Psoriasis	74
	Reiter's syndrome	75
	Stevens–Johnson disease	83
	Toxoplasmosis	89
	Varicella (chickenpox)	95

continued

TABLE 6–3. (Cont.)

Anterior Segment Manifestation	Specific Systemic Disorder(s)	Number on Top 100 Chart (Table 6–1)
Hemorrhage	Anemia(s)	9
	Hemophilia	32
	Hypertension	40
	Leukemia(s)	48
	Occlusive arterial disease	67
	Periarteritis nodosa	71
	Pneumonia	72
	Septicemia	80
Hyperemia	Allergies	6
	Fabry's disease	25
	Louis–Barr syndrome	51
	Polycythemia vera	73
	Sickle cell disease	81
	Systemic lupus erythematosus	86
Hypoxia (pallor)	Anemia(s)	9
	Occlusive arterial diseae	67
Lumps and bumps	Amyloidosis	8
	Breast cancer	13
	Gaucher's disease	28
	Kaposi's sarcoma	47
	Lung cancer	53
	Melanoma	58
Pigmentary changes	Addison's disease	2
	Alkaptonuria	5
	Hypervitaminosis	42
	Melanoma	58
Xerosis	Hyperparathyroidism	39
	Hypervitaminosis	42
	Malnutrition	55
	Vitamin deficiencies	96
Sclera and episclera		
Episcleritis	Periarteritis nodosa	71
	Sturge–Weber syndrome	84
	Systemic lupus erythematosus	86
Pigmentary changes	Ehlers–Danlos syndrome	24
	Liver disease	50
	Marfan's syndrome	56
	Nevus of Ota	66
	Osteogenesis imperfecta	69
Sclerouveitis	Gout	30
	Rheumatoid arthritis	76
Cornea		
Arcus	Cardiovascular disease	14
	Hypertension	40
	Lipidoses	49
Clouding	Gaucher's disease	28
	Mucopolysaccharidosis	60
	Rubella (congenital)	77
	Turner's syndrome	92
Changes in size/shape	Ehlers–Danlos syndrome	24
	Facial deformity syndrome	26
	Turner's syndrome	92
Deposits	Amyloidosis	8
	Gout	30
	Multiple myeloma	61
Erosion	Diabetes mellitus	21
Infiltrates	Chlamydial disease	16
	Cogan's syndrome	17

continued

TABLE 6–3. (Cont.)

Anterior Segment Manifestation	Specific Systemic Disorder(s)	Number on Top 100 Chart (Table 6–1)
Infiltrates (cont.)	Fabry's disease	25
	Syphilis	85
Keratitis	Acne rosacea	1
	Behçet's disease	12
	Chlamydial disease	16
	Dermatitis	19
	Herpes simplex	33
	Herpes zoster	34
	Hyperthyroidism	41
	Influenza	46
	Liver disease	50
	Mumps	63
	Pemphigoid	70
	Pneumonia	72
	Reiter's syndrome	75
	Scleroderma	79
	Sjögren's syndrome	82
	Stevens–Johnson disease	83
	Systemic lupus erythematosis	86
	Tuberculosis	91
Keratoconus	Downs' syndrome	22
Keratopathy	Cardiovascular disease	14
	Hyperparathyroidism	39
	Hypervitaminosis	42
	Malnutrition	55
	Rheumatoid arthritis	76
Pigmentary changes	Alkaptonuria	5
	Wilson's disease	100
Prominent nerves	Neurofibromatosis	97
Ulceration	Gonorrhea	29
	Herpes simplex	33
	Herpes zoster	34
	Pneumonia	72
	Rheumatoid arthritis	76
	Sjögren's syndrome	82
	Wegener's granulomatosis	98
Anterior Chamber		
Brushfeld's spots	Downs' syndrome	22
Glaucoma	(All steroid therapy)	
	Amyloidosis	8
	Lowe's syndrome	52
	Osteogenesis imperfecta	69
	Neurofibromatosis	97
Hyphema	Behçet's disease	12
	Herpes simplex	33
	Melanoma	58
Iris abnormalities	Multiple myeloma	61
	Rubella (congenital)	77
	Wilms' tumor	99
Pupil abnormalities	Marfan's syndrome	56
	Myasthenia gravis	65
Rubeosis iridis	Diabetes mellitus	21
	Occlusive venous disease	68
Uveitis	Ankylosing spondylitis	10
	Behçet's disease	12
	Crohn's disease	18
	Gonorrhea	29
	Herpes zoster	34
	Leukemia(s)	48
	Lymphoma(s)	54

TABLE 6–3. (Cont.)

Anterior Segment Manifestation	Specific Systemic Disorder(s)	Number on Top 100 Chart (Table 6–1)
Uveitis (cont.)	Mononucleosis	59
	Periarteritis nodosa	71
	Reiter's syndrome	75
	Rheumatoid arthritis (and JRA)	76
	Sarcoidosis	78
	Septicemia	80
	Stevens–Johnson disease	83
	Syphilis	85
	Systemic lupus erythematosus	86
	Temporal arteritis	87
	Toxoplasmosis	89
	Ulcer (peptic)	93
	Ulcerative colitis	94
Lens		
Cataract	Alport's syndrome	7
	Downs' syndrome	22
	Eczema	23
	Galactosemia	27
	Homocystinuria	38
	Hypervitaminosis	42
	Hypoparathyroidism	43
	Hypothyroidism	44
	Lowe's syndrome	52
	Rubella (congenital)	77
	Turner's syndrome	92
	Wilson's disease	100
Dislocation	Homocystinuria	38
	Marfan's syndrome	56
Lenticonus	Alport's syndrome	7
	Lowe's syndrome	52

XIV. Self-assessment Questions

Match the objective findings (1 to 10) in column A with their associated systemic disorders in column B. Then match the pathological classifications (11 to 20) in column C with the disorders in column B:

Column A
1. Port wine stain
2. Comma-shaped conjunctival vessels
3. Anterior uveitis
4. Proptosis
5. Lid or conjunctival edema
6. Loss of lateral one third of eyebrows
7. Corneal crystals
8. Blue sclera
9. Recurrent chalazia
10. Brushfeld's spots

Column B
a. Downs' syndrome
b. Gout
c. Hives (urticaria)
d. Acne rosacea
e. Osteogenesis imperfecta
f. Leukemia
g. Sickle cell anemia
h. Ankylosing spondylitis
i. Sturge–Weber syndrome
j. Hypothyroid

Column C
11. Dermatological
12. Collagen vascular
13. Metabolic
14. Endocrine
15. Allergic
16. Chromosomal
17. Neoplastic
18. Phakomatoses
19. Musculoskeletal
20. Hematological

For answers, refer to Appendix 6.

REFERENCES

1. Browning DJ, Proia AD: Ocular rosacea in blacks. Am J Ophthalmol 101:441, 1986

2. Tierney DW: Basal cell epithelioma. J Am Optom Assoc 58:307, 1987

3. Cooper M: Epidemiology of herpes zoster. Eye 1:413, 1987

4. Rubinstein MD: Diabetes, the anterior segment and contact lens wear. Contact Lens J 15:5, 1987
5. Gorum C: Ophthalmopathy of Grave's disease. N Engl J Med 308:453, 1983
6. Cooper DS: Subclinical hypothyroidism. JAMA 258:246, 1987
7. Cockburn DM: Wilson's disease (hepatolenticular degeneration). Clin Exp Optom 70:20, 1987
8. Auran JD, Starr MB, Jakobiec FA: Acanthamoeba keratitis: A review of the literature. Cornea 6:1, 1987

ANNOTATED REFERENCES

Braunwald E, et al (eds): Harrison's Principles of Internal Medicine, ed 11. New York, McGraw-Hill, 1987
Definitive source regarding systemic medical conditions and care. Comprehensive work on all disease categories, with in-depth discussion on each area and condition.
Harley RD: Pediatric Ophthalmology, ed 2. Philadelphia, WB Saunders, 1983
Specific and comprehensive in the area of ocular syndromes of congenital or developmental nature. Comprehensive descriptions, tables, and care for each condition.
Kanski JJ: The Eye in Systemic Disease. London, Butterworths, 1986
Well-organized text of major systemic conditions with ocular involvements. Brief tabular information on each condition with excellent photographs.
Krupp MA, Chatton MJ, Tierney LM: (eds): Current Medical Diagnosis and Treatment 1986. Los Altos, Lange Medical, 1986
Quick, in-office reference source for common systemic diseases in all categories. Short descriptions, listings, and differential diagnostic considerations with standard current treatment approaches.
Roy FH: Ocular Syndromes and Systemic Diseases. Orlando, FL, Grune & Stratton, 1985
Two-part book, one of short descriptions of most systemic diseases and ocular syndromes and one of differential diagnoses categorized by common subjective symptoms and objective signs. Good quick reference resource.

7

Contact Lens-related Anterior Segment Care

Chapter Outline

I. Prefit Considerations and Care

A. RISK FACTOR GUIDELINES IN CONTACT LENS CARE

1. Explanation of contact lens (CL) risk factors

Risk Factor	Relative to Clinical Condition
0	No direct or indirect adverse effects on CL wear
1+	Possible indirect adverse effect on CL wear
2+	Probable indirect adverse effect on CL wear
3+	Possible direct adverse effect on CL wear
4+	Probable direct adverse effect on CL wear

2. Management guidelines relative to contact lens risk factors
   a. Reduce prefit risk factors, whenever possible, with prefit care
   b. Prefit risk factors of 0 to 2+ can usually be fit with or without prefit care
   c. Prefit risk factors of 3 to 4+ should always receive prefit considerations
   d. Prefit risk factors reduced with prefit care by 25 percent or less should be followed every 3 to 4 months or PRN
   e. Postcare (after prefit care) risk factors should be managed as follows:

TABLE 7–1. CONTACT LENS PREFITTING GUIDE: CONDITIONS OF THE EYELIDS AND ASSOCIATED STRUCTURES

Clinical Condition	Contact Lens Wear Risk Factor	Prefit Care (Need)	Treatment Highlights
Allergic blepharitis	3+	Valuable	Remove cause; cold packs; oral antihistamine/decongestants; steroids (?)
Basal cell carcinoma	0	Optional	Counsel and advise; photodocument; refer to dermatology
Bell's palsy	1+	None	Advise; refer to medicine or neurology
Blepharitis (see specific cause)	2–4+	Valuable	Treat specific cause
Blepharospasm	1+	Optional	Reassurance; antihistamines (?)/biofeedback (?)
Blowout fracture	0	Optional	Oral antibiotics and decongestants; refer to oculoplastics
Burns of eyelid	1+	Valuable	Treat per tissue involvement and degree
Cellulitis			
Orbital	4+	Essential	Refer stat to medicine
Preseptal	4+	Essential	Oral antibiotics; hot packs
Chalasis	1+	Optional	Reassure; photodocument, refer to oculodermatology
Chalazion	3+	Essential	Hot packs; surgical excision; steroid infection, reassure
Coloboma	1+	None	Reassure; lubricate cornea if necessary
Contusion of eyelid	3+	Valuable	R/O ocular involvement, crepitus, blowout fracture
Dacryocystitis	4+	Essential	Antibiotics (topical/oral); dilate/irrigate
Dacryostenosis	3+	Valuable	Dilate and irrigate; heat
Demodex blepharitis	3+	Valuable	Lid scrubs; hot packs, mercuric oxide ointment (hs); AM wash
Districhiasis	2+	None	Epilate; counsel and advise
Ecchymosis	1+	Valuable	(See Contusion); 24-hr cold packs; 3–5 days hot packs
Ectropion	3+	Optional	Lubricate; tape lid (?); refer to oculoplastics
Edema of eyelid(s)	2+	Valuable	Determine cause; treat cause; cold packs
Entropion	2+	Valuable	Soft contact lens; tape lid (?); refer to oculoplastics

Postcare
Risk Factor	Management Care
0 to 1+	Routine or PRN
2+	Every 3 months or PRN
3+	Very close follow (if fit)
4+	Do not fit!

    f. Apply these conditions to the risk factors found in the contact lens prefitting guides that follow

B. CONDITIONS OF THE EYELIDS AND ASSOCIATED STRUCTURES[1]

Please refer to Table 7–1

C. CONDITIONS OF THE NONCORNEAL OCULAR SURFACE[1]

Please refer to Table 7–2

D. CONDITIONS OF THE CORNEA[1]

Please refer to Table 7–3

E. ANTERIOR SEGMENT-RELATED ANOMALIES[1]

Please refer to Table 7–4

Follow-up Period Before Contact Lens Fit	Postcare Risk Factor	Risk Factor Reduction (%)	Postcare Fitting Considerations
10–14 days	2+	33	GPH or low water
None	0	N/A	Fitter's choice
None	1+	0	Large soft with lubricant
Per condition	0–2+	50	Per condition
None	1+	0	Fitter's choice
30 days	0	N/A	Fitter's choice
10–14 days	0	100	Fitter's choice
Per consultant	1+	75	Soft and loose
14–21 days	0	100	Fitter's choice
None	1+	0	Soft or GPH
To resolution	1+	66	Soft
None	1+	0	Soft and large
14–21 days	0	100	Fitter's choice
14–21 days	1+	75	Fitter's choice
7 days	2+	33	GPH
10–14 days	1+	66	Low water or GPH
None	2+	0	Large diameter, soft
14–21 days	0	100	Fitter's choice
None	1+	66	Low water or GPH
7–14 days	1+	50	Soft
None	1+	50	Large soft

continued

TABLE 7–1. (Cont.)

Clinical Condition	Contact Lens Wear Risk Factor	Prefit Care (Need)	Treatment Highlights
Epiblepharon	1+	None	Treat complications; counsel, reassure
Epicanthus	1+	None	R/O strabismus; reassure and advise
Epiphora	2+	Valuable	Determine cause; treat cause
Erythema of eyelids	3+	Valuable	Determine cause; treat cause
Herpes simplex	3+	Valuable	Supportive skin therapy; acyclovir; prophylax eye (if indicated)
Herpes zoster	4+	Essential	Supportive skin therapy; steroids (oral and topical?) Refer to dermatology
Hordeolum	3+	Valuable	Hot packs; antistaphylococcal ointment
Impetigo	3+	Valuable	Topical and oral erythromycin; hygiene
Insect bites/stings	3+	Valuable	Remove stinger; cold packs; oral antihistamine–decongestant; steroids (?)
Keratoses	0	Optional	Ointment lubrication (early stages); treat complication, advise
Laceration of eyelid	4+	Essential	Clean wound and treat per nature and degree of laceration
Lagophthalmos	1+	None	Lubricate; soft contact lens; tape lids (?)
Madarosis	2+	Valuable	Lid scrubs; hot packs, antistaph ointment
Meibomianitis	4+	Essential	Hot packs; topical (and oral?) antistaphylococcal therapy
Molluscum contagiosum	1+	Optional	Alcohol preparation; curette contents; squeeze out; alcohol wipe
Papilloma	0	Optional	Remove (if requested and small); refer to ophthalmic surgeon or dermatology
Pediculosis	3+	Essential	Kwell shampoo or eserine ointment
Poliosis	2+	Valuable	Lid scrubs; hot packs, antistaphylococcal ointment
Ptosis	1+	Optional	Congenital; reassure; acquired; refer to appropriate specialist
Sebaceous cyst	0	Optional	Drain if requested (and superficial)
Seborrheic blepharitis	3+	Valuable	(Same as staphylococcal blepharitis), reduce fatty foods
Sinusitis	3+	Essential	Oral decongestants and dichloxacillin
Squamous cell carcinoma	2+	Essential	Refer to oculoderm.
Staphylococcal blepharitis	4+	Essential	Hygiene; lid scrubs; hot packs, antistaphylococcal ointment
Streptococcal blepharitis	4+	Essential	Topical and oral antibiotics; hot packs
Subcutaneous cilia	1+	Valuable	Remove cilia; prophylax (1 ×)
Sudoriferous cyst	1+	Valuable	Drain (if requested); reassure
Trichiasis	3+	Valuable	Epilate; soft contact lenses
Tylosis	3+	Optional	Lid scrubs; hot packs, antistaphylococcal/steroid combination ointment
Verrucae	1+	Optional	No treatment if asymptomatic; refer to oculodermatology
Xanthalasma	0	Optional	Counsel; reassure; refer to oculodermatology (if requested)

Follow-up Period Before Contact Lens Fit	Postcare Risk Factor	Risk Factor Reduction (%)	Postcare Fitting Considerations
None	1+	0	Fitter's choice
None	1+	0	Fitter's choice
None	1+	50	High water
7–14 days	1+	66	Soft or GPH
30 days	2+	33	GPH
Per consultant	2+	50	Soft and loose
14–21 days	0	100	Fitter's choice
14–21 days	1+	66	Low water or GPH
7–14 days	0	100	Fitter's choice
None	0	N/A	Fitter's choice
30 days	1+	75	Large soft
None	1+	0	Extended-wear soft
7–14 days	1+	50	Low water or GPH
None	0	N/A	Fitter's choice
20–30 days	2+	50	Low water or GPH
None	1+	0	Low water or GPH
None	0	N/A	Fitter's choice
14–21 days	0	100	Fitter's choice
7–14 days	1+	50	Low water or GPH
None	1+	0	Soft or GPH
None	0	N/A	Fitter's choice
7–10 days	1+	66	Low water or GPH
14–21 days	1+	66	Soft or GPH
None	1+	50	Fitter's choice
14–21 days	1+	75	Low water or GPH
14–21 days	0	100	Fitter's choice
None	0	100	Fitter's choice
None	0	100	Fitter's choice
None	1+	66	Large soft
7–14 days	2+	33	GPH
None	1+	0	Low water or GPH

TABLE 7–2. CONTACT LENS PREFITTING GUIDE: CONDITIONS OF THE NONCORNEAL OCULAR SURFACE

Clinical Condition	Contact Lens Wear Risk Factor	Prefit Care (Need)	Treatment Highlights
Allergic conjunctivitis	3+	Valuable	Remove cause; cold packs; topical and oral antihistamine/decongestant; steroids(?)
Argyrosis	2+	Valuable	Remove cause (silver)
Axenfeld's loops	0	None	No treatment, reassure
Bacterial conjunctivitis	4+	Essential	Hot packs; irrigation; topical antibiotic
Bitot's spots	1+	Optional	Swab; lubricate; remove cause; vitamin A supplement
Blue sclera	0	None	Counsel; reassure
Conjunctivitis (see cause)	2–4+	Valuable	Per condition
Dermoid	1+	Optional	Reassure; refer to oculoplastics
Episcleritis	1+	Valuable	Hot packs; topical steroids; aspirin
Epithelioma	3+	Essential	Refer for removal and biopsy
Giant papillary conjunctivitis	4+	Valuable	Remove lens; lubricate; aspirin and antihistamines (?)
Granuloma	2+	Optional	Hot packs or surgical excision if indicated
Hyaline plaque	0	None	No treatment; reassure
Hyperacute conjunctivitis	4+	Essential	Culture; topical (and oral) antibiotic; hot packs
Icteria (jaundice)	0	Systemic	Refer to physician for (liver) evaluation
Inclusion cyst	1+	Optional	Reassure; attempt drainage if requested; refer to ophthalmic surgery
Keratinization	1+	Optional	Lubricate; decongest; reassure
Laceration of conjunctiva	3+	Optional	Irrigate; prophylax with topical antibiotic
Lithiasis	2+	Optional	Reassure; remove if symptomatic; prophylax (1×)
Lymphangectasia	1+	Valuable	Drain, if requested
Lymphangioma	1+	Valuable	R/O lymphoma; reassure
Melanosis, acquired	1+	Optional	R/O melanoma; reassure, counsel
Melanosis, congenital	0	None	Reassure; counsel
Melanosis, scleral	0	None	R/O blue sclera; reassure
Nevus of Ota	0	None	(See melanosis, sclera)
Ochronosis	3+	Systemic	Counsel; refer to medicine
Papilloma of conjunctiva	2+	Optional	R/O neoplasia; reassure; refer to ophthalmic surgery (if requested)
Pharyngoconjunctival fever	3+	Valuable	(Same as viral conjunctivitis)
Pigmentations	2+	Valuable	Determine cause; treat cause
Pinguecula	1+	Optional	Decongest; lubricate; reassure
Pseudomembrane	4+	Valuable	Remove with swab or forceps
Scleritis	4+	Essential	Refer to ophthalmology and medicine
Staphyloma	1+	None	Reassure; counsel
Subconjunctival hemorrhage	1+	None	Attempt to determine cause; reassure; hot or cold packs (placebo?)
Telangectasia	0	None	Document; reassure
Toxic conjunctivitis	2+	Valuable	Lubricate or zinc oxide ointment

TABLE 7–3. CONTACT LENS PREFITTING GUIDE: CONDITIONS OF THE CORNEA

Clinical Condition	Contact Lens Wear Risk Factor	Prefit Care (Need)	Treatment Highlights
Adenovirus	2+	Valuable	Supportive and palliative measures
Anterior mosaic dystrophy	0	None	Monitor changes
Arcus senilis	0	None	R/O serum lipids
Band keratopathy	2+	Optional	Monitor or chelate

Follow-up Period Before Contact Lens Fit	Postcare Risk Factor	Risk Factor Reduction (%)	Postcare Fitting Considerations
10–14 days	2+	33	Low water or GPH
None	0	100	Fitter's choice
None	0	N/A	Fitter's choice
14–21 days	0	100	Fitter's choice
None	1+	0	GPH
None	0	N/A	Fitter's choice
Per condition	0–2+	50	Per condition
None	0	100	Fitter's choice
20–30 days	0	100	Fitter's choice
Postsurgical	1+	66	Soft and loose
20–30 days	3+	25	Change material
None	1+	50	Soft or GPH
None	0	N/A	Fitter's choice
20–30 days	1+	75	Low water or GPH
None	0	N/A	Fitter's choice
None	0	100	Fitter's choice
None	1+	0	Soft or GPH
30 days	0	100	Fitter's choice
None	0	100	Fitter's choice
None	0	100	Fitter's choice
None	0	100	Fitter's choice
None	1+	0	Soft or GPH
None	0	N/A	Fitter's choice
None	0	N/A	Fitter's choice
None	0	N/A	Fitter's choice
Per consultant	1+	66	GPH
None	0	100	Fitter's choice
14–21 days	0	100	Fitter's choice
None	0	100	Fitter's choice
None	1+	0	Small soft or GPH
20–30 days	1+	75	Soft or GPH
Per consultant	3+	25	Don't fit
None	1+	0	Soft or GPH
7–14 days	0	100	Fitter's choice
None	0	N/A	Fitter's choice
14–21 days	1+	50	High water or GPH

Follow-up Period Before Contact Lens Fit	Postcare Risk Factor	Risk Factor Reduction (%)	Postcare Fitting Considerations
14–21 days	1+	50	Soft or GPH
None	0	N/A	Fitter's choice
None	0	N/A	Fitter's choice
None	1+	50	High water, large

continued

Table 7– 3. (Cont.)

Clinical Condition	Contact Lens Wear Risk Factor	Prefit Care (Need)	Treatment Highlights
Bullous keratopathy	2+	Essential	Bandage soft lens
Central cloudy dystrophy	0	None	Monitor changes
Chlamydia	4+	Essential	Topical and oral tetracycline or venereal
Cogan's microcystic dystrophy	2+	Valuable	Hypertonics or soft lenses
Congenital hereditary endothelial dystrophy	N/A	Essential	Refer to pediatric ophthalmologist
Corneal			
Abrasion, deep	4+	Essential	Abrasion protocol
Abrasion, superficial	2+	Optional	Lubricants, prophylax (+/−)
Burns	4+	Essential	Per degree
Contusion	3+	Valuable	R/O complications
Degeneration	1–2+	Variable	Monitor changes
Dystrophy	2–4+	Variable	Specific diagnosis by layer
Erosion, recurrent	2+	Essential	Lubrication, hypertonics or soft lenses
Farinata	0	None	Monitor changes
Foreign bodies	4+	Essential	Diagnosis, depth of penetration
FBT	1+	Optional	Remove cause and lubricate, prophylax (+/−)
Removal of	2+	Essential	Use most comfortable, efficient procedure
Guttata	1+	None	Monitor endothelial and epithelial changes
Pigmentations	0	None	Remove cause and treat complications
Crocodile Shagreen	0	None	Monitor changes
Dellen (Gaule spot)	2+	Valuable	Lubricant or soft lens
Dry-eye syndrome	3+	Valuable	Lubrication therapies
Endothelial disorders	3+	Optional	Monitor endothelium and epithelium
EKC	4+	Valuable	Supportive and palliative; steroids if severe
EBMD	3+	Valuable	Lubricants, hypertonics, or soft lenses
Fleck dystrophy	0	None	Monitor changes
Fuchs' dystrophy	3+	Essential	Multiple antiedema procedures
Fungal disease	4+	Essential	Refer to corneal specialist
Granular dystrophy	3+	Optional	Monitor changes
Hassle Henle bodies	1+	None	Monitor changes
Hemosiderosis (rust)	3+	Valuable	Remove completely
Herpes simplex	3+	Essential	Treat aggressively with antiviral agents
Dendriform	4+	Essential	Treat aggressively with antiviral agents
Disciform	3+	Essential	Steroids required (refer to corneal specialist)
Metaherpetic	4+	Essential	Antivirals (with guarded prognosis)
Primary	4+	Essential	Antivirals (with pediatric consult)
Recurrent	4+	Essential	Monitor epithelial and stromal changes
Stromal (interstitial)	4+	Essential	Refer to corneal specialist (for steroids)
Herpes zoster	4+	Essential	Treat ocular complications appropriately

Follow-up Period Before Contact Lens Fit	Postcare Risk Factor	Risk Factor Reduction (%)	Postcare Fitting Considerations
None (SL therapy)	1+	50	High water, large
None	0	N/A	Fitter's choice
30 days	0	100	Fitter's choice
None (SL therapy)	1+	50	High water, large
None	3+	N/A	Don't fit
7–10 days	1+	75	Soft or GPH
3–5 days	0	100	Fitter's choice
14–21 days	1+	75	High water, large
7–14 days	1+	66	Soft or GPH
None	0–1+	50	Per condition
None	0–2+	50	Per condition
None (SL therapy)	0	100	High water, EW
None	0	N/A	Fitter's choice
7–10 days	1+	75	Soft or GPH
3–5 days	0	100	Fitter's choice
7–10 days	0	100	Fitter's hoice
None	1+	0	High water or GPH
None	0	N/A	Fitter's choice
None	0	N/A	Fitter's choice
None (SL therapy)	0	100	Large, soft
None (SL therapy)	1+	66	Low water with lubricants
None (SL therapy)	1+	66	High water or GPH
30 days	1+	75	Soft or GPH
None (SL therapy)	1+	75	High water, large, EW
None	0	N/A	Fitter's choice
None (SL therapy)	1+	66	High water, large, loose
Per consultant	3+	25	Don't fit
None	2+	33	Soft or GPH
None	1+	0	High water, loose
7–10 days	0	100	Fitter's choice
30 days	2+	33	Soft
30 days	2+	50	Soft
Per consultant	3+	0	Don't fit
30–60 days	2+	50	Soft
30 days	1+	75	Soft
30 days	2+	50	Soft
Per consultant	3+	25	Don't fit
Per consultant	2+	50	Soft

continued

Table 7–3. (Cont.)

Clinical Condition	Contact Lens Wear Risk Factor	Prefit Care (Need)	Treatment Highlights
Keratoconus	2+	Valuable	Contact lens (firm) and monitor
Posterior	4+	None	Refer for genetic counseling
Keratitis	3+	Variable	
Atopic	3+	Valuable	Topical steroids
Dendriform	4+	Essential	Antiviral (if herpetic); lubricant (if infiltrative)
Filamentary	3+	Valuable	Remove filaments and lubricate or soft lens
Marginal	4+	Essential	Combination antibiotic/steroid (lids and eye)
Neurotropic	3+	Essential	Lubrication therapies
Sicca	4+	Essential	Lubrication therapies
Striate	2+	Optional	Treat cause and complications
Stromal	4+	Essential	(see also Herpes)
Viral	3–4+	Valuable	(see also Herpes)
Kruchenburg's spindle	0	None	R/O chronic uveitis or pigment dispersion syndrome
Lattice dystrophy	2+	None	Monitor changes
Limbal girdle of Vogt	0	None	No treatment
Macular dystrophy	2+	None	Monitor changes
Marginal furrow degeneration	1+	None	Monitor changes
Meesman's dystrophy	1+	None	Monitor changes
Megalocornea	1+	None	R/O increased IOP
Microcornea	2+	None	R/O syndromes; refer to pediatrics
Mooren's ulcer	4+	Essential	Refer to corneal specialist
Pellucid marginal degeneration	4+	Essential	Usually steroids when active
Phlyctenular keratoconjunctivitis	4+	Essential	Combination antibiotics and steroid
Posterior amorphous dystrophy	0	None	Monitor changes
Pre-Descemet's dystrophy	0	None	Monitor changes
Pterygium	3+	Valuable	Measure advancement toward pupil
Reis–Buckler's dystrophy	2+	None	Monitor changes
Sclerocornea	1+	None	No treatment
Sjögren's syndrome	3+	Valuable	Monitor dry eye syndrome
SPK	2–4+	Variable	Remove cause and lubricate, prophylax (+/−)
of Thygeson	3+	Valuable	Lubricate and/or soft lenses
Staphylococcal	4+	Essential	Antistaph therapy and lubrication
Viral	3–4+	Valuable	Supportive and lubrication
Subepithelial infiltrates	2+	Optional	Remove cause; steroid when dense or anterior stromal
Superior limbic keratoconjunctivitis	4+	Valuable	D/C thimerosol or soft lenses; steroids(?), silver nitrate, cromolyn sodium
Terrien's degeneration	4+	Essential	Steroids and prophylax
Ulcers, corneal	4+	Essential	Refer to corneal specialist
Bacterial	4+	Essential	Refer to corneal specialist
Dendriform	4+	Essential	Antiviral therapy (if herpetic)
Fungal	4+	Essential	Refer to corneal specialist
Gonococcal	4+	Essential	Refer to corneal specialist
H. flu	4+	Essential	Refer to corneal specialist
Mooren's	4+	Essential	Refer to corneal specialist

Follow-up Period Before Contact Lens Fit	Postcare Risk Factor	Risk Factor Reduction (%)	Postcare Fitting Considerations
None (SL therapy)	1+	50	GPH
Per consultant	4+	0	Don't fit
Per condition	1+	66	Per condition
To resolution	2+	33	High water, large
30 days	2+	50	Soft
None	1+	66	High water, loose
14–21 days	2+	50	Soft or GPH
None (SL therapy)	1+	66	Large soft
None (SL therapy)	1+	75	Low water with lubricant
14–21 days	1+	50	Soft or GPH
Per consultant	3+	25	Don't fit
30 days	1–2+	50	Per condition
None	0	N/A	Fitter's choice
None	2+	0	High water, loose
None	0	N/A	Fitter's choice
None	2+	0	High water, loose
None	1+	0	Large soft or GPH
None (SL therapy)	1+	0	Soft or GPH
None	1+	0	Large soft or GPH
None	2+	0	GPH (Beware!)
Per consultant	3+	25	Don't fit
30 days	3+	25	Fit only with keratoconus
20–30 days	2+	50	Large soft or GPH
None	0	N/A	Fitter's choice
None	0	N/A	Fitter's choice
Post surgical	1+	66	GPH
None (SL therapy)	2+	0	High water, loose, EW
None	1+	0	Large, soft or GPH
None (SL therapy)	1+	66	Low water with lubricants
Per condition	1–2+	50	Per condition
None (SL therapy)	1+	66	Large soft
14–21 days	2+	50	Soft or GPH
30 days	1–2+	50	Per condition
30 days	1+	50	Monitor cornea closely
20–30 days	2+	50	No thimeresol
Per consultant	3+	25	Don't fit
Per consultant	1+	75	Soft, loose
Per consultant	1+	75	Soft, loose
30 days	2+	50	Soft, loose
Per consultant	3+	25	Don't fit
Per consultant	1+	75	Soft, loose
Per consultant	1+	75	Soft, loose
Per consultant	3+	25	Don't fit

continued

TABLE 7–3. (Cont.)

Clinical Condition	Contact Lens Wear Risk Factor	Prefit Care (Need)	Treatment Highlights
Pseudomonas	4+	Essential	Refer to corneal specialist
Serpiginous	4+	Essential	Refer to corneal specialist
Staphylococcal	4+	Essential	Refer to corneal specialist
Toxic	4+	Essential	Antistaphylococcal agents and steroids
Streptococcal	4+	Essential	Refer to corneal specialist
Vernal keratoconjunctivitis	4+	Essential	Steroids, antihistamines, aspirin, cromolyn sodium
Wessely ring	2+	Valuable	Remove cause and steroids

TABLE 7–4. CONTACT LENS PREFITTING GUIDE: ANTERIOR SEGMENT-RELATED ABNORMALITIES

Clinical Condition	Contact Lens Wear Risk Factor	Prefit Care (Need)	Treatment Highlights
Acne rosacea	4+	Essential	Topical tetracycline and steroids; oral tetracycline
Adie's tonic pupil	0	None	R/O neurological disease
Albinism	1+	None	Monitor ocular abnormalities
Anemia	0	Systemic	Counsel and refer to medicine
Anterior uveitis, acute	3+	Valuable	Cycloplege and dilate; topical steroids
Anterior uveitis, chronic	3+	Essential	Cycloplege and dilate; steroids; medical referral
Axenfeld's anomaly	0	None	Monitor IOP closely
Cancer (metastatic)	0	Systemic	R/O ocular involvement; counsel
Cardiovascular disease	0	Systemic	Monitor ocular signs; counsel
Cerebrovascular disease	0	Systemic	Monitor ocular signs; counsel
Collagen vascular disease	2+	Systemic	Monitor ocular complications; counsel
Congenital syndromes	1+	None	Monitor ocular complications; counsel
Dermatitis, chronic	3+	Valuable	Refer to dermatologist
Dermatoses	1+	Valuable	Topical (see cause); refer to dermatology (+/−)
Diabetes	2+	Systemic	Monitor ocular complications; counsel
Downs' syndrome	1+	None	Monitor ocular complications; counsel
Glaucoma, acute closure	4+	Essential	2–4% pilocarpine q10min, oral glycerine or Diamox
Glaucoma, chronic marrow	2+	Essential	Refer to ophthalmology
Glaucoma, COAG	1+	Essential	Anti glaucoma therapies
Glaucoma, secondary	2+	Essential	Refer to ophthalmology (glaucoma specialist)
Hyphema	2+	Valuable	Immobilize and monitor for complications
Hypopyon	4+	Essential	Treat cause (usually corneal ulcer)
Marfan's jsyndrome	1+	None	Monitor ocular signs; counsel
Migraine, classic	3+	Optional	R/O neuro-ocular disease; refer to medicine
Migraine, common	3+	Optional	R/O neuro-ocular disease; refer to medicine
Multiple sclerosis	0	None	Refer to neurology; monitor ocular signs
Neurological disease	0–2+	Systemic	Refer to neurology
Neurosis	2+	Optional	Refer to psychology; counsel
Ocular hypertension	0	Systemic	Monitor ocular signs; counsel
Osteogenesis imperfecta	0	None	Monitor ocular signs; counsel

Follow-up Period Before Contact Lens Fit	Postcare Risk Factor	Risk Factor Reduction (%)	Postcare Fitting Considerations
Per consultant	1+	75	Soft, loose
Per consultant	3+	25	Don't fit
Per consultant	1+	75	Soft, loose
14–21 days	2+	50	Soft or GPH
Per consultant	1+	75	Soft, loose
5–10 years	3+	25	Don't fit
30 days	1+	50	Soft or GPH

Follow-up Period Before Contact Lens Fit	Postcare Risk Factor	Risk Factor Reduction (%)	Postcare Fitting Considerations
10–15 years		25	Don't fit
None		N/A	Fitter's choice
None		0	Soft or GPH
None		N/A	Fitter's choice
14–21 days		100	Fitter's choice
6–12 weeks		33	Soft, loose
None		N/A	Fitter's choice
None		N/A	Fitter's choice
None		N/A	Fitter's choice
None		N/A	Fitter's choice
None		50	Soft or GPH
None		0	Per syndrome
30 days		33	Soft or GPH
To resolution		0	Soft or GPH
None		0	High water soft
None		0	Soft, EW
Postsurgical		75	Soft (loose) or GPH
Per consultant		50	Soft (loose) or GPH
To IOP control		0	Soft or GPH
Per consultant		50	Soft or GPH
30 days		100	Fitter's choice
30 days		75	Soft or GPH
None		0	Soft or GPH
Per consultant		0	Soft
Per consultant		0	Soft
Per consultant		N/A	Fitter's choice
Per consultant	0–2+	0	Per condition
Per consultant	1+	50	Soft
None	0	N/A	Fitter's choice

continued

TABLE 7–4. (Cont.)

Clinical Condition	Contact Lens Wear Risk Factor	Prefit Care (Need)	Treatment Highlights
Peter's anomaly	4+	Valuable	Refer to pediatric ophthalmology
Phakamatoses	2+	Optional	Monitor ocular signs; refer to medicine
Posterior embryotoxon	0	None	Monitor IOP
Psychosis	4+	Essential	Refer to psychiatry
Reiger's syndrome	2+	None	Monitor IOP closely
Stevens–Johnson syndrome	4+	Valuable	Monitor ocular complications; refer to medicine
Strabismus	0	Valuable	Treat functionally or refer to ophthalmology
Systemic manifestations	0–4+	Valuable	Monitor ocular complications; refer to medicine
Temporo mandibular joint syndrome	0	Valuable	Refer to oral surgery
Thyroid eye disease	3+	Essential	Monitor ocular signs; refer to medicine
Tic doloureaux	3+	Valuable	Refer to neurology
Trachoma	4+	Essential	Refer (active) to ophthalmology
Traumatic iritis	3+	Valuable	Cycloplege and dilate; topical steroids
Venereal disease	2+	Essential	Monitor ocular complications; refer to medicine
Vitiligo	0	Optional	Reassure; refer to dermatology (+/−)
Wilson's disease	1+	Essential	Refer to neurology

II. Postfit Considerations and Care

A. MAJOR CONTACT LENS COMPLICATIONS BY ETIOLOGY

Please refer to Table 7–5

B. CONTACT LENS COMPLICATIONS (BY SOAP)

1. Bedewing

Subjective

- No discomfort
- Photophobia
- Reduced visual acuity with prolonged or extended wear

Objective

- Hazy ground-glass appearance to epithelium
- Diffuse to periphery
- No positive staining
- Stroma clear (no edema)

Assessment

- Mechanical
  1. Poor PMMA surface or edges
  2. Poor lathe cut soft
  3. Debris entrapment in EW

- Physiological
  1. Associated with endothelial changes
  2. No movement in soft lens fit
  3. Red eye reaction

Plan

- Mechanical
  1. Repolish PMMA
  2. Replace soft
  3. Loosen EW soft
- Physiological
  1. Loosen fit
  2. D/C EW temporarily or permanently

Follow-up

- Return check (RTC) 1 week after corrective measures
- If problem persists, refit
- If problem resolves, schedule routine follow-up

2. Cells or Flare

Subjective

- Dull aching pain
- Photophobia
- No immediate improvement on lens removal

Follow-up Period Before Contact Lens Fit	Postcare Risk Factor	Risk Factor Reduction (%)	Postcare Fitting Considerations
None	0	N/A	Fitter's choice
Per consultant	2+	50	Soft, large
None	2+	0	Per condition
None	0	N/A	Fitter's choice
Per consultant	3+	25	Don't fit
None	2+	0	Soft or GPH
Per consultant	3+	25	Don't fit
None	0	N/A	Fitter's choice
Per ocular involvement	0–4+	Variable	Per condition
Postdental care	0	N/A	Fitter's choice
None	2+	33	Soft
Per consultant	2+	33	Soft
Per consultant	2+	50	Soft or GPH
14–21 days	0	100	Fitter's choice
Per consultant	1+	50	Fitter's choice
None	0	N/A	Fitter's choice
Per consultant	0	100	Fitter's choice

TABLE 7–5. MAJOR CONTACT LENS COMPLICATIONS BY ETIOLOGY

Contact Lens Complications	Possible Etiologies				
	Infectious	Immunological	Mechanical	Physiological	Other
Bedewing			X	X	
Cells or flare	X	X	X		
Conjunctival hyperemia	X	X	X	X	X
Endothelial changes				X	
Epithelial breakdown	X	X	X	X	
Giant papillary conjunctivitis		X	X		
Keratoconjunctivitis	X	X		X	X
Limbal engorgement			X	X	
Microcystic edema			X	X	
Microcysts (vesicles)			X	X	X
Mucous debris/buildup		X	X		X
Neovascularization	X	X	X	X	
Pannus	X	X	X	X	
Pseudodendrites	X	X		X	
Stippling			X		X
Striate keratitis	X			X	X
Stromal edema	X		X	X	X
Stromal infiltrates	X	X			
Subepithelial infiltrates	X	X			
Superficial punctate keratitis	X	X	X	X	X
Superior limbic keratoconjunctivitis		X	X		X
Toxic keratitis	X	X			X
Ulceration (corneal)	X	X	X	X	X

Objective

- Cloudy, turbid aqueous (protein)
- White or pigmented cells in aqueous
- Occasional debris on posterior cornea

Assessment

- Infectious
  1. Associated with other infectious signs
  2. Common in ulcers
- Immunological
  1. Produced from keratitis (prostaglandin) response
  2. Superficial irritation
- Mechanical
  1. Prominent perilimbal flush
  2. Circumcorneal soft lens edge binding

Plan

- Infectious
  1. D/C lens immediately
  2. Topical antibiotics
  3. Cycloplege/dilate
- Immunological
  1. D/C lens
  2. Topical steroids
  3. Cycloplege/dilate
- Mechanical
  1. Refit loose SL or GPH
  2. Hot packs

Follow-up

- RTC 24 to 48 hours after corrective measures
- If problem persists, increase dosages
- If problem resolves, RTC 3 to 6 weeks

3. Conjunctival Hyperemia[2]

Subjective

- No pain involved
- Pain would mean corneal involvement (keratoconjunctivitis)
- Itchy or nonspecific irritation/congested feeling

Objective

- Pinkish to meaty red injection
- Mild to moderate chemosis
- Associated lid congestion or hyperemia

Assessment

- Infectious
  1. Bacterial signs
  2. Viral signs
- Immunological
  1. Irritation, itching
  2. Solution (?)
- Mechanical
  1. Poor surfaces
  2. Debris buildup or entrapment
- Physiological
  1. Tight lens
  2. Corneal edema
- Other
  1. Hygiene
  2. Compliance

Plan

- Infectious
  1. D/C lens temporarily
  2. Antibiotics
- Immunological
  1. Enzymatic cleaning
  2. Change solutions
- Mechanical
  1. Clean lenses
  2. Loosen lenses
- Physiological
  1. Loosen lens
  2. D/C EW temporarily
- Others: Reinstruct on procedure and wear

Follow-up

- RTC 3 to 5 days after corrective measures
- If problem persists, treat alternate etiologies
- If problem resolves, RTC 3 months

4. Endothelial Changes

Subjective

- Usually no symptoms
- May notice a slight AM blur
- Occasional AM discomfort (mild)

Objective

- Reduced endothelial count (dropout)
- Increased corneal guttata
- Polymegathism (change in cell shape)

Assessment

- Physiological
  1. Tight lens
  2. Secondary edema (epithelial and stromal)

Plan

- Physiological
  1. Refit loose lens
  2. D/C EW

Follow-up

- RTC 1 to 2 weeks after corrective measures
- If problem persists, discontinue (D/C) contact lens wear for 2 to 4 weeks
- If problem resolves, RTC 4 to 6 weeks

5. Epithelial Breakdown

Subjective

- Foreign-body sensation
- Irritation and discomfort
- Variable visual acuity (VA) reaction
- Usually sudden onset of symptoms
- No immediate relief on lens removal

Objective

- Corneal epithelial disruption
- Diffuse epithelial decompensation
- Small or large focal epithelial erosions
- Secondary epithelial edema

Assessment

- Infectious
  1. Bacterial signs
  2. Viral signs
  3. Focal erosion
  4. Stromal and endothelial involvement
- Immunological
  1. Local pockets of debris
  2. Peripheral decompensation
  3. Red eye associated
- Mechanical
  1. History of recent insertion/removal
  2. Foreign body on posterior lens
- Physiological
  1. Advanced endothelial changes
  2. Tight lens

Plan

- Infectious
  1. D/C lens (temporarily)
  2. Antibiotics
  3. Lubricants
  4. Cycloplege/dilate
- Immunological
  1. D/C lens (temporarily)
  2. Enzymatic
  3. Lubricants
  4. Antibiotic (+/−)
- Mechanical
  1. D/C lens (temporarily)
  2. Antibiotic
  3. Clean lens
- Physiological
  1. Loosen lens
  2. D/C EW
  3. Lubricate

Follow-up

- RTC 24 to 48 hours after corrective measures
- If problems persists, increase dosages and RTC 24 to 48 hours
- If problem resolves, RTC 7 to 10 days

6. Giant Papillary Conjunctivitis (GPC)[3,4]

Subjective

- Bilateral irritation and discomfort
- Superior conjunctival hyperemia
- Giant papillae on tarsal palpebral conjunctiva

Objective

- Excess protein buildup on lens surfaces
- Superior conjunctival hyperemia
- Giant papillae on tarsal palpebral conjunctiva

Assessment

- Immunological
  1. Increased mucous debris
  2. Complete tarsal papillae coverage
- Mechanical
  1. Minimal mucoid debris
  2. Papillae greatest at zone 3 of tarsus

Plan

- Immunological
  1. D/C lenses temporarily
  2. Optional drugs: topical steroids, topical and oral antihistamines/decongestants, lubricants, aspirin, Opticrom
  3. Refit different material or diameter
- Mechanical
  1. D/C lenses temporarily
  2. Lubricants
  3. Refit new lens design

Follow-up

- RTC 2 to 3 weeks after initial therapies
- If GPC persistent, RTC 2 to 3 weeks or add drugs
- If GPC resolved, refit material or design

7. Keratoconjunctivitis[5]

Subjective

- Scratchy irritation
- Mild to moderate VA reduction
- Photophobia
- Mild symptom reduction on lens removal

Objective

- Conjunctival hyperemia (red eye)
- Diffuse, regional or focal SPK
- Usually specific etiological signs

Assessment

- Infectious
  1. Bacterial signs
  2. Viral signs
  3. Diffuse or inferior SPK

- Immunological
  1. Toxic reactions
  2. Solution problems
  3. Peripheral or superior SPK
- Physiological
  1. Associated edema
  2. Tight lens signs
  3. Epithelial or stromal edema
- Other
  1. Hygiene
  2. Stiff lens
  3. Compliance

Plan

- Infectious
  1. D/C lens temperature
  2. Antibiotics
  3. Lubricants
- Immunological
  1. D/C lens (temporarily)
  2. Change solutions
  3. Steroids (optional)
- Physiological
  1. Hypertonic solutions
  2. Loosen lens
  3. D/C EW temporarily
- Other
  1. Reinstruct
  2. Replace lens
  3. Advise

Follow-up

- RTC 5 to 7 days after corrective measures
- If problem persists, treat alternate etiologies
- If problem resolves, RTC 4 to 6 weeks

8. Limbal Engorgement[6]

Subjective

- No pain or discomfort
- Insidious onset
- Appearance persists on removal

Objective

- Circumcorneal flush
- Prominent limbal arcades
- Conjunctival drag
- Superficial vessel segmenting or engorging

Assessment

- Mechanical
  1. Edges binding at limbus
  2. No edge movement
  3. Edge banging at prominent limbal vessels
- Physiological
  1. Tight lens fit

2. Deep limbal engorgement
3. Neovascularization

Plan

- Mechanical
  1. Change to GPH
  2. Increase SL diameter
- Physiological
  1. Loosen fit
  2. D/C until neovascular tufts reduceHypertonic solutions

Follow-up

- RTC 1 week after corrective measures
- If problem presists, D/C wear until quiet
- If problem resolves, schedule routine follow-up

9. Microcystic Edema[7]

Subjective

- No discomfort
- Photophobia
- Slight VA reduction AM

Objective

- Epithelial "glistening" and increased density on direct illumination
- Greater in central corneal region
- May be associated with stromal thickening or endothelial straie

Assessment

- Mechanical
  1. Central touch or rubbing
  2. Lens unstable on eye
- Physiological
  1. Tight lens fit
  2. Anoxic cornea

Plan

- Mechanical
  1. Steeper base curve
  2. Larger lens
  3. GPH
- Physiological
  1. Loosen fit
  2. D/C EW temporarily
  3. Hypertonic solutions

Follow-up

- RTC 1 week after corrective measures
- If problem persists, decrease wearing time or extended wear (EW)
- If problem resolves, RTC 3 to 4 weeks

10. Microcysts (Pseudocysts or Vesicles)

Subjective

- May have no symptoms
- May have AM syndrome
- Advanced cases have irritation and VA reduction[8]

Objective

- Intraepithelial cysts (<1 mm) or blebs best seen on retroillumination
- Discrete vesicles from few to 50 to 60 central-ward
- Positive staining AM (possibly erosion)

Assessment

- Mechanical
  1. Increase over months to year with rigid material
  2. Follows CL-related or other injury
- Physiological
  1. Greater in diabetics
  2. Tight lens fit
  3. Present with microcystic edema
- Other
  1. Map–Dot degeneration in 20–60-yr-old (greater in women)
  2. Aggravated in rigid lenses or adverse conditions

Plan

- Mechanical
  1. Refit SL
  2. Advise patient
- Physiological
  1. Loose in diabetics
  2. Loosen lens
  3. Hypertonic solution hs
- Other
  1. Hypertonics with RGP
  2. Loose EW

Follow-up

- RTC 1, 2, and 4 weeks after corrective measures
- If problem persists, high water, thin, loose EW
- If problem resolves, RTC every 3 months

11. Mucous Debris or Buildup

Subjective

- Itchy, burny irritation
- Possible VA reductions
- Immediate relief on lens removal

Objective

- Buildup on lens surfaces
- Lens slippage
- Lens stiffening
- Secondary toxic epithelial responses (peripheral)
- Red eye reaction
- Stippling of epithelium (central)

Assessment

- Immunological
  1. Itchy or foreign-body irritation
  2. Epithelium breakdown (peripheral)
  3. Red eye
  4. Infiltrates
- Mechanical
  1. Posterior lens debris and entrapment
  2. Positive staining
  3. Stippling (central)
  4. Lens surface irregularities
- Other
  1. Stiff lens syndrome
  2. Patient allergies
  3. Sinus congestion
  4. Hygiene

Plan

- Immunological
  1. Enzyme clean
  2. Low water or GPH refit
  3. D/C temporarily
- Mechanical
  1. Enzyme clean
  2. Replace lens every 6–12 months
- Other
  1. Replace lens every 6–12 months
  2. Oral and topical antihistamine–decongestants

Follow-up

- RTC 1 week after corrective measures
- If problem persists, increase enzyme, peroxide, or replace lenses
- If problem resolves, instruct and RTC 4 to 6 weeks

12. Neovascularization[9]

Subjective

- No symptoms
- No VA reduction

Objective

- Corneal vascularization (stromal depths) terminating in spike, twigs, branches, or loops greater than 1.5 mm
- May show whole blood circulation or ghost vessels
- May be point foci or any circumferential width up to 360 degrees

Assessment

- Immunological
  1. Secondary to inflammatory disease
  2. Usually 5–90°
  3. May be more extensive
  4. Acne rosacea
- Mechanical
  1. Aggravation of prominent limbal arcade
  2. Usually sectorial
  3. Sclerocornea
  4. Limbal engorgement
- Physiological
  1. Usually 360°
  2. Secondary edema
  3. Tight lens signs
  4. Circumferential ≥1 mm

Plan

- Immunological
  1. Monitor for reactivation
  2. Fit loose
  3. Do not fit acne rosacea
- Mechanical
  1. Document prominent limbal vessels in prefit examination
  2. Large diameter soft or GPH
- Physiological
  1. Monitor 1 mm circumferential vessels closely
  2. Fit loose
  3. D/C EW

Follow-up

- RTC 1 week, 1 month after corrective measures
- If problem advances, D/C all lens wear (temporarily)
- If problem arrests or resolves, RTC 6 to 12 weeks

13. Pannus[10]

Subjective

- No subjective symptoms
- Cosmetic awareness
- Aggravated appearance with lens wear (or over-wear)

Objective

- Superficial vessel tufts onto corneal surface
- Range from 10 to 180 degrees at limbus
- Great inferior (staphylococcal toxin) at 4 and 8 o'clock positions

Assessment

- Immunological
  1. Toxic (staphylococcal) response from lids
  2. Secondary inflammatory disease

- Mechanical
  1. Aggravation of prominent limbal arcade
  2. Usually sectorial
  3. Sclerocornea
  4. Limbal engorgement
  5. Dellen formations
- Physiological
  1. Tight lens
  2. Secondary edema
  3. Larger (>90°) pannus areas

Plan

- Immunological
  1. Fit large diameter or RGP
  2. Monitor for activity
- Mechanical
  1. Document prominent limbal vessels in prefit examination
  2. Large diameter soft or RPG
  3. Add lubricant
- Physiological
  1. Fit loose
  2. GPH
  3. D/C EW

Follow-up

- RTC 1 to 2 weeks after corrective measures
- If problem advances, D/C wear temporarily
- If problem arrests or resolves, RTC every 3 months

14. Pseudodendrites[11]

Subjective

- No symptoms
- May affect VA (especially when central)

Objective

- Arborizing, variable branching infiltrative lesion on epithelial surface
- Usually peripheral
- May be <2 mm or sinuous and 3 to 6 mm

Assessment

- Immunological
  1. Infiltrative
  2. No terminal buds (herpetic)
  3. Rebound after topical steroids

Plan

- Immunological
  1. D/C lens temporarily
  2. D/C chemical cleaning
  3. No steroids

Follow-up

- RTC 5 to 7 days after corrective measures
- If problem persists, R/O herpetic dendrite (again)
- If problem resolves, rewear, heat disinfect, RTC (3 to 4 weeks)

15. Stippling (Dimple Veiling)

Subjective

- Usually no symptoms
- May produce reduced VA
- Resolves in minutes to hours on removal

Objective

- Dimples or small (<1 mm) depression on central corneal epithelium
- No positive staining
- Usually debris entrapment under lens
- May be bubbles under lens

Assessment

- Mechanical
  1. Static tear interchange
  2. Tight or steep rigid lens
  3. Debris or bubbles trapped
- Other
  1. Poor hygiene of rigid lenses
  2. Overwear of rigid lenses

Plan

- Mechanical
  1. Flatten lens
  2. Loosen lens
  3. Lubricants
- Other
  1. Instruct on hygiene
  2. Fit soft or GPH

Follow-up

- RTC 1 to 2 weeks after corrective measures
- If problem persists, D/C wear temporarily
- If problem resolves, schedule routine follow-up

16. Striate Keratitis[12,13] (Color Plate 97)

Subjective

- Frequent VA reduction
- Edematous symptoms
- Greater in AM

Objective

- Thin (or dense) lines in deep stroma or posterior cornea
- Usually vertically oriented
- Associated with other signs of stromal or epithelial edema

Assessment

- Infectious
  1. Associated with advanced corneal infection
  2. Corneal ulcer
- Physiological
  1. Tight lens
  2. Reduce during day
  3. Seen occasionally in first weeks or months of EW
- Other
  1. Congenital striae
  2. Interstitial keratitis

Plan

- Infectious
  1. D/C lenses immediately
  2. Refer to corneal specialist
- Physiological
  1. Loosen lens
  2. Monitor closely
- Other: Prefit evaluation and documentation

Follow-up

- RTC 24 to 48 hours after corrective measures
- If problem persists, monitor closely or refit
- If problem resolves, RTC every 3 to 6 weeks

17. Stromal Edema[4]

Subjective

- Reduced VA
- Usually worse in AM

Objective

- Cloudy stroma
- Thickened cornea
- Greatest central
- Increased myopia

Assessment

- Infectious
  1. Associated with advanced infection
  2. Corneal ulcer
- Mechanical: contusive (blunt) injury to eye
- Physiological
  1. Tight lens
  2. Vertical striae
  3. Secondary epithelial edema
- Other
  1. Dystrophy (central)
  2. Degeneration (peripheral)

Plan

- Infectious
  1. D/C lenses immediately
  2. Refer to corneal specialist

- Mechanical: D/C lens wear temporarily
- Physiological
  1. Loosen fit
  2. D/C wear temporarily
- Other: prefit examination documentation

Follow-up

- RTC 48 to 72 hours after corrective measures
- If problem persists, D/C wear and refit
- If problem resolves, RTC 6 to 12 weeks

18. Stromal Infiltrates

Subjective

- May have no symptoms
- Symptoms associated with primary cause

Objective

- Anterior stromal small (0.5 to 2 mm) foci of whitish-gray inflammatory cell accumulations
- Borders may be well defined or hazy
- May be dense or pale
- May be one or many central, peripheral, or diffuse

Assessment

- Infectious
  1. Viral origin: central
  2. Chlamydial: peripheral/superior
  3. Diffuse scars of previous infection
- Immunological
  1. Usually peripheral
  2. Solution related
  3. SPK of Thygeson
  4. SLK
  5. Pseudodendrites (?)

Plan

- Infectious
  1. D/C lens temporarily
  2. Treat orally
  3. Prefit examination documentation
- Immunological
  1. Change solutions
  2. Monitor closely
  3. D/C in SLK and pseudodendrites temporarily

Follow-up

- RTC 5 to 7 days after corrective measures
- If problem persists, RTC weekly for 4 to 6 weeks
- If problem resolves or stabilizes, RTC every 6 to 12 weeks

19. Subepithelial Infiltrates

Subjective

- May have no symptoms
- Symptoms associated with primary cause

Objective

- Level of Bowman's layer
- 0.5 to 1 mm foci of whitish-gray inflammatory (WBC) accumulations
- Borders are usually well defined
- May be dense or pale
- Number few to many
- Regions associated are diffuse, peripheral, superior, or inferior

Assessment

- Infectious
  1. Viral origin: central
  2. Chlamydial: peripheral superior
  3. Diffuse scars of previous infection
- Immunological
  1. Peripheral region: solutions or toxic debris
  2. SPK of Thygeson: diffuse and fine to coarse
  3. SLK: superior

Plan

- Infectious
  1. D/C lens temporarily
  2. Treat orally
  3. Prefit examination documentation
- Immunological
  1. Change solutions
  2. Refit soft or GPH
  3. D/C lenses temporarily
  4. Change material (?)

Follow-up

- RTC 5 to 6 days after corrective measures
- If problem persists, RTC weekly for 4 to 6 weeks
- If problem resolves or stabilizes, RTC every 6 to 12 weeks

20. Superficial Punctate Keratitis (SPK)

Subjective

- Mild to moderate foreign-body irritation
- Moderate VA reduction (depending on region)
- Symptoms persist for minutes to hours on removal

Objective

- Variable degrees of SPK
  1. Mild: fine and sparse
  2. Moderate: coarse or dense
  3. Severe: coarse and dense, and focal confluence
- Variable regions or corneal surface
  1. Diffuse: viral, SPK of Thygeson, poor procedures
  2. Peripheral: immune response, lens edges, physiological edema

3. Central: flat lens, physiological edema
4. Superior: SLK, *Chlamydia*, GPC
5. Inferior: *Staphylococcus*, tight lid, solution/preservative response
6. Focal: bacterial, viral, fungal, or sterile ulcer

Assessment

- Infectious
  1. Inferior or diffuse = staphylococcal
  2. Diffuse = viral
  3. Focal = ulcer
- Immunological
  1. Peripheral
  2. Diffuse = SPK of Thygeson
  3. Superior = SLK, *Chlamydia*, GPC
  4. Focal = sterile ulcer
- Mechanical
  1. Peripheral = edges
  2. Central = flat
  3. Inferior = tight lid
- Physiological
  1. Central to midperiphery
- Other
  1. Inferior = Solutions and preservatives
  2. Anywhere = poor procedure

Plan

- D/C lens temporarily, treat cause, lubricate (and prophylax +/−)

Follow-up

- RTC within 1 week of completion of corrective measures
- If problem persists, continue or increase therapy
- If problem resolves, RTC 3 to 4 weeks or PRN

21. Superior Limbic Keratoconjunctivitis (SLK)[15]

Subjective

- Bilateral foreign-body irritation and burning
- Usually no substantial VA reduction
- Symptoms resolve slowly on removal

Objective

- Superior conjunctiva hyperemic and chemotic
- Superior cornea moderate to severe SPK
- Cornea elsewhere may show SPK, subepithelial or stromal infiltrates and edema

Assessment

- Immunological
  1. Reaction to lens material
  2. Reaction to thimerosal

- Mechanical
  1. Reaction to lens edges or design
  2. Lens movement
- Other: SLK of Theodore, unknown etiology

Plan

- Immunological
  1. Change material
  2. D/C all thimerosal
  3. Lubricants
  4. D/C wear temporarily
- Mechanical
  1. Refit, RGP
  2. Tighten lens (?)
  3. Lubricants
  4. D/C wear temporarily
- Other
  1. Cromolyn sodium (?)
  2. Fit large-diameter soft lens

Follow-up

- RTC 5 to 7 days (or PRN) after corrective measures
- If problem persists, add steroids
- If problem diminishes, follow every week to resolution

22. Toxic Keratitis

Subjective

- Mild to moderate irritation and burning
- Increasing lens intolerance
- History of chronic or subacute lid problems
- Moderate reduction of symptoms on removal

Objective

- Variable patterns of SPK
- Occasional peripheral infiltrates
- Occasional inferior pannus or neovascularization

Assessment

- Infectious
  1. Inferior SPK = staphylococcal
  2. Diffuse SPK = viral or staphylococcal
- Immunological
  1. Peripheral SPK
  2. Diffuse SPK = solution response
- Other
  1. Debris entrapment with secondary SPK
  2. Nonspecific SPK or subepithelial infiltrates

Plan

- Infectious
  1. Lid scrubs, etc.
  2. Lubricate
  3. Irrigation

- Immunological
  1. D/C or refit lens
  2. Lubricate
  3. Change solutions
- Other
  1. Enzyme clean
  2. Lubricate
  3. Monitor closely

Follow-up

- RTC 1 to 2 weeks after corrective measures
- If problem persists, add short-term steroids
- If problem resolves, RTC 2 to 4 weeks

23. Corneal Ulceration[16-20]

Subjective

- Foreign-body irritation of rapid onset
- History of recent lens handling "episode"
- Possibility of immune-compromised patient

Objective

- Three to 4+ conjunctival hyperemia (crimson red)
- Focal epithelial defect ≥1 to 2 mm
- Mucopurulence over or around lesion
- Stromal infiltration
- Posterior corneal response (KP, striae, fibrin)
- One to 3+ anterior chamber reaction (cells and flare)

Assessment

- Infectious
  1. Pseudomonas within 24–48 hr
  2. Other gram +/− bugs
  3. Local SPK
- Immunological
  1. Sterile: in compromised pattern
  2. Proteolytic response
- Mechanical
  1. Lens manipulation
  2. Fingernail abrasion
  3. Erosion
- Physiological
  1. Chronic edema
  2. Tight lens with secondary infection
- Other
  1. Poor hygiene
  2. Poor procedures
  3. Noncompliant (esp. EW)

Plan

- Infectious: refer immediately to corneal specialist
- Immunological
  1. Monitor closely
  2. Enzyme clean
- Mechanical
  1. Careful history
  2. Refer immed. to corneal spec.
- Physiological: fit loose lenses

TABLE 7–6. CONTACT LENS MANAGEMENT AND PATIENT EDUCATION MNEMONICS

"I'M A PSYCHO" (from fitting contact lenses)

I = Infectious/inflammatory reactions
M = Mechanical response
A = Allergic/hypersensitivity/immune reactions
P = Physiological response (tight lens syndrome)
S = Solution reactions
Y = Yearly replacement (6–12 months)
C = Compliance with instructions, wear, procedures
H = Hygiene: hands, lids, lenses, and case
O = Others: secondary systemic manifestations, sinus

Instruct all your contact lens patients on (Stan) "Yamane's Yardstick" or (Joe) "Soper's Invitation"

Every morning look in your mirror and ask three simple questions about your eyes and your contact lenses:

Do I (my eyes and contacts)

1. Feel good? (No irritation or burning?)
2. Look good? (No red or watery eyes?)
3. See good? (Check each eye individually)

"Invite" your contact lens patients to **"RSVP"**

R = Redness (return if any redness occurs)
S = Sun sensitivity (return if light sensitivity occurs)
V = Vision variations (return if vision changes in any way)
P = Pain (return immediately if any pain develops)

TABLE 7–7. PRIORITIZING CARE IN EXTENDED-WEAR COMPLICATIONS

Treatment	Folds in Descemet's Membrane	Defects in Epithelium (Staining)	Anterior Uveitis	Epithelial Edema	Neovascularization	Corneal Infiltrates	Corneal Ulcer	Endophthalmitis
				Clinical Condition				
Monitor	First	First		First	First	First	(Eighth)	(Eighth)
Loosen fit	Fourth		Third		Third	Fourth	(Seventh)	(Seventh)
Tighten fit		Fourth		Fourth				
Replace lens		Third						
Increase O_2	Third			Third	Second	Third	(Sixth)	(Sixth)
Eliminate preservatives		Fifth		Fifth		Sixth		
Wetting drops	Second	Second		Second		Second		
Antibiotics							Third	Third
Steroids			First			Fifth	(Fifth)	(Fifth)
Dilate and cycloplege			Second				Fourth	Fourth
Culture eye							Second	Second
Hospitalize							First	First

- Other
  1. Instruct
  2. No EW for noncompliant patients

Follow-up

- RTC and refit per consultant
- Routine follow-up every 3 months or PRN

C. MANAGEMENT AND PATIENT EDUCATION MNEMONICS[21]

Please refer to Table 7–6

D. PRIORITIZING CARE IN EXTENDED-WEAR COMPLICATIONS

Please refer to Table 7–7

III. Therapeutic Contact Lens Care

A. INTRODUCTION

1. Long and dynamic history associated with material and design advancements
   a. Scleral haptics
      i. Cosmetic fits (with scarring)
      ii. Keratoconus
   b. PMMA
      i. Cosmetic fits (with scarring)
      ii. Keratoconus
      iii. Orthokeratology (experimental)
   c. Hydrophilic and gas-permeable materials[22]
      i. Cosmetic fits (with scarring)
      ii. Keratoconus
      iii. Corneal surface abnormalities
         - Bandaging epithelial defects
         - Hydrating or dehydrating epithelium
         - Mechanical protection
         - Pain reduction
         - Promotion of healing
         - Visual improvement over irregular surfaces
      iv. Drug reservoirs
         - Chronic conditions
         - Glaucomas
         - Infectious keratitis

2. The more common categories and specific disease entities are managed by the primary eye care practitioner
   a. Congenital or acquired disfigurement and anomalies
   b. Persistent epithelial defects
   c. Mechanical irritations to the cornea
   d. Chronic edema problems
   e. Drying and erosive conditions

3. Outline considerations for each category and specific disorders
   a. Diagnostic highlights
   b. Goals in fitting
   c. When to fit
   d. What to fit
   e. How to fit
   f. How to follow
   g. Complications to watch out for

B. CONGENITAL AND ACQUIRED DISFIGUREMENTS AND ANOMALIES[23,24]

1. **Aniridia**
   a. Diagnostic highlights
      i. Lack of iris structure
      ii. Always remnant on gonioscopy
      iii. Photo aversion
      iv. Secondary nystagmus
      v. Usually strabismic
      vi. Often cataracts
      vii. Hypoplasia of the macula common
   b. Goals in fitting
      i. Cosmetic relief
      ii. Visual improvement (in limited cases)
   c. When to fit
      i. At earliest possible age to prevent deprivation of the visual system
      ii. To enhance proper stimulation to avoid the secondary and sensory nystagmus and degradation of form and abnormal binocular interaction
   d. What to fit
      i. An opaque artificial iris
      ii. Gel or gas permeables
      iii. Availability
         • Narcissus foundation
         • Custom tint
         • Titmus Eurocon
         • Igel
         • Caprice (rigids)
   e. How to fit
      i. Usually before the age of 2 years general anesthesia is needed
      ii. Look for good centration and align along the optical axis with a 3- to 5-mm pupil (iris is needed)
      iii. Extremely early ages (before the age of 1 year) use about 10-mm iris
      iv. After the age of 1 year, a normal 11- to 12-mm iris is needed

   v. Appropriate refractive error components can be included
   vi. Coloboma, corectopia, and dyscoria may require Neo-Synephrine or 0.5 percent tropicamide (Mydriacyl) for dilation to align the visual axis with the center of the artificial pupil
   f. How to follow
      i. Every 3 to 6 months
      ii. Earlier fittings follow more frequently
      iii. Patient has to be followed closely because subjective response cannot be relied on with infants
   g. Complications
      i. Power determination can be difficult
         • There is usually plus acceptance
         • Hyperopia due to lamination
      ii. The painted irides, if fused, can be a problem that could induce neovascularization and other complications similar to soft lenses
      iii. Thick soft hydrogel lenses
      iv. Avoid ointments, pilocarpine, epinephrine, low-molecular-weight sodium fluorescein, Goniosol
      v. With aniridia, one must always be concerned with renal congenital neoplasm
      vi. Wilms' tumor and glaucoma are always a concern because of angle problems

2. **Albinism**
   a. Diagnostic highlights
      i. Transillumination of the iris
      ii. Several forms of ocular albinism
      iii. Usually congenital triad
         • With the rule astigma
         • Albinotic fundus
         • Secondary (sensory) nystagmus due to poor binocular development as well as hypoplasia of the macula
   b. Goals in fitting: same as aniridia
   c. When to fit: same as aniridia
   d. How to fit: same as aniridia
   e. How to follow: same as aniridia
   f. Complications: same as aniridia

3. **Traumatic Postsurgical Disfigurements (Color Plates 98 and 99)**
   a. Diagnostic highlights

i. Any keratopathy or iris defect

ii. Disfigurements range from dense leukomas (pthisical) to a distracting nebulae

b. Goals in fitting

i. Cosmetic relief

ii. Visual improvement (in limited cases)

c. When to fit

i. Photoaversion

ii. Cosmetic concern

d. What to fit

i. A translucent or opaque gel lens, depending on the severity of disfigurement

ii. If the eye is pthisical, a ring of translucent color makes it look somewhat larger bordering the periphery

iii. The hydrogels seem to tract better than corneal or haptic lenses although each is still used only on occasion

e. How to fit

i. Conventional methods with good centration and movement

ii. With blind eyes, may consider extended wear

iii. One must be concerned at all times with monocular patients with disfigured eyes and the fact that it never matches the other eye exactly

iv. Use prism (in eyeglasses) to align strabismic patients, to make it cosmetically more acceptable

f. How to follow

i. Initially see patients on a weekly basis for about 1 month

ii. Then, every 3 months thereafter, unless concomitant factors are involved that would necessitate close monitoring for other conditions

g. Complications

i. Many problems are associated with diseased prosthesis (e.g., diabetics)

ii. Color match because of the anterior chamber depth on monocular cases

iii. Aphakics (owing to the high plus systems) have problems with centration at times

iv. There is always more plus needed with the lamination because of

flexure problems (less plus effectivity)

4. Diplopia and Amblyopia

a. Diagnostic highlights

i. Intractable diplopia (usually fit as a last resort)

ii. Either before or after straightening (surgical) procedures have been tried

iii. After prism and occlusion has been attempted, unless cosmetics are a big factor

b. Goals in fitting

i. Visual improvement

ii. Occlusion therapy

c. When to fit

i. Amblyopia; usually after 5 or 6 years of age, little benefit is gained

ii. Have to be fit early and take the place of occlusion therapy if a large enough pupil is used and the cosmetics are good

iii. You must have an understanding parent

d. What to fit

i. A hydrogel or haptic for diplopia

ii. Availability through the Narcissus Foundation primarily and custom tint

iii. You can use a clear or tinted area for color match

iv. Extended-wear option through Igel 77 (London)

e. How to fit

i. A large pupil is needed

ii. Sometimes as large as 9 to 10 mm because of dilation and light scattering and for complete deprivation of the eye in amblyopia therapy

f. How to follow

i. Every month generally to monitor the lens as well as the effectiveness in amblyopia therapy

ii. Diplopia every 6 months, unless other medical consideration

g. Complications

i. If the lens is not totally opaque, will not be effective

ii. Normal sequelae seen with gels must be monitored

iii. Parental consent can be a factor

iv. Difficulty in fitting these patients

v. Usually when amblyopia is diagnosed between the ages of 2 to 5, general anesthesia may be needed

vi. Cosmetics can be a problem with a large black opaque pupil (compared with the other eye)

5. Color Anomalies

a. Diagnostic highlights

   i. Color testing with the Farnsworth D-15 seems most effective

   ii. Poor macular function with monochromats and subjective complaints of pseudophotoaversion

b. Goal in fitting: visual improvement

c. How to fit

   i. Must educate the patients

   ii. Essentially any color anomaly can be attempted
   - Total rod monochromats
   - Severely colorblind
   - Mildly colorblind

   iii. Seem to be most effective with red–green anomalies

d. What to fit

   i. The X- chrome available through a number of sources

   ii. The Hydrogel lens through Igel in England and the Narcissus Foundation in California

e. How to fit

   i. Conventional

   ii. Nondominant eye is generally fitted

   iii. The fellow eye is usually best suited for brown or gray lens

f. How to follow

   i. Poor results, especially at night (the patient should be discouraged from wearing the lenses at night)

   ii. Cosmetics can be a factor, especially with the soft lenses

   iii. Thickness is a critical factor in the absorption and cloudiness of the lens

C. PERSISTENT EPITHELIAL DEFECTS

1. Epithelial Basement Membrane Disorders

a. Diagnostic highlights

   i. AM syndrome

   ii. Maps–dots–fingerprints

   iii. Epithelial erosions

   iv. History of trauma (e.g., fingernail)

b. Goals in fitting

   i. Bandage

   ii. Dehydration

   iii. Pain reduction

   iv. Promote healing

   v. Visual improvement

c. When to fit

   i. Chronic pain

   ii. Recurrent erosion

   iii. VA reduction below 20/40

d. What to fit

   i. High water content soft lens[25]

   ii. Possibly RGP

e. How to fit

   i. Large diameter, thin, loose lens

   ii. Extended-wear preferable

f. How to follow

   i. Gentamicin drop bid or tid (optional)

   ii. RTC every 4 to 6 weeks or PRN

   iii. Attempt D/C extended wear after 3 to 4 months

g. Complications

   i. Corneal edema with folds
   - Must add lubricant drops up to every 2 hours, especially first week of therapy
   - This complication tends to resolve after 1 month
   - For stubborn cases, lens may need to be refit to increase oxygen supply to cornea

   ii. Anterior uveitis
   - Must consider risk–benefit ratio
   - Add homatropine bid and 1 percent prednisolone qid and watch every day for improvement
   - Consider different fit (either looser, higher water content or thinner)

   iii. Infiltrates
   - Discontinue contact lens therapy
   - Rule out corneal ulcer via negative stain with sodium fluorescein
   - Add steroids up to every 2 hours
   - Re-evaluate lens fit as well as related solution problems when infiltrates resolve

   iv. Corneal ulcer

2. Recurrent Corneal Erosion (RCE) (Color Plates 79 and 100)
  a. Diagnostic highlights
    i. History of tangential abrasion
    ii. AM syndrome following patching therapy
  b. Goals in fitting
    i. Bandage
    ii. Dehydration
    iii. Pain reduction
    iv. Promote healing
  c. When to fit
    i. Chronic re-erosion
    ii. Severe AM syndrome
  d. What to fit: high water content soft lens
  e. How to fit
    i. Large diameter, thin, loose lens
    ii. Extended wear
  f. How to follow
    i. Hypertonics AM and hs
    ii. Gentamicin drops bid or tid
    iii. RTC every 3 to 4 weeks or PRN
    iv. Attempt D/C extended wear after 3 to 4 months
  g. Complications to watch for
    i. Aberrant regeneration of corneal epithlium
    ii. All extended-wear complications as related to coexisting conditions

3. Cogan's Microcystic Degeneration
  a. Diagnostic highlights
    i. Older males
    ii. Large (1 to 2 mm) microcysts
  b. Goals in fitting
    i. Bandage
    ii. Dehydration
    iii. Pain reduction
    iv. Promote healing
  c. When to fit
    i. Chronic pain
    ii. Recurrent erosion
  d. What to fit: high water content soft lens
  e. How to fit
    i. Large diameter, thin, loose lens
    ii. Extended wear preferable
  f. How to follow
    i. Gentamicin drop bid or tid (optional)
    ii. RTC every 4 to 6 weeks or PRN
    iii. Attempt D/C extended wear after 3 to 4 months
  g. Complications: same as EBMD

D. MECHANICAL IRRITATIONS

1. Entropion and Trichiasis
  a. Diagnostic highlights
    i. Foreign-body sensation
    ii. Foreign-body tracking
    iii. Lashes turned inward
  b. Goals in fitting
    i. Bandage for protection of cornea
    ii. Pain reduction
  c. When to fit
    i. Inability or refusal to repair
    ii. Chronic irritation
  d. What to fit
    i. Low water content soft lenses
    ii. Durable or cheap
  e. How to fit
    i. Daily wear if possible
    ii. Extended wear if problem causes incomplete lid closure
  f. Follow-up
    i. Every 1 to 3 months as schedule allows
    ii. Remove lashes at each visit
    iii. May need to replace lens at each visit (especially extended wear)
  g. Complications
    i. Lens spoilage
    ii. Corneal anesthesia or relative anesthesia can delay treatment of abrasions, ulcers
    iii. All problems of extended wear (therefore, move to daily wear early as risk–benefit ratio dictates)

2. Other Mechanical Irritations
  a. Diagnostic highlights: epithelial insult resulting in defect
  b. Goals in fitting: variable
  c. When to fit
    i. Persistent epithelial defects or filamentary keratitis
    ii. Can be used to prevent symblepharon formation in particular alkaline burns
    iii. Complications when dryness occurs as a result of other complications
  d. What to fit
    i. A Hydrogel lens with plano or thin design
    ii. Low to medium water content lens

e. How to fit
  i. Good centration with minimal but adequate movement for good flushing
  ii. Cycloplegics and antibiotics for prophylaxis are usually indicated
f. How to follow
  i. Daily for the first few days
  ii. Then every 3 to 4 days
  iii. Then 4 to 5 weeks thereafter until condition is resolved
g. Complications
  i. Superinfection and secondary iritis
  ii. The traditional noninfectious complications of wearing Hydrogel lenses

E. CHRONIC EDEMA

1. Fuchs' Endothelial Dystrophy
a. Diagnostic highlights
  i. AM syndrome
  ii. Dense guttata
  iii. Bullous keratopathy
  iv. Neovascularization and scarring
b. Goals in fitting
  i. Bandage
  ii. Dehydration
  iii. Pain reduction
  iv. Promote healing
  v. Possible vision impairment in certain cases
c. When to fit
  i. Severe AM syndrome
  ii. Bullous keratopathy
d. What to fit: high water content soft lens
e. How to fit
  i. Large diameter, thin, loose
  ii. Extended wear preferable
f. How to follow
  i. Add hypertonics when necessary
  ii. Follow daily-wear patients every 3 to 6 months
  iii. Follow extended-wear patients every 2 to 3 months
g. Complications
  i. In extended-wear, watch for all the same complications as epithelial basement membrane dystrophy, but move to daily wear at first sign of problems as there is a much different risk–benefit ratio
  ii. Watch for tight lens syndrome (keep it loose)
  iii. Watch for neovascularization, a sign of hypoxia, as well as progression of the dystrophy

2. Bullous Keratopathy
a. Diagnostic highlights
  i. Severe pain
  ii. Full-thickness epithelial blebs
  iii. More common in postsurgery or post-trauma
b. Goals in fitting
  i. Bandage
  ii. Dehydration
  iii. Pain reduction
  iv. Promote healing
  v. Promote vascularization (experimental)
c. When to fit
  i. Nonresponsive to hypertonics
  ii. Recurrence
  iii. With favorable risk–benefit ratio
d. What to fit
  i. High water content soft lens
  ii. Medium water content or CSI lens
e. How to fit
  i. Extended-wear lens almost always
  ii. Large diameter, thin, and loose
f. How to follow
  i. Add hypertonic solution
  ii. Add steroids with fibrosis
  iii. Watch IOP (add glaucoma medications aggressively)
  iv. Watch inflammation
g. Complications
  i. Condition aggravated by even moderately high intraocular pressure (IOP) (must keep pressure low)
  ii. Condition aggravated by uveitis (if steroids are not enough, add atropine)
  iii. Neovascularization may not be a bad complication unless a graft is under consideration. It may clear central cornea (carefully analyze risk–benefit ratio)
  iv. Watch out for all extended wear complications as noted previously
  v. Irreversible fibrin formation under bullae possible in delayed treatment

3. Physiological Edema
a. Diagnostic highlights (broken down into anterior and posterior forms)

i. Anterior
- Subjective response would be halos
- Biomicroscopic evaluation would include granular epithelium with clouding
- General haze with NaFl staining
- Little effect subjectively on visual acuity

ii. Posterior
- Endothelial decompensation
- Biomicroscopically shows folds, striae, and endothelial buckling and dropout
- Severe forms of edema
  Dystrophy
  Guttata
  Bullous keratopathy
  Aphakia or pseudophakia

b. Goals in fitting
   i. Dehydration
   ii. Pain reduction

c. When to fit
   i. Severe morning (AM) syndrome
   ii. Severe or chronic pain
   iii. Bullous changes
   iv. Recurrent erosions
   v. When there is an irregular anterior surface where a wicking phenomenon will facilitate the effects of hypertonic solution
   vi. To compensate temporarily for a leaking endothelium
   vii. To avoid aphakic corneal edema secondary to epithelial downgrowth

d. What to fit
   i. High water content soft lens
   ii. Thin design

e. How to fit
   i. Large diameter, loose lens
   ii. Not too loose to cause mechanical problems
   iii. Extended wear preferable

f. How to follow
   i. Generally 24 hours after fitting, 2 to 3 days later, then 1 week, 1 month, and then every 3 months or PRN
   ii. Hypertonics AM and hs

g. Complications
   i. Superinfection
   ii. Noninfectious complications are neovascularization and lens deposits
   iii. A soft lens sequelae seen as frequent lens loss

iv. Often minimal visual improvement

F. DRYING AND EROSIVE SYNDROMES

1. Dry Eye – Keratoconjunctivitis Sicca Syndrome

a. Diagnostic highlights
   i. Late-day irritation
   ii. Positive rose bengal, band-region SPK
   iii. Conjunctival thickening and hyperemia
   iv. Accompanying blepharitis (staphylococcal)

b. Goals in fitting
   i. Bandage
   ii. Hydration
   iii. Pain reduction
   iv. Promote healing

c. When to fit
   i. When cornea involved with superficial punctate keratopathy
   ii. Unresponsive to all lubricants
   iii. Unresponsive to acetylcysteine
   iv. First try punctal occlusive techniques

d. What to fit
   i. Low water content lenses
   ii. Silicone elastomer lenses

e. How to fit
   i. Extended wear (cautiously!)[27]
   - Large silicone lens 12.5 mm diameter
   - Low water content lens as thick as possible
   - Keep it loose
   ii. Daily wear
   - Low to medium water content lenses
   - Large and thick
   - Not as loose as extended wear

f. How to follow
   i. Add wetting drops up to every hour, but watch for preservative toxicity
   ii. Watch for mucous plaques that may lead to mucous clog syndrome

g. Complications
   i. All extended-wear complications have a higher incident of infection
   ii. Move to daily wear early in complicated cases
   iii. Lens spoilage is high and may be alleviated through the use of sili-

cone elastomer extended-wear lenses or daily-wear lenses

    iv. As this syndrome is usually accompanied by blepharitis, there is a high incidence of staphylococcal ulcers

- Called triple S syndrome

    Staphylococcus

    Seborrhea

    Sicca

- Antistaphylococcal therapy

2. **Exposure Keratitis***

  a. Diagnostic highlights

    i. Foreign-body sensation

    ii. Band SPK

    iii. Rose bengal staining

  b. Goals in fitting

    i. Bandage

    ii. Mechanical protection

    iii. Pain reduction

    iv. Promote healing

  c. When to fit

    i. Nonresponsive to lubricants

    ii. Secondary complications

  d. What to fit

    i. Low to medium water content lenses

    ii. Durable or deposit resistant

  e. How to fit

    i. Extended-wear lens in most cases

    ii. If daily wear, must tape eye closed at night

  f. How to follow

    i. Twenty-four hours, 1 week, 2 weeks, 1 month, 3 months

    ii. May need to follow more often to replace lenses

    iii. Must monitor causative condition and try to discontinue bandage lens when condition improves

  g. Complications

    i. Lens spoilage and loss

    ii. Extended-wear complications

    iii. Corneal anesthesia

3. **Neuroparalytic Keratitis**

  a. Diagnostic highlights

    i. Decreased vision

    ii. Band SPK with epithelial sloughing

    iii. No pain

    iv. Diminished or absent touch reflex

---

*Bell's Palsy, coloboma, hyperthyroidism, lagophthalmos, postblepharoplasty.

  b. Goals

    i. Bandage protection

    ii. Promote healing

  c. When to fit

    i. When patching is unsuccessful

    ii. When tarsorrhaphy is impractical (i.e., one-eyed patient)

  d. What to fit: any bandage soft lens material as indicated by other factors (e.g., dry eye, edema)

  e. How to fit

    i. Large to very large

    ii. As loose as possible

    iii. Almost always extended wear

    iv. Daily wear only if extended wear fails; the eye must then be patched when not wearing the lens

  f. How to follow

    i. Very closely (12 hours, 24 hours, 2 days, 1 week, 2 weeks, monthly)

    ii. Watch for tight lens syndrome

    iii. Replace lens when surface deposits affect performance of lens

    iv. Add wetting drops, antibiotics, steroids aggressively

  g. Complications

    i. Ulcers and endophthalmitis are common

    ii. All extended-wear lens complications occur, and they occur much faster

    iii. Lens spoilage is a consideration

    iv. Must reassess risk–benefit ratio frequently

4. **Filamentary Keratitis**

  a. Diagnostic highlights

    i. Moderate to severe irritation

    ii. Adherent buds or threads on corneal surface

  b. Goals in fitting

    i. Mechanical protection

    ii. Pain reduction

    iii. Promote healing

    iv. Stabilize precorneal tear film

  c. When to fit

    i. When course of removing filaments and 5 percent sodium chloride fails

    ii. When course of lubricants or acetylcysteine fails

  d. What to fit

    i. Low water content if secondary to dry eye or if dry eye is coexistent

    ii. High water content lens otherwise

  e. How to fit

    i. Extended wear

ii. Extra loose for dry-eye problems
f. How to follow
    i. Twenty-four hour, 1 week, 2 weeks, 1 month
    ii. Try to discontinue lens in 1 month
    iii. May need to continue indefinitely
g. Complications
    i. All those previously mentioned in any extended-wear lens
    ii. Extra caution as many of these patients have dry eyes and are subject to tightening of the lenses with secondary infectious complications

5. Dellen
a. Diagnostic highlights
    i. Local depression caused by an adjacent elevation
    ii. Usually do not stain but rather accumulate into a pool
    iii. Adjacent elevation may show negative stain
b. Goals in fitting: hydration
c. When to fit
    i. Rarely—overnight pressure patch will usually solve problem
    ii. If elevation is secondary to inflammation, steroids may be helpful with or without bandage
    iii. Fit soft lens only in stubborn or recurring cases
d. What to fit
    i. Any soft lens (low to medium H₂O)
    ii. Must be extended wear
e. How to fit
    i. As large a diameter as possible (15.5 or 16.0 mm)
    ii. Must obtain a good fit
f. How to follow
    i. Twenty-four hours, 1 week
    ii. Attempt to discontinue lens
g. Complications
    i. All previously mentioned extended-wear complications
    ii. Lens may increase inflammation and cause elevated area to worsen (if this is the case, add steroids)

G. KERATOCONUS

1. Diagnostic highlights
a. Early differential diagnosis is difficult and often times confusing, especially with hard lens molding syndromes
b. Can be confused with other pseudo-conditions
    i. Pellucid degeneration
    ii. Noninflammatory thinning disorders, which would include keratoglobus and even posterior keratoconus in early stages
c. Irregular astigmatism is usually present
    i. Difference between keratoconus and hard lenses molding
        • K readings rarely correspond to the spectacle cylinder axis in early keratoconus
        • More closely aligned to the K readings with hard lens molding
d. Age is generally in the late teens or 20s
e. There is usually a blur with increased astigmia
f. Frequent spectacle changes
g. Glare
h. Photoaversion
i. Occasionally polyopia
j. Objective finding
    i. Retinoscopy
        • Myopic astigmatism (usually)
        • Scissors reflex with yawning motion
    ii. Slit-lamp examination and externals
        • Central to inferior corneal protrusion (Munson's sign)
        • Stromal thinning (early sign: some believe optical illusion)
        • Fleischer's ring: basal layer of the epithelium that demarcates the base of the cone
        • Fibrillary lines that are subepithelial or anterior stromal clearing lines
        • Scarring at any level, primarily Bowman's or anterior stromal
        • Prominent nerves and stress lines in the pre-Descemet's area and usually in a vertical or oblique fashion (Vogt's lines)
        • Increased endothelial light reflex
    iii. Keratometry
        • Irregular or inclined mires
        • Inferior steepening increasing over the course of time
    iv. Other signs
        • Ruzzuti's light reflex (from the side you see a peaked light reflex)

- Complications would include corneal hydrops (3 percent)
- Perforation is rare

2. Goals in fitting
   a. Visual improvement
   b. Attempting to reduce, retard, or arrest cone progress
3. When to fit
   a. A bandage lens can be used in corneal hydrops as an adjunct to therapy for the purpose of visual acuity
   b. Rigid lenses only seem to be sufficient in moderate or severe cases
      i. In early cases, spectacles and soft lenses can be tried first
      ii. Early soft lenses are encouraged, as hard lenses can create sequelae and are believed to exacerbate thinning
4. What to fit
   a. The soft lens is indicated in certain cases
   b. A rigid lens only in the form of gas-permeable materials should be attempted
      i. Single cuts
      ii. Aspheric designs
      iii. Soper bicurve designs
      iv. Modified McGuire techniques using very small optic zones (OZ) with multiple peripheral curves can be used
5. How to fit
   a. Vault the apex
      i. Not often accomplished because of the steepness of the cornea
      ii. Sometimes have to compromise with divided support with primary bearing off the apex
   b. A modified McGuire technique with a very small OZ
      i. Usually a diameter of 8.4 and OZ of 2 to 2.5 mm less than the overall diameter
      ii. The secondary radius is usually 1.7 to 2 mm flatter than the base curve, with gradual dropoff in multiple peripheral curves out toward the periphery
      iii. High powers certainly necessitate lenticular cuts in most cases
      iv. Flat-fitting lenses notoriously give great comfort and great vision and are tempting to fit in such a fashion, but the sequelae have to be of concern
6. How to follow

   a. Generally seen every 3 months after successful fitting
   b. Depends on progression of condition
7. Complications
   a. As long as there is continued steepening, you are going to have plus acceptance with apical bearing on each visit
      i. These findings should be tipoffs that a steeper lens is needed
      ii. Alter power to a certain point, as the corneal tear–film relationship does not hold because of all the bearing involved
   b. Nodular scarring can occur from a flat-fitting lens or frequent rubbing of the eye
   c. Neovascularization is rare, except in haptic lenses, where there is also broadening of the cone
   d. Epithelial staining is fairly common
      i. Swirl or whirl pattern with occasional erosion
      ii. Vortex staining is also fairly common
   e. Some hard gas-permeable lenses could produce transient impressions
      i. Secondary radius
      ii. Decrease the OZ
      iii. Alter the base curve
      iv. Even change the material since pervaporation plays a role
   f. Edema can be common even with the gas-permeable lenses

H. APHAKIA

1. Diagnostic highlights
   a. The patient has no lens
   b. Can be accompanied by the whole spectrum of coexisting conditions
2. Goals in fitting
   a. Vision rehabilitation
   b. As related to coexisting conditions
3. When to fit
   a. Monocular aphakia
   b. High risk for intraocular lens
   c. Spectacle rejection
   d. As indicated by coexisting conditions
4. What to fit
   a. Extended wear
      i. If no other factors, a medium to high water content lens with good optics and durability
      ii. Any coexisting conditions will affect choice of materials and designs

b. Daily wear
  i. Gas-permeable hard contact lenses
  ii. Daily-wear soft only in rare cases, i.e., young aphake with excellent dexterity
5. How to fit
  a. Extended-wear lens is first choice
  b. Depends more on coexisting factors than on aphakic condition alone
6. How to follow
  a. Standard extended-wear follow-up (24 hours, 1 week, 1 month, every 3 to 4 months thereafter)
  b. Teach insertion and removal when appropriate
  c. Risk–benefit ratio is affected by the fact that, without a contact lens, the patient is an "optical cripple"
  d. In difficult management cases, consider a secondary intraocular lens when appropriate
7. Complications
  a. All complications of extended wear
  b. Patient may delay treatment in complications because of concerns of ageriatric population, i.e., transportation, living alone, and confusion over dangerous warning signs

I. OTHER CONSIDERATIONS

1. Diabetes[28]

a. Diagnostic highlights
  i. History of diabetes (weakened basal lamina)
  ii. Associated anterior segment problems
    • Tangential injuries
    • Recurrent erosion
    • Epithelial basement membrane dystrophy
  iii. Recent surgery as lensectomy, vitrectomy, retinal detachment (RD) repair, endophotocoagulation, silicone oil replacement, all with corneal epithelial loss
  iv. Associated with neurotropic keratitis
b. Goals in fitting
  i. Bandage
  ii. Promote healing
  iii. Assessment of visual potential for further surgical procedures
  iv. Supply best vision for the remainder of the shortened life span
c. When to fit
    i. Progressive epithelial basement membrane dystrophy
    ii. Retarded epithelial healing rate
    iii. Chronic epithelial syndromes
    iv. Chronic or frequent re-erosion
d. What to fit
    i. Any of the extended-wear lens materials, depending on other considerations (e.g., dry eye, edema, aphakia)
    ii. Try to stick to Hydrogels if there is an epithelial problem caused by minimal trauma to the epithelium
e. How to fit
    i. Extended-wear lenses in most cases in which epithelium is abnormal
    ii. Fitting depends on other factors, as diabetes can cover the whole range of considerations
    iii. If the epithelium is "normal" and a rigid lens is considered, it must be a gas-permeable material
f. How to follow
    i. Conservatively, as anything can go wrong with these patients
    ii. See the patient more often
    iii. React more quickly to problems and assess risk–benefit ratio more frequently
g. Complications
    i. Corneal anesthesia that brings on all of the sequelae of neurotrophic keratitis
    ii. All extended-wear complications
    iii. Lens spoilage
    iv. The risk–benefit ratio is completely different in these patients owing to the life span considerations

2. Microwounds

a. Diagnostic highlights
    i. Immediate postoperative period of anterior segment surgery with limbal wound
    ii. Flat chamber
    iii. Zero to low IOP
    iv. Negative Seidel test
    v. Choroidal detachment
b. Goals
    i. Seals microwound leak
    ii. Stabilize anterior segment
c. When to fit: when surgical reintervention is not indicated
d. What to fit: low to medium water content soft contact lens

   e. How to fit: extended-wear lens

   f. Follow-up

      i. Every 12 to 24 hours, until chamber reforms

      ii. Every 5 to 7 days, until choroid resolves

   g. Complications

      i. All extended-wear complications

      ii. Higher risk of infection

      iii. Retinal detachment

3. Viral Disease

   a. Diagnostic highlights

      i. Herpes simplex recurrent SPK at first can result in ulceration

      ii. Infiltrates and stain indicate that there is activity

   b. Goal in fitting: promote healing

   c. When to fit

      i. Nonhealing herpetic ulcers (simplex)

        • May eliminate the need for prolonged patching

        • Conjunctival flap

        • Tarsorrhaphy

      ii. When a leaking descemetocele is present

      iii. It may buy time for penetrating keratoplasty on an inflamed eye

      iv. Usually wait to fit these patients until dendrite heals

      v. If epithelium breaks down, you can use lens

      vi. Also indicated in neurotrophic conditions as in post-herpes zoster

      vii. Can also serve as an adjunct before conjunctival flap if melting of the stroma is eminent

   d. How to fit

      i. First should culture

      ii. Insert on first try and avoid touching concave surface

   e. What to fit

      i. High water lens (if loss is a problem, go to a thinner low water lens)

      ii. Should consider thin low water lens with limbal ulceration to promote neovascularization, which is greater and faster with a low water lens, to aid the inflammatory response

   f. How to follow

      i. Initially almost every day

      ii. Then every 2 to 3 days, 1 week, until epithelium and the lens can be removed

   g. Complications

      i. Superinfection

      ii. Other complications, including noninfectious sequelae

      iii. The potential of stromal melting with any herpetic condition

      iv. With chronic use of prophylactic medications, resistance and intolerance can develop

        • Timoptic with the lens has proved to be an epithelial toxin

        • Toxicities have been noted with EDTA, thimerosol, chlorabutanol, and benzylkonium chloride as preservatives in antibiotics

4. Corneal Grafting

   a. Diagnostic highlights

      i. Penetrating keratoplasty

      ii. Lamellar or thermal keratoplasty

      iii. Some of the new surgical refractive procedures, including epikeratophakia

      iv. For penetrating injury, perform Seidel test

   b. Goals in fitting

      i. Bandaging defects

      ii. Mechanical protection

      iii. Promote healing

      iv. Visual enhancement

   c. When to fit

      i. Dellen or minor irritating plateau paracentral drying effect of the graft

      ii. With slight dehiscence if the anterior chamber reforms, for visual acuity purposes

   d. What to fit

      i. A rigid lens for vision

      ii. In therapeusis, a high water lens usually does best

      iii. May need a rigid (gas-permeable) bitoric lens, especially if there is marked astigmia, a tilted graft, or an uneven host–graft junction

   e. How to fit

      i. Try to avoid bearing on the host–graft junction

      ii. Ideally, it would be nice to fit within the grafted tissue, but large lenses are usually needed for centration

 iii. In penetrating injuries, "splint" where you fit the lens quite steep to promote swelling of stroma in hope of sealing the leak

f. How to follow

 i. Daily until the anterior chamber is formed

 ii. Three days, then 1 week until condition is normal

 iii. May need a suture in the cornea if cornea does not seal with a bandage lens

 iv. See patient every 3 months after successful fitting

g. Complications

 i. For penetrating injuries, you have to be concerned about flat anterior chambers

 ii. Grafts produce concern for neovascularization, scarring, edema, and signs of rejection

- Always monitor for epithelial and endothelial rejections
- There is no proof that a contact lens will cause immunological graft rejection, but it certainly may exacerbate the situation, if present
- Soft lenses can increase leukocytic potential for infiltration and graft rejection

5. Immunological Considerations

 a. SLK of Theodore

  i. Diagnostic highlights
- Not soft lens related
- Bilateral
- Upper lid mild papillary hypertrophy and inflammation
- Sharply circumscribed ("corridor") injection of upper bulbar conjunctiva with edema

TABLE 7–8. SUMMARY OF THERAPEUTIC CONTACT LENS INDICATIONS AND FITTING OPTIONS

Therapeutic Contact Lens Indication	Large Diameter	Medium Diameter	Small Diameter	Standard	Thin	Thick	Daily Wear	Extended Wear	Loose	Regular	Tight	Low H₂O Soft	Medium H₂O Soft	High H₂O Soft	Silicone	RGP	PMMA
Aphakia	X	X	X	X	X	X	Second	First	X	X	X	X	X	X	X	X	X
Bullous	X					X	Second	First	X					X			
Dellen	X				X		First	Second	X	X		X	X				
Diabetes	X	X		X	X	X	First	Second	X	X		X	X	X	X	X	
Disfigurement	X	X		X		X	First	Second	X	X				X		X	X
Dry eye	X	X		X	X		First	Second	X				X		X		
EBMD	X				X	X	Second	First		X			X	X			
Entropion/trichiasis	X			X	X		First	Second		X		X			X		
Exposure	X			X	X		First	Second	X	X		X	X				
Filament	X				X	X	First	Second	X			X		X			
Fuchs'	X	X				X	Second	First	X					X			
Neurotropic	X			X	X	X	Second	First	X			X	X	X			
Recurrent erosion	X			X	X	X	—	First	X			X	X	X			
Theodore	X			X	X		First	Second		X		X	X				
Thygeson	X	X		X	X	X	Second	First	X	X		X	X	X			

TABLE 7 – 9. SUMMARY OF THERAPEUTIC CONTACT LENS GOALS AND OPTIONS

Therapeutic Fitting Goal	Standard Diameter	Large Diameter	Thin Center	Standard Thickness	Low H_2O	Medium H_2O	High H_2O	Daily Wear	Extended Wear	Loose Fit	Tight Fit	RGP	PMMA
Aphakia	X	X	X		X	X	X	X	X	X		X	X
Cosmetic		X		X	X	X	X	X			X		X
Epithelial bandage		X	X			X	X	X	X	X		X	
Epithelial dehydration (edema control)		X	X			X	X	X	X	X			
Epithelial hydration	X	X		X	X	X	?	X		X			
Keratoconus	X		X									X	
Mechanical protection		X		X	X	X		X	X	X		X	
Orthokeratology	X			X						X		X	X
Pain reduction	X	X	X			X	X	X	X	X			
Promote healing		X	X			X	X		X	X			
Visual improvement over irregular surface	X	X	X	X	X	X	X	X		X		X	X

TABLE 7–10. SUMMARY OF CONSIDERATIONS IN FITTING AND FOLLOWING THERAPEUTIC CONTACT LENS PATIENTS

Clinical Condition	Diagnostic Highlights	Goals in TX Fitting	When to Fit
Aphakia	No crystalline lens	Visual improvement	Especially monocular
Bullous keratopathy	Severe pain, bullae	Bandage, pain reduction	Severe pain
Cogan's degeneration	Large microcysts	Bandage, pain reduction	Chronic pain
Dellen	Peripheral cup	Hydration	Non response to lubricants
Diabetes	Systemic history	Bandage, promote healing	Progressive EBMD
Disfigurement	Gross anomaly	Cosmetic relief	On request
Dry-eye keratitis sicca	Positive rose bengal	Hydration	Nonresponse to lubricants
EBMD	Maps, dots, erosions	Bandage	Re-erosions
Edema	Bedewing, microcystic	Dehydration	Bullae, erosions
Entropion/trichiasis	Inturning lash(es)	Mechanical protection	Chronic irritation
Exposure keratitis	Band SPK	Mechanical protection	Nonresponse to lubricants
Filamentary keratitis	Adherent buds or threads	Promote healing	Nonresponse to lubricants
Fuchs' dystrophy	Dense guttata	Bandage, dehydration	Severe symptoms
Keratoconus	Central corneal thinning	Bandage, visual	Reduced best VA
Recurrent erosion	AM syndrome	Bandage, dehydration	Chronic
SLK of Theodore	Superior SPK and injection	Mechanical	Nonresponsive to medications
SPK of Thygeson	Diffuse SPK and SEI	Bandage	Chronic irritation

- SPK of cornea and superior limbus
- Positive staining with rose bengal
- One third of cases have filamentary formation
- Superior bulbar conjunctival limbal lexity (sagging)
- Occasional superior pannus

ii. Goals in fitting
  - Mechanical protection
  - Reduce pain

iii. When to fit
  - If 5 percent silver nitrate fails
  - If vasoconstrictors fail
  - In recurrent cases
  - Before surgical intervention is considered
  - Topical steroids are contraindicated in this condition
  - Cromolyn drops are of questionable value

iv. What to fit
  - Low to medium water contact lenses
  - Standard thickness

v. How to fit
  - Large diameter
  - Daily wear if possible

vi. How to follow
  - Try oral antihistamine–decongestant and aspirin or ibuprofen

- Return every 1 to 2 weeks, until objective signs resolve
- If wear discontinued, reinstitute upon exacerbation

vii. Complications
  - This condition may worsen as a result of bandage lens therapy
  - This condition may be self-limiting if left alone
  - If the extended-wear modality is used, all extended-wear complications are a concern

b. SPK of Thygeson
  i. Diagnostic highlights
    - Central bilateral SPK with epithelial (raised) infiltrates
    - History of exacerbations and remissions
    - No stromal involvement or anterior chamber reaction
    - White eye presentation "keeping no company"

  ii. Goals in fitting
    - Bandage
    - Pain reduction
    - Improve VA

  iii. When to fit
    - If low-dose steroids are ineffective or contraindicated
    - If nonsteroidal anti-inflammatory drops or lubricants are ineffective

What to Fit	How to Fit	How to Follow	Highest-Risk Complications
Medium/high H$_2$O or GPH	Extended wear (EW) if possible	Every 3–4 months	Infection
High H$_2$O soft	Large, thin, loose (EW)	Every 6–8 weeks	Infection
High H$_2$O soft	Large, thin, loose (EW)	Every 4–6 weeks	Infection
Low/medium H$_2$O	Large diameter	Every week	Physiological
Medium H$_2$O or GPH	Large, loose on K	Every 2–3 months	Mechanical
Cosmetic lens	Large and tight	Every 2–3 months	Physiological
Low/medium H$_2$O	Loose, daily wear	Every 2–3 months	Infection
High H$_2$O or GPH	Large, thin loose (EW)	Every 4–6 weeks	Infection
High H$_2$O soft or GPH	Large, thin loose (EW)	Every 6–8 weeks	Physiological
Low/medium H$_2$O	Standard thickness	Every 3 months	Infection
Low/medium H$_2$O	Extended wear	Every 6–12 weeks	Infection
Low/medium H$_2$O	Large diameter	Every week	Physiological
High H$_2$O soft	Large, thin loose (EW)	Every 4–6 weeks	Infection
GPH	On K or slightly flat	Every 2–3 months	Mechanical
High H$_2$O soft	Large, thin loose (EW)	Every 3–4 weeks	Infection
Low to medium H$_2$O	Large, daily wear	Every 1–2 weeks (initially)	Immunological
Low to medium H$_2$O	Daily or extended wear	Every 4–6 weeks	Immunological

- If vision is reduced
  iv. What to fit: low to medium water content soft contact lenses
  v. How to fit
    - Extended wear
    - Daily wear if necessary
  vi. How to follow
    - Normal extended-wear follow-up, but try to discontinue the lens when epithelium is clear or in 6 months
    - Because this disease "waxes and wanes," the bandage soft lens may prolong the active phase; therefore, it should be discontinued after 6 months in either case
  vii. Complications
    - Condition may not respond or even worsen with soft lens bandage
    - If extended wear consider all associated complications

J. SUMMARY OF THERAPEUTIC CONTACT LENS INDICATIONS AND FITTING OPTIONS

Use Table 7–8 to consider specific therapeutic lens materials and designs appropriate for specific conditions

K. SUMMARY OF THERAPEUTIC CONTACT LENS GOALS AND OPTIONS

Use Table 7–9 to assess general fitting considerations for bandage lenses in specific conditions

L. SUMMARY OF CONSIDERATIONS IN FITTING AND FOLLOWING THERAPEUTIC CONTACT LENS PATIENTS

Use Table 7–10 to review management decisions in use of therapeutic contact lenses as bandages for specific conditions

---

IV. Self-assessment Questions

For each of the contact lens complications (1 through 20) listed below, select one of the following (lettered) drug categories that *might* be considered the most effective first drug of choice.

Drug Categories
  a. Anti-infectives (e.g., antibiotics)
  b. Anti-inflammatories (steroids or NSAIDs)
  c. Antiedema therapies (e.g., hypertonic salines)
  d. Withold all drugs for at least 5 to 7 days of discontinued wear or until definitive diagnosis

Contact Lens Complications
  1. _____ Bedewing
  2. _____ Cells or flare
  3. _____ Conjunctival hyperemia
  4. _____ Endothelial changes
  5. _____ Epithelial breakdown
  6. _____ Giant papillary conjunctivitis (GPC)
  7. _____ Keratoconjunctivitis
  8. _____ Microcystic edema
  9. _____ Microcysts (vesicles)
  10. _____ Neovascularization
  11. _____ Pannus
  12. _____ Pseudodendrites
  13. _____ Stippling
  14. _____ Striate keratitis
  15. _____ Stromal edema
  16. _____ Stromal infiltrates
  17. _____ Subepithelial infiltrates (SEIs)
  18. _____ Superficial punctate keratitis (SPK)
  19. _____ Superior limbic keratoconjunctivitis (SLK)
  20. _____ Corneal ulceration

For answers, refer to Appendix 6

REFERENCES

1. Catania LJ: A categorical approach to pre and post fit contact lens conditions. J Am Optom Assoc 58:10, 1987
2. McMonnies C, Chapman-Davies A: Assessment of conjunctival hyperemia in contact lens wearers. Am J Optom Physiol Opt 64:251, 1987
3. Allansmith MR, Korb DR, Greiner JV, et al: Giant papillary conjunctivitis in contact lens wearers. Am J Ophthalmol 83:697, 1977
4. Adler RJ, Wenderoth FA: Sodium cromolyn eyedrops in allergic soft lens users. Contact Lens Forum 11:36, 1986

5. McMonnies C, Chapman-Davies A: Assessment of conjunctival hyperemia in contact lens wearers. Am J Optom Physiol Opt 64:251, 1987

6. Korb DR, Greiner JV: Prevalence of conjunctival changes in wearers of hard contact lenses. Am J Ophthalmol 90:336, 1980

7. Efron N: Clinical management of corneal edema. Contact Lens Spect 1:13, 1986

8. Rubinstein MD: Diabetes, the anterior segment and contact lens wear. Contact Lens J 15:5, 1987

9. McMonnies C: Contact lens induced corneal vascularization. J Br Contact Lens Assoc 7:154, 1984

10. Udell M, Mannis MJ, Meisler DM, et al: Pseudodendrites in soft contact lens wearers. Contact Lens Association of Ophthalmology 11:51, 1985

11. Holden B, Efron N, Sweeney D, et al: Effects of long-term extended contact lens wear on the human cornea. Invest Ophthalmol 26:1489,1985

12. Chaston J, Fatt I: Corneal oxygen uptake under a soft contact lens in phakic and aphakic eyes. Invest Ophthalmol 23:234, 1982

13. Efron N: Clinical management of corneal edema. Contact Lens Spect 1:13, 1986

14. Stenson S: Soft on lens-related superior limbic keratoconjunctivitis. Contact Lens Forum 11:22, 1986

15. Mondino BJ, Weissman BA, Farb MD, et al: Corneal ulcers associated with daily wear and extended wear contact lenses. Am J Ophthalmol 102:58, 1986

16. Stenson S: Soft contact lenses and corneal infection. Arch Ophthalmol 102:58, 1986

17. Cohen E, Laibson P, Arentsen JJ, et al: Corneal ulcers associated with cosmetic extended wear soft contact lenses. Ophthalmology 94:109, 1987

18. Chalupa H, Swarbrick HA, Holden BA, et al: Severe corneal infections associated with contact lens wear. Ophthalmology 94:17, 1987

19. Amerod LD, Smith RE: Contact lens-associated microbial keratitis. Arch Ophthalmol 104:79, 1986

20. Collins M, Carney L: Patient compliance and its influence on contact lens wearing problems. Am J Optom Physiol Opt 63:952, 1986

21. Thoft RA: Bandages for bad corneas. Aud Dig 25:1, 1987

22. Key J, Mobley C: Cosmetic hydrogel lenses for therapeutic purposes. Contact Forum 12:18, 1987

23. Morrison R, Shovlin J: A review of the use of bandage lenses. Met Pediatr Syst Ophthalmol 6:117, 1982

24. Kaufman HE, Baldone JA: Soft contact lenses and clinical disease. (Letter.) Am J Ophthalmol 95:851, 1983

25. Kaufman ME: Bullous keratopathy. Contact Lens Association of Opthalmology 10:232, 1984

26. Efron N, Carney LG: Oxygen levels beneath the closed eyelid. Invest Ophthalmol 18:93, 1979

27. Rubinstein MD: Diabetes, the anterior segment and contact lens wear. Contact Lens J 15:5, 1987

ANNOTATED REFERENCES

Aquavella JV, Rao GN (eds): Contact Lenses. Philadelphia, JB Lippincott, 1987
Short but relevant text regarding current concepts and approaches to contact lens, fitting complications and therapeutic uses.

Cohen EJ (ed): Contact lenses and external disease, in International Ophthalmology Clinics, Boston, Little, Brown, 1986
Comprehensive presentations on major categories by experts in the field regarding contact lens related disease. Each area covered in detail with clinical discussions and new concepts in care.

Hamano M, Kaufman ME: The physiology of the Cornea and Contact Lens Applications. New York, Churchill Livingstone, 1987
In-depth detailed discussion of corneal physiology and its relationship to contact lens wear. Valuable information for understanding and fitting contact lenses on the cornea and dealing with their effects.

Larke JR: The Eye in Contact Lens Wear. London, Butterworths, 1985
Well-organized book dealing with each anatomical structure affected by contact lens wear and the theoretical (scientific) and clinical considerations of the relationship between the lens and the eye.

Stenson SM (ed): "Contact Lenses: A Guide to Selection, Fitting and Management of Complications." E. Norwalk, CT, Appleton & Lange, 1987
Current approaches, concepts, and care regarding contact lens fitting and complications. Information on management of complications provides most recent thinking in the field.

Case Reports with Color Plates

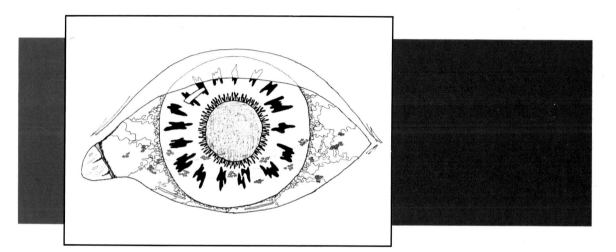

Section Outline

I. Case Reports with Color Plates

43. Fuchs' endothelial dystrophy (guttata)
44. Bullous keratopathy
45. Filamentary keratitis
46. Pterygium
47. Hudson–Stahli line
48. Kaiser–Fleisher ring (Wilson's disease)
49. Maps (in EBMD)
50. Dots (in EBMD)
51. Microcysts (in EBMD)
52. Fingerprints (in EBMD)
53. Negative NaFl staining
54. Diffuse superficial punctate keratitis
55. Focal inferior SPK "Patch"
56. Marginal keratitis
57. Marginal infiltrate with diffuse NaFl staining
58. Gonococcal corneal ulcer
59. Corneal ulcer with exudate
60. Pseudomonal corneal ulcer
61. Mild pseudomembrane
62. Moderate pseudomembrane
63. Severe pseudomembrane
64. Subepithelial infiltrates in EKC
65. Dendrites in recurrent HSV keratitis
66. NaFl ulceration test
67. Metaherpetic ulcer
68. Ocular rosacea keratitis
69. Superior limbic keratoconjunctivitis
70. Keratitis sicca with rose bengal staining
71. Band-region SPK
72. Foreign-body tracking

73. Corneal abrasion (superficial)
74. Corneal abrasion (deep to basement membrane)
75. Superficial corneal foreign body
76. Corneal foreign body with Coate's white ring
77. Stromal penetration
78. Hemosiderosis (rust ring)
79. Recurrent corneal erosion syndrome
80. Acute anterior uveitis
81. Cells and flare
82. Mutton fat KP
83. Kruckenburg's spindle
84. Posterior synechiae
85. Seclusio pupillae
86. Hyphema
87. Iris atrophy
88. Iris tumor (?)
89. Persistent pupillary membrane
90. Rubeosis iridis
91. Ectopia lentis (Marfan's syndrome)
92. Acne rosacea
93. Herpes zoster ophthalmicus
94. Psoriatic lid lesion
95. Band keratopathy (hyperparathyroidism)
96. Port-wine stain (Sturge–Weber syndrome)
97. Folds in Descemet's membrane (striate keratitis)
98. Leukomatous corneal scarring
99. Dense physiological edema
100. Recurrent erosion with bandage soft contact lens

II. **Self-assessment Questions**

I. Case Reports with Color Plates

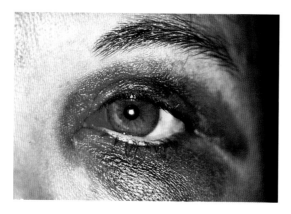

1. ECCHYMOSIS

Blunt injury to the left lid produced superior lid edema and whole-blood accumulation in its lateral aspect, with diffuse hemorrhaging and edema in the inferior lid as well. Palpation indicated no crepitation (air in the tissue) nor subjective or objective indication of fracture.

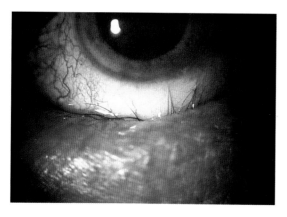

2. ENTROPION

This 68-year-old man presented with constant irritation (scratchy feeling) for more than 1 year. His lower lid folded inward, causing constant rubbing of his lashes over an irregular, probably partially numbed, inferior corneal surface. Lid surgery relieved problem completely.

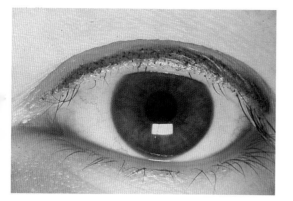

3. MADAROSIS

This young adult woman presented with a history of recent emotional trauma (sudden death of her husband) and subsequent patchy loss and thinning of lashes. Antistaphylococcal therapy (bacitracin ointment) produced moderate improvement in the condition over a 6-month period. *Post hoc ergo propter hoc* ("After this, therefore because of this")—a risky conclusion in diagnosis and treatment!

4. TRICHIASIS

This 62-year-old man presented with a transient history of foreign-body sensation and chronic "sandy, gritty feeling" in his left eye. Slit-lamp evaluation of the cornea demonstrated irregular staining of the inferior temporal aspect being caused by isolated (two or three) lashes turning inward and causing abrasion.

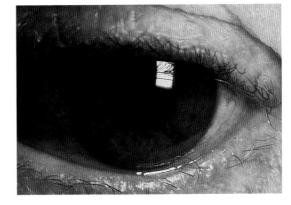

5. CHRONIC BLEPHARITIS

Longstanding (>3-month duration) marginal lid hypertrophy, crustation (rosettes), patchy madarosis, and a superior temporal epithelial ulceration in a typical chronic, staphylococcal, marginal blepharitis.

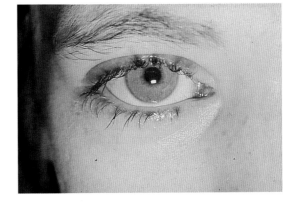

6. SUBACUTE MARGINAL BLEPHARITIS

This 17-year-old girl was cosmetically distressed by the recurring hyperemic appearance to her lid margins (bilaterally). Antistaphylococcal treatment with bacitracin ointment at bedtime for 6 weeks and ongoing weekly maintenance therapy eliminated recurrences completely.

7. PRESEPTAL CELLULITIS

Periorbital erythema and tenderness in this 58-year-old man proved (radiologically) to be secondary to acute sinusitis. A critical differential diagnosis (by history and clinical presentation) must rule out orbital cellulitis.

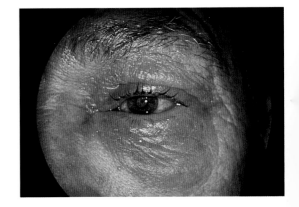

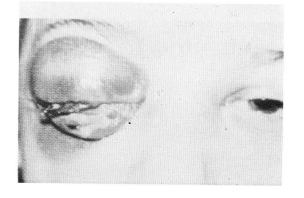

8. ORBITAL CELLULITIS

One of the most serious, life-threatening ocular manifestations of systemic disorders is an orbital cellulitis. The proptosis noted in this plate is usually associated with constitutional symptoms, diplopia, frozen globe, and relatively gross ocular tissue congestion (e.g., chemosis).

9. HERPES SIMPLEX BLEPHARITIS

A series of diffuse pustules are noted on this moderately tender inferior lid surface of a young man with recurrent herpes simplex. The entire surrounding skin is erythematous, and the lateral lesions appear softer than the harder, crusty medial pustules.

10. ALLERGIC BLEPHARITIS

During a seasonal change (winter to spring), this child presented with an immediate (type 1) allergic reaction (within hours) to his right superior eyelid after playing outdoors. This is typical of a contact-type reaction responsive to cold packs and antihistamines and decongestants.

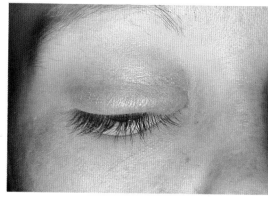

11. EARLY BASAL CELL CARCINOMA

This small nodule on the skin adjacent to the lower lid was noted during general examination. A patient history of (1) extensive exposure to the sun, (2) previous history of basal cell, (3) observation of vascularized central depression to nodule, and (4) loss of skin texture over nodule surface triggered referral for biopsy that proved positive.

12. ADVANCED BASAL CELL CARCINOMA

This pigmented lesion in an elderly woman had all the classic signs of basal cell carcinoma: raised, hardened borders and umbilicated, pigmented central ulceration, accompanied by similar lesions elsewhere on the face, neck, and forearms.

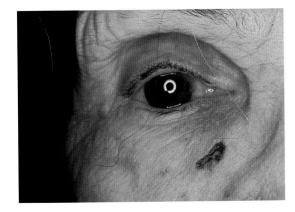

13. EXTERNAL CHALAZION

This common "lump" extending through the temporal aspect of this patient's superior lid was firm and painless on palpation. A negative history of irritation and mild signs of inflammation are typical in the chalazion presentation. Heat therapy for 3 weeks shrunk this 8- to 9-mm granuloma down to a reasonable, noncosmetically observable lid nodule.

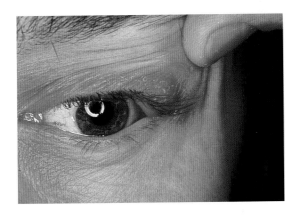

14. DERMOID

This mass in the right superior temporal brow region had been noted by the patient for many years before presenting for general examination. Being a common position for dermoid formations the benign congenital tumor has been observed periodically (annually) as a standard precautionary measure.

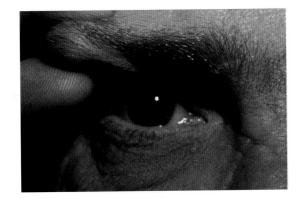

15. EXTERNAL HORDEOLUM

This self-diagnosed stye was seen primarily due to its cosmetic affectation. It had developed over a 5-day period with increasing superficial suppuration and mild irritation over a 48-hour period. Slight secondary edema and the erythematous base of the hordeolum resolved rapidly over hot packs and polysporin ointment (tid × 5 days).

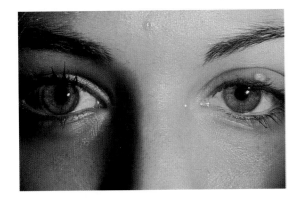

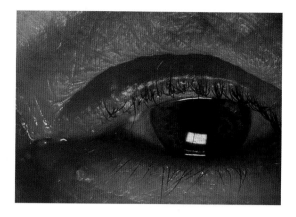

16. INTERNAL HORDEOLUM

Exquisite pain on palpation at the medial aspect of this superior lid indicated an internal hordeolum buried in a relatively dramatic erythematous swollen lid presentation. The pointing suppuration noted at the lid margin was a definite sign of early meibomian gland abcess.

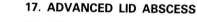

17. ADVANCED LID ABSCESS

This child went without treatment for 2 weeks, for an internal hordeolum in his right superior lid, resulting in a large meibomian lid abscess. This degree of involvement usually will not respond to topical or oral antibiosis and requires surgical incision and drainage.

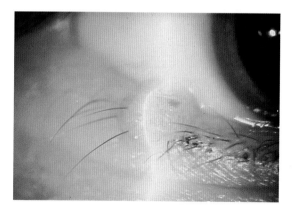

18. AMELANOTIC PAPILLOMA

A quiet, asymptomatic mass at the inferior mucocutaneous border of the lid margin was reported during general examination. Note the eyelashes growing directly through epithelial overgrowth.

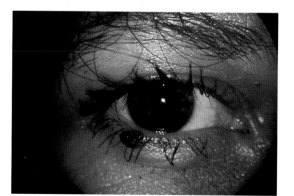

19. PIGMENTED PAPILLOMA

This inferotemporal heavily pigmented papilloma was noted in a darkly pigmented Caucasian male. Lesion was stable and asymptomatic.

20. SUPERFICIAL SEBACEOUS CYST

An older woman presented with an enlarging caseous filled superficial cyst of approximately 5 to 6 mm at the superior nasal palpebral sulcus. Upon request, the cyst was lanced and expressed of its contents.

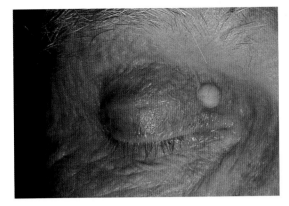

21. DEEP SEBACEOUS CYST

This large subcutaneous cyst of approximately 10 mm was found at the inner canthus during a general examination in an older man who denied concern for the longstanding lesion and refused treatment. Note the prominent overlying capillary vessels.

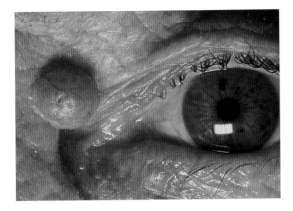

22. SUDORIFEROUS CYST

This patient presented with an asymptomatic clear fluid-filled cyst recently noticed on her right outer canthal lid margin. Drainage relieved cyst immediately.

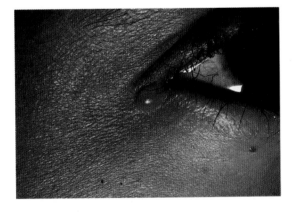

23. VERRUCA DIGITALA

The pedal-like (digitated) brownish mass emanating from this patient's superior lid margin is typical of the rather common verruca digitala found in older patients. The proximity of this viral papillomatous lesion to the ocular surface may be reason for its occasional association with viral keratoconjunctivitis.

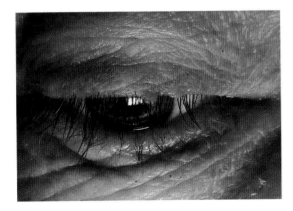

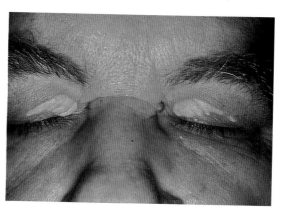

24. XANTHALASMA

Superior, bilateral, yellowish plaques following the medial sulcus of the superior lid is the most common presentation for xanthalasma. Lesions often appear simultaneously at the inferior medial aspect as well. These familial lesions were showing insidious increase in size and color but, upon reassurance and counseling, the patient chose to forego cosmetic surgical excision for the time being.

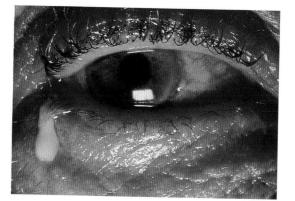

25. HYPERACUTE BACTERIAL CONJUNCTIVITIS

This unilateral presentation of a meaty red hyperemic bulbar conjunctiva with associated mucopurulent discharge (overflowing) developed during 48-hour period with no contributory history. Irrigation and erythromycin ointment q4h reversed the condition within 72 hours.

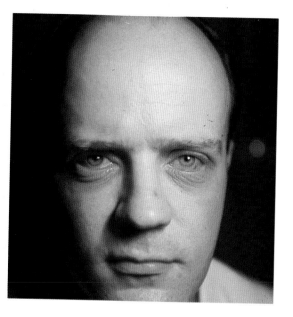

26. BILATERAL (HEMORRHAGIC) CONJUNCTIVITIS

This patient presented with bilateral hyperacute conjunctivitis with small petechial and subconjunctival hemorrhages scattered on the bulbar conjunctiva (greater inferiorly), secondary lid erythema, and moderate purulent discharge. There was a systemic history of a recent streptococcal infection reported.

27. FOLLICLES

These small, pale, discrete mounds of infiltrative cells (high-lighted by NaFl) were present on the inferior palpebral conjunctiva in an acute viral conjunctivitis. No prominent vascular pattern was noted on their surface or at their base.

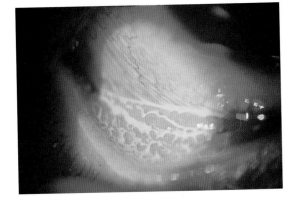

28. VIRAL CONJUNCTIVITIS

The diffuse purplish-pinkish bulbar hyperemia usually associated with viral conjunctivitis is depicted. Whereas this particular presentation shows diffuse injection, the patient will frequently present with more pronounced changes at the inner canthal region. Also note the "rugae" folds in the inferior cul-de-sac formed by abundant follicles and an early pseudomembranous formation.

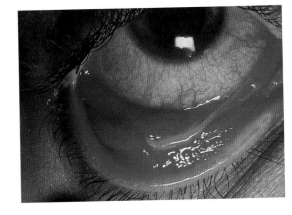

29. ALLERGIC CONJUNCTIVITIS WITH CHEMOSIS

Allergic conjunctivitis, particularly the immediate type 1 response, produces subconjunctival infiltrative edema giving a raised, "puffy" appearance to the bulbar conjunctiva. Such a distinct objective sign associated with a subjective history of "itching" invariably equals an allergic reaction.

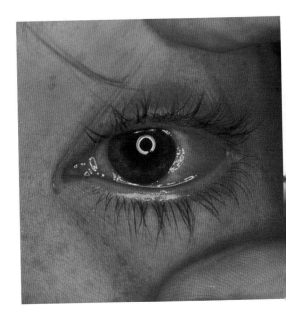

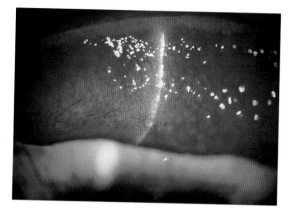

30. GIANT PAPILLARY CONJUNCTIVITIS

This superior palpebral conjunctival reaction was witnessed in a 20-year-old white woman experiencing discomfort with her soft contact lens. This common complication to hydrophilic lenses is typical of the papillae (note the prominent vascular tufts) observed in hypersensitivity, autoimmune reactions.

31. CHRONIC CONJUNCTIVITIS

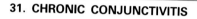

Dry eye was the diagnosis for this low-grade nonspecific conjunctivitis presentation. In the absence of discharge, follicles, edema, and other problems, with positive rose bengal staining (conjunctiva) and reduced BUT supported the diagnosis and the need for heavy lubrication therapy.

32. EPISCLERITIS

This 38-year-old white woman presented with a second occurrence of unilateral episcleritis (first occurrence, 2 years earlier) in her left eye. Tenderness over the sector of deep injected vessels (no nodules) was not severe and the area responded to warm packs and topical steroids qid within 2 weeks.

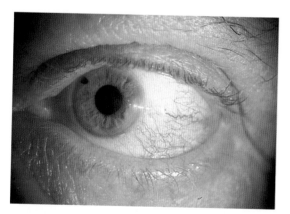

33. NODULAR EPISCLERITIS

This 23-year-old woman presented with a tender, large sector of episcleritis, including a raised central nodule (slightly obscured by the overlying hyperemic tissue) of 10 days duration. Completely negative history and good health ruled out systemic associations; on topical steroids and oral ibuprofen 1600 mg/day q4h, the eye resolved (slowly) over a 3-week period with no etiology established.

34. PALPEBRAL CONJUNCTIVAL GRANULOMA

These common masses are often seen emanating from the palpebral conjunctiva and "climbing" over the lid into prominent view. The outer side (away from the ocular surface) is characterized by the typical spongy vascularized appearance of granulomatous tissue, while the rear side assumes the smooth continuous contour of the ocular surface itself.

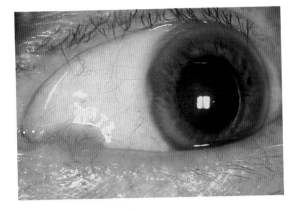

35. PALPEBRAL CONJUNCTIVAL GRANULOMA (BLEEDING)

This patient reported concern regarding recent bleeding over the surface of a slowly enlarging mass in the palpebral conjunctival area of the right eye. The vascularized spongy mass was referred for excision, primarily because of the acquired bleeding and doctor and patient were reassured by the anticipated pathology report of granuloma.

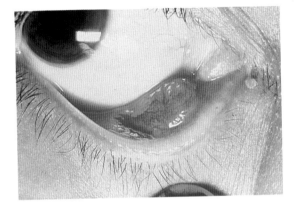

36. SUBCONJUNCTIVAL HEMORRHAGE WITH TELANGIECTASIA

In this subconjunctival hemorrhage, a round, circumscribed, focal elevation at the superior border of the hemorrhage is noted. This is typical of a dilated telangiectatic vessel associated with (and probable cause of) subconjunctival hemorrhaging.

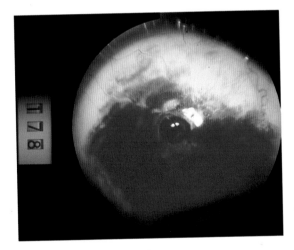

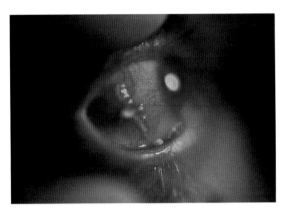

37. LYMPHANGIECTASIA

This is an elongated multiply dilated lymphangiectasia in an adult male who presented with relative concern over this lesion of 2-months duration. Upon specific request, simple piercing of the dilated areas (single or multiple) with a 22- or 25-gauge needle and gentle finger massage over the closed lid, immediately collapses these thin-walled lymphatic cysts. Any prophylaxis or follow-up is optional.

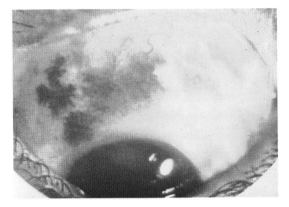

38. BENIGN ACQUIRED MELANOSIS

This 36-year-old white man, examined for general care, showed superficial patches of "clean," nonvascularized, gray-black pigment on the superior bulbar conjunctiva of his right eye. The history indicated no other pigmentary changes on the body and close management (every 6 months) showed no substantial increase in this acquired melanosis for 4-years duration.

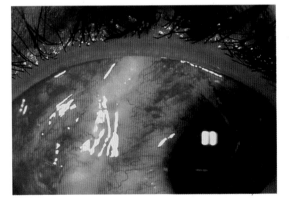

39. CONJUNCTIVAL LACERATION

A dramatic conjunctival laceration secondary to a vertically oriented "clothesline" injury caused considerable subconjunctival hemorrhaging in this very concerned, yet mildly symptomatic young woman. After ruling out scleral penetration or intraocular injury, the bare scleral (white) area and the redundant, edematous, "bloody" conjunctival tissue were copiously lavaged and examined for any foreign matter. Self-resolution of the lacerated tissue under q4h anti-infective ointment prophylaxis, irrigation, and warm packs began to produce improvement in 5 to 7 days with complete healing over a 4-week period.

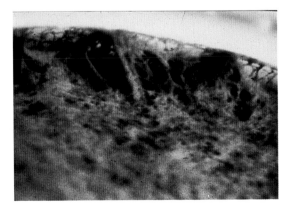

40. AXENFELD'S ANOMALY

This 13-year-old boy presenting for general examination was found to have a rather prominent Schwalbe's line (posterior embryotoxon) under slit-lamp examination. Upon gonioscopy, rather dense iris processes attached to the posterior cornea (at Schwalbe's line) plus a normal IOP confirmed the A/R syndrome, Axenfeld's anomaly.

41. REIGER'S SYNDROME

Iris hypoplasia is demonstrated dramatically under pupillary dilation in this patient with raised intraocular pressure (IOP) and other A/R syndrome findings (e.g., posterior embryotoxon, iris strands) and dentition (palatine) deformities typical of Reiger's syndrome. Note the lack of response of the sphincter pupillae muscle versus radial fibers.

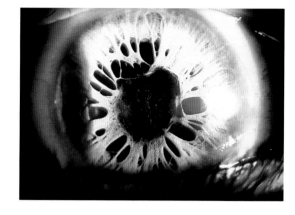

42. CONGENITAL TEARS IN DESCEMET'S MEMBRANE

During general examination, these vertical opaque lines were noted (under slit lamp) in the left eye of this 32-year-old black man. Best correctable vision was 20/30, and the patient reported a "weak left eye" since birth. Assumed cause was birth trauma (leading cause of vertical folds or tears in Descemet's, especially left eye).

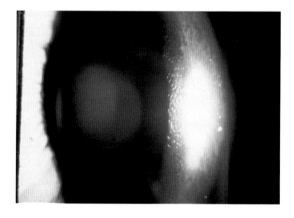

43. FUCHS' ENDOTHELIAL DYSTROPHY (GUTTATA)

Specular reflection (and retroillumination) is the most effective way of examining corneal endothelial guttata. Occasionally, guttata increase with age (especially in women) unveiling Fuchs' endothelial dystrophy, with its multiple signs and symptoms. When sparse or increasing (sometimes termed endothelial dystrophy in younger age ranges), monitor annually and watch for accumulation of pigment on guttata walls.

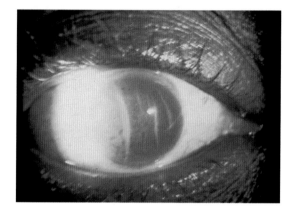

44. BULLOUS KERATOPATHY

A frequent complication of Fuchs' endothelial dystrophy is advanced epithelial edema, leading to "bubbling" of the epithelium into bullae formations (note separations of epithelium from base on anterior slit beam, to right), producing severe pain and risk of fibrotic scarring on corneal surface. Effective therapy for maintenance and pain control includes soft contact lens bandaging.

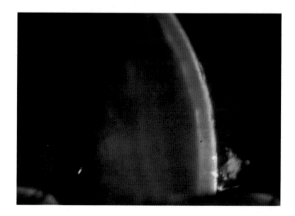

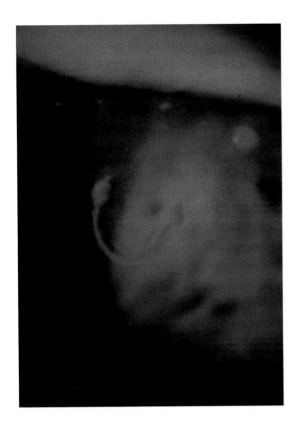

45. FILAMENTARY KERATITIS

This 48-year-old woman, complaining of a distinct foreign-body sensation under her right upper lid, was noted to have small (1-mm) immovable mucoid plugs on the superior cornea, with some generating trailing filamentary strands. This filamentary keratitis condition responded to heavy lubrication therapy over a 2- to 3-week period.

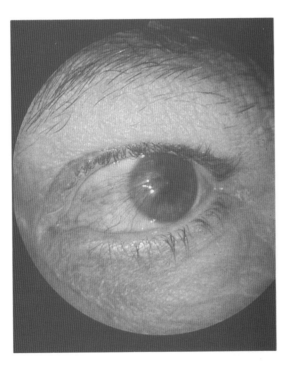

46. PTERYGIUM

A rather thick, fleshy, large, vascularized pterygium is shown in the nasal (usual) aspect of a left eye. Its triangular shape with apex toward pupil and base toward canthus is well defined. While the pupil is not dilated, it can be appreciated, with dim illumination, that the leading edge of the pterygium will definitely interfere with mid-dilation. Surgery will probably add another millimeter of scar interference. Consider these issues in your management or referral decisions.

47. HUDSON–STAHLI LINES

Brownish-orange (ferric ion) pigment lines at the level of Bowman's approximating the position of closed lid margins are nonpathological Hudson–Stahli lines found with increasing age. Incidence relative to years: age 20 = 20 percent, age 30 = 30 percent, age 60 to 80 plus = 100 percent). Three presentations are common: (a) light segmented lines; (b) light to dense continuous line (limbus to limbus); (c) lines with surrounding whitish/yellow deposits.

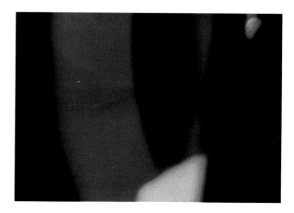

48. KAYSER–FLEISHER RING (WILSON'S DISEASE)

A neurologist referred this 32-year-old woman for confirmation of his tentative diagnosis of Wilson's hepaticolenticular disease. The classic (rare) finding of a brownish-orange (copper) ring on the posterior peripheral cornea confirmed the neurologist's suspicions. Penacillamine treatment resolved condition and reduced ring.

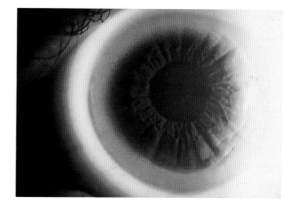

49. MAPS (IN EBMD)

Retroillumination of some rather obvious map configuration in a corneal EBM. More subtle, smaller patterns of geographic, amorphous, circular, linear shapes and sinuous lines are best (if not exclusively) observed by retroillumination (with a good slit lamp). Suggestive symptoms, negative staining, trauma, aging, and so forth, warrant a careful search for diagnosis of EBMD and appropriate management.

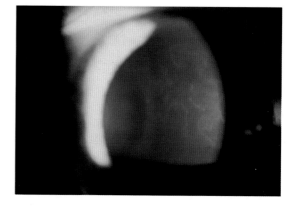

50. DOTS (IN EBMD)

The left eye of this asymptomatic 74-year-old patient shows obvious gray dots surrounded by amorphous map patterns in the pupillary zone. Vision was slightly reduced (perhaps lens and retinal changes contributing), but the asymptomatic nature warranted no treatment other than advisement of potential symptoms and PRN of 6 to 12 months recall.

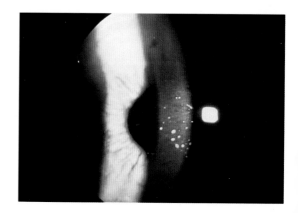

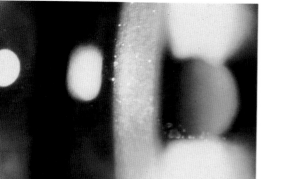

51. MICROCYSTS (IN EBMD)

Microcysts (really pseudocysts) form intraepithelially as clear fluid filled or grayish (putty-colored) cysts in EBMD. They range in size from pinpoint (and difficult to spot without retroillumination) to about 1 mm and are obvious even with direct illumination. They are usually in small groupings of multiple-sized dots, usually central, sometimes symptomatic —especially AM (morning) syndrome—and almost always produce negative staining.

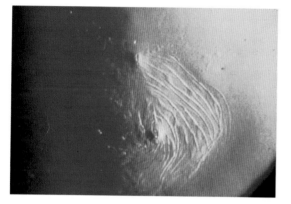

52. FINGERPRINTS (IN EBMD)

Whereas maps, dots, and microcysts are frequent in EBMD, fingerprints are less common, if not less noticeable, under slit-lamp examination. Easily described as having a "thumbprint" appearance on the cornea, they may be rather large or only present in small (2 mm) regions in the central cornea. Found more in older corneas, their subjective and objective signs and symptoms are similar to maps and dots.

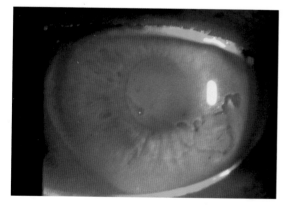

53. NEGATIVE NAFL STAINING

"Negative" in this term does not mean "no pattern." It means that NaFl stain does not disperse or spread evenly over a specific area upon blinking, as opposed to BUT (tear breakup time), which is random and delayed (2 to 10 seconds) Negative staining is focal and instant, usually suggesting an epithelial or epithelial basement membrane disorder. Note the typical cascading effect produced by the fluorescein breakup.

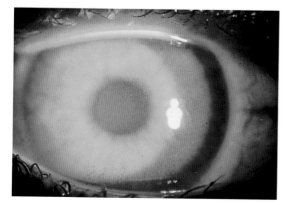

54. DIFFUSE SUPERFICIAL SPK

This young woman presented with a "sandy, gritty burning" irritation to her right eye. No viral signs were noted in conjunction with the diffuse punctate staining, but an active chronic marginal blepharitis and positive response to lid therapy supported a presumptive diagnosis of staphylococcal SPK.

55. LOCAL INFERIOR SPK "PATCH"

When SPK becomes sufficiently dense in a focal area, it will stain with NaFl as a "patch" rather than distinct punctata. This is often seen at the inferior 4 and 8 o'clock positions and may well be a precursor (and diagnostic indicator) or impending staphylococcal, toxic, infiltrative, marginal keratitis.

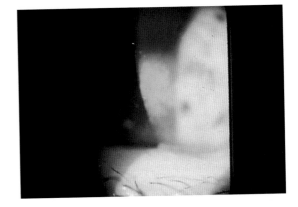

56. MARGINAL KERATITIS

This 48-year-old woman complained of frequent superficial irritation on waking culminating in this acute painful red eye. A marginal infiltrate at about the 4 o'clock position on her inferior corneal border (a midperipheral "island") with a thickened inferior lid margin (tylosis) supported a staphylococcal origin.

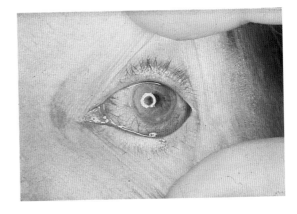

57. MARGINAL INFILTRATE WITH DIFFUSE NAFL STAINING

Because of the intensity of this toxic reaction, this marginal infiltrate was surrounded by dense, circumscribed epithelial and anterior stromal edema and scattered SPK. Such surrounding edema can suggest a bacterial (versus sterile) corneal ulceration, unless carefully examined for the interval of Vogt and other sterile infiltrative keratitic signs.

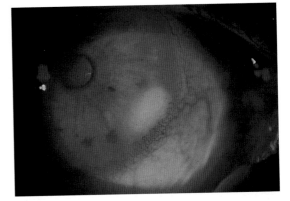

58. GONOCOCCAL CORNEAL ULCER

This 29-year-old man presented 48 hours after noncompliant treatment (prescribed by another practitioner) for a hyperacute red eye. An inferior, mid-peripheral ulceration of approximately 4 mm was observed in the 360-degree crimson red left eye. Rapid advancement, deep surrounding infiltration, 3+ anterior chamber reaction, and copious mucopurulence suggested a gram-negative organism, as confirmed by laboratory workup as *Neisseria gonorrhoea*. In spite of the most aggressive treatment, the ulcer perforated the inferior cornea.

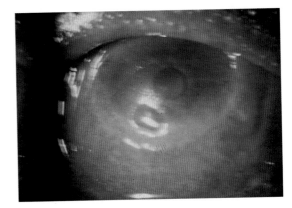

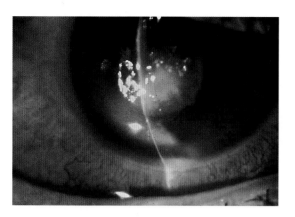

59. CORNEAL ULCER WITH EXUDATE

This 32-year-old mother was unable to receive care after a fingernail abrasion for 72 hours because of a snowstorm (in Rochester, NY). Upon examination, an exudative mucous plug over a deep central corneal lesion indicated bacterial ulceration of the defect. Cultures revealed gram-negative *Serratia Marcesans*. Post-treatment BVA was 20/200.

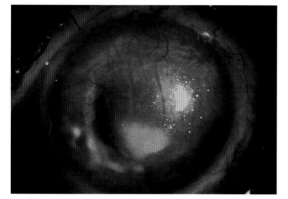

60. PSEUDOMONAL CORNEAL ULCER

Three days after an untreated corneal abrasion, this 24-year-old woman reported increasing pain and reduced vision in her right eye. A hazy, circumscribed, opaque lesion in the inferior pupillary zone with dense superior stromal infiltration and corneal striae proved to be a secondary pseudomonal ulceration upon scraping and cultures.

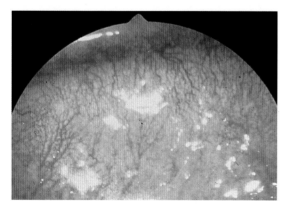

61. MILD PSEUDOMEMBRANE

The development of a transparent "slimy" film over the palpebral conjunctiva in an ocular infection (viral or bacterial) indicates infiltrative debris combined with fibrin material, forming a pseudomembrane.

62. MODERATE PSEUDOMEMBRANE

A fibrinous accumulation on the inferior palpebral conjunctiva was noted during examination of a hyperacute bacterial conjunctivitis. The accumulation was loosely attached and was successfully removed by manipulation with a wetted cotton-tipped applicator. No bleeding or subjective irritation was noted.

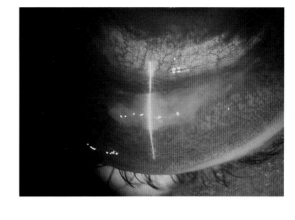

63. SEVERE PSEUDOMEMBRANE

This dense pseudomembrane covered the superior and inferior palpebral conjunctiva in an extremely virulent EKC presentation. Peeled off (very uncomfortable, even with topical anesthesia) with jeweler's forceps, the material came off in multiple small to large sheets.

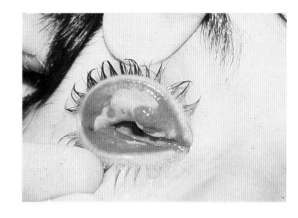

64. SUBEPITHELIAL INFILTRATES IN EKC

These SEIs were observed on the fifteenth day of a classic EKC (rule of 8s) clinical presentation. Being subepithelial, they stained negatively (NaFl breakup over area), but they were not anterior stromal, hence blanched completely (without steroids) in 6 weeks. Vision reduced to 20/30 for 2 weeks.

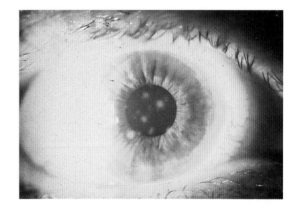

65. DENDRITES IN RECURRENT HSV KERATITIS

Two classic dendritic ulcers in a known (three times) recurrent HSV epithelial keratitis patient. Note the distinct branches with terminal end buds and staining vividly with NaFl (and rose bengal). (They all should be so easy!)

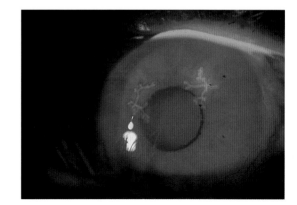

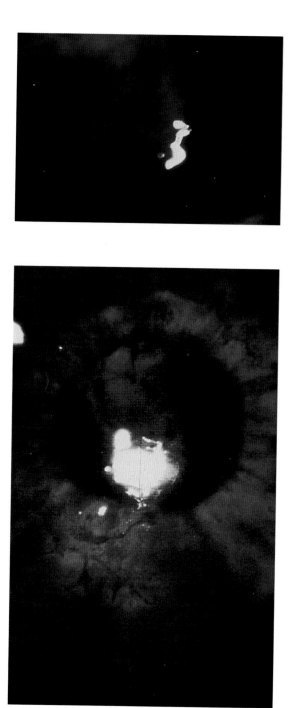

66. NAFL ULCERATION TEST

Three minutes after staining of this dendritic lesion, it shows NaFl spreading underneath surrounding epithelium in a geographic or amorphous pattern. Only HSV dendrites are ulcerative and produce this subepithelial undermining effect. All other dendriform keratites are infiltrative and will shed NaFl (to a threadlike pattern) in 2 to 3 minutes.

67. METAHERPETIC ULCER

After 14 days of antiviral treatment (with Viroptic), these dendrites had not resolved and showed persistent rose bengal staining. Raised, "rolled" edge development, plus increasing anterior stromal infiltration suggested early metaherpetic (indolent) ulcer formation. Referral to ophthalmology and subsequent course of clinical signs confirmed the diagnosis.

68. OCULAR ROSACEA KERATITIS

Often uncontrollable (with oral tetracycline), acne rosacea will produce increasing circumcorneal changes, ranging from limbal engorgement to peripheral SPK, anterior stromal involvement to peripheral pannus and neovascular changes (as pictured). Topical therapies including steroids are indicated in the presence of rosacea-related keratitis.

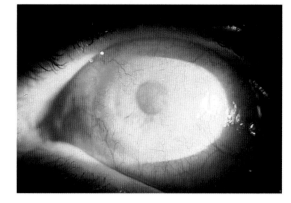

69. SUPERIOR LIMBIC KERATOCONJUNCTIVITIS (SLK)

This patient demonstrates superior limbic keratoconjunctivitis with the pathonumonic sign of corridor hyperemia of the superior bulbar conjunctiva along the insertion of the superior rectus muscle.

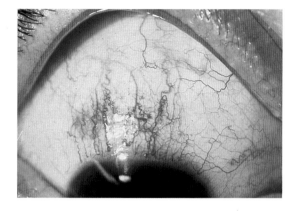

70. KERATITIS SICCA WITH ROSE BENGAL STAINING

This 56-year-old woman in good health reported late-day chronic irritation, burning, and "dryness" of her eyes bilaterally. Slit-lamp evaluation of the cornea demonstrated band-region SPK, which produced positive rose bengal staining. Note also the positive rose staining of the exposed (triangular) bulbar conjunctival areas.

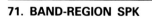

71. BAND-REGION SPK

This 53-year-old woman reported nonspecific irritation in the late day and evening. Band-region staining with fluorescein and rose bengal confirmed a definitive diagnosis of dry eye syndrome that responded within 2 weeks to heavy lubrication therapy.

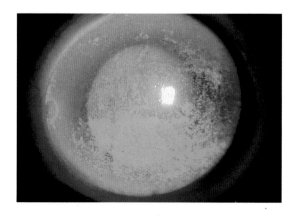

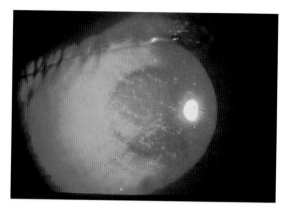

72. FOREIGN-BODY TRACKING

A 16-year-old girl presented with a history of a windblown particle entering her left eye while driving. Although the patient was certain it was still "in her eye," examination demonstrated diffuse FBT in the absence (on cornea, conjunctiva or lid, through double eversion) of any foreign matter. Condition resolved with irrigation and lubrication in 24 hours.

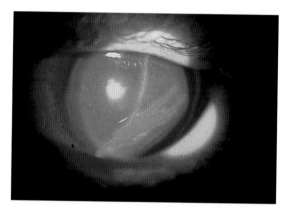

73. CORNEAL ABRASION (SUPERFICIAL)

This 9-year-old boy was brought in as an emergency patient after a tree branch "sprang" across his right eye. Geography: 15 percent cornea, 0 percent pupil, inferotemporal; depth: 6 × 2 mm squamous, 3 × 1 mm basal, no basement membrane involvement; edge: 1 × 0.5 mm inferior flap; edema: 1/2 circumferential mild.

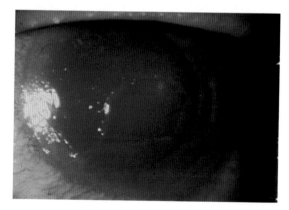

74. CORNEAL ABRASION (DEEP TO BASEMENT MEMBRANE)

This mechanic presented under workers compensation with a history of a machine part hitting his left eye. Geography: 20 percent cornea, 25 percent pupil, central (inferior); depth: 7 × 5 mm squamous, 6 × 5 mm basal, 6 × 5 mm basement membrane; edge: 1-mm loose flap 360; edema: 1-mm infiltrative ring.

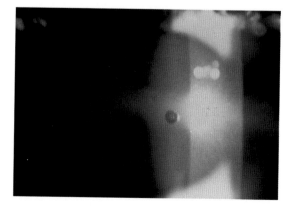

75. SUPERFICIAL CORNEAL FOREIGN BODY

This nonmetallic (probably sand) foreign body was noted on the epithelial surface of a 13-year-old boy presenting with a history of left eye irritation following a day at the beach. A crisp, noninfiltrative superficial foreign-body appearance was shown best by retroillumination. Removal was simple with one flick of a needle; treatment was that for superficial corneal abrasion.

76. CORNEAL FOREIGN BODY WITH COATE'S WHITE RING

A cinder flew into this patient's eye during heavy winds. Irritation was minimal but persistent over a 3-day period. Upon examination, an infiltrative, edematous ring (Coate's white ring) was noted with direct and indirect illumination around the embedded particle. Removal was quick and easy with jeweler's forceps; treatment was that for a deep corneal abrasion with complete healing in 2 to 3 days and resolution of the "ring" in 1 week.

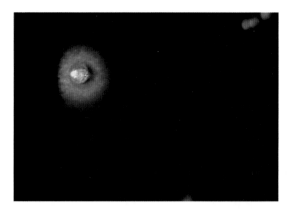

77. STROMAL PENETRATION

This 11-year-old boy presented as an emergency patient with a pine needle "stuck in his cornea." Removal by an emergency physician resulted in a collapsed chamber and "wrinkled cornea" that filled and reshaped completely in 6 hours. The injury caused a thin opaque channel through the stroma (note associated thickening) and endothelial disruption. Topical and oral medications quieted the eye, with resultant scar.

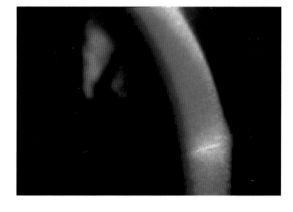

78. HEMOSIDEROSIS (RUST RING)

After getting a piece of rust in his eye while working under his car 3 days earlier, this 25-year-old man called emergently (at 3:00 AM) with increasing pain and discomfort. Upon removal (at 8:00 AM) this rust ring was also noted and required removal as well. Because of the delay in care (3 days), hemosiderosis caused permanent staining to Bowman's layer directly beneath the area of epithelial involvement.

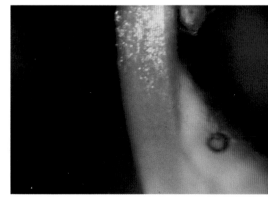

79. RECURRENT CORNEAL EROSION SYNDROME

Following treatment, resolution, and dismissal for a deep corneal abrasion, this 28-year-old woman called one morning (2 weeks later) with severe discomfort in the same (right) eye. Upon examination, a recurrent erosion of epithelium had produced a corneal abrasion with surrounding edema somewhat larger than the original traumatic abrasion. Treatment was that for deep corneal abrasion with "forceful" instructions to comply with hypertonic ointments at bedtime for at least 6 weeks after resolution.

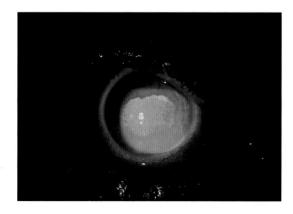

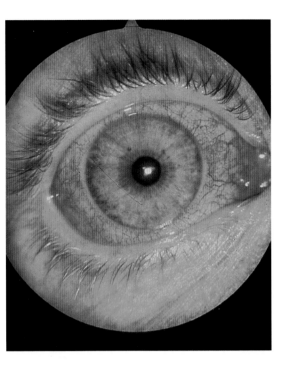

80. ACUTE ANTERIOR UVEITIS

This 48-year-old white woman reported throbbing pain inside her right eye during her workday (near tasks). Although the pain diminished in the evening, the photophobia and redness persisted. First presentation responded quickly to standard therapy.

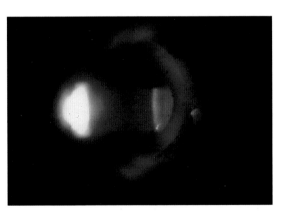

81. CELLS AND FLARE

One of the most difficult clinical signs to spot easily. When other uveitic signs are present (history, subjective, objective), focus on the aqueous for as long as it takes to view the discrete cells or the turbidity of an aqueous flare.

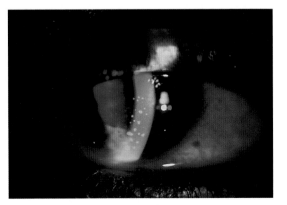

82. MUTTON FAT KP

These inferior, large, waxy KPs are typically noted in chronic, recurring uveitis. Vigorous steroid therapy will usually reduce increasing density but will not necessarily dissolve existing lesions. Counting the KPs becomes a useful management tool for control (i.e., increasing number means activity).

83. KRUCKENBURG'S SPINDLE

When pigmented KPs are present in a uveitic response, they often form a vertical line (or "spindle") at the inferior posterior corneal surface as a result of the convection currents in the aqueous. The differential diagnosis should be pigment dispersion syndrome.

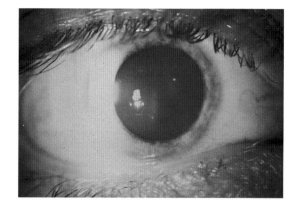

84. POSTERIOR SYNECHIAE

Multiple posterior synechiae on and behind the pupil border producing a corectopic pupil. Attempt to break as many of these fibrous adhesions as possible (with dilation) to reduce long-term risks.

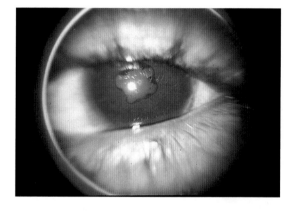

85. SECLUSIO PUPILLAE

An advanced and potentially dangerous level of posterior synechiae formation is this 360-degree involvement. Its presence frequently produces buildup of aqueous pressure behind the iris, resulting in iris bombi and secondary glaucoma. Such complications require surgical intervention.

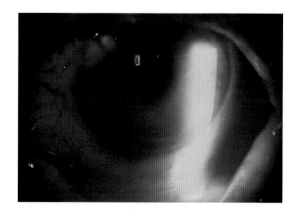

86. HYPHEMA

After contusion injury, this patient presented with a 2-mm hyphema consisting of whole red blood in the inferior anterior chamber. Although the recovery and reabsorption were uneventful (without rebleed) 1 week reduced activity and 30-degree head elevation during sleep, the long-range prognosis for secondary glaucoma is guarded because of greater than 180 degrees of angle recession.

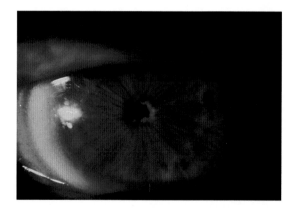

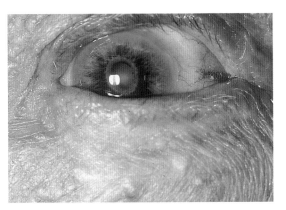

87. IRIS ATROPHY

This 64-year-old man experienced a contusive injury to his left eye 2 years prior to this examination. Although recovery from the injury proved uneventful (as reported), and the cornea, IOP, and angle appeared normal, a unilateral (ipsilateral) iris atrophy was presumed secondary to trauma.

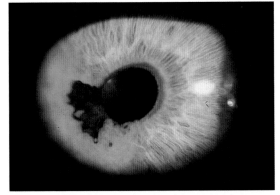

88. IRIS TUMOR(?)

This iris (pupil border)-pigmented mass was noted during general examination. Almost never metastatic and infrequently malignant, photo-documentation is used in following any suspicious iris nevus. The irregular pupil shape (corectopia) in this presentation made it more suggestive of melanoma. Close observation (every 3 months) over 2 years has produced no changes.

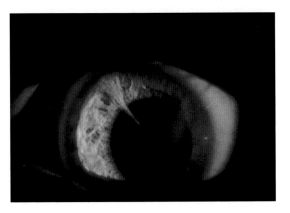

89. PERSISTENT PUPILLARY MEMBRANE

This embryologically produced persistent pupillary membrane can be differentiated from posterior synechiae by its origin from the collarette versus the pupil border, its elastic versus fibrous nature, and its presence in a healthy, non-uveitic eye.

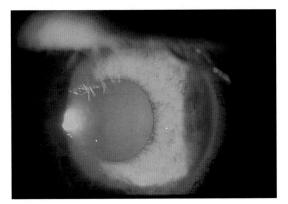

90. RUBEOSIS IRIDES

Neovascularization of the iris is a secondary complication occurring in many systemic conditions (e.g., diabetes, vascular occlusive disease) as well as specific ocular conditions. This neovascular network was produced by an advanced, intractable glaucoma.

91. ECTOPIA LENTIS (MARFAN'S SYNDROME)

This 27-year-old white man was found to have high myopia and a superior temporal displaced crystalline lens in his left eye during general eye examination. His tall stature, long fingers (arachnodactyly), and extremely long arms (wider than his height) made his (prediagnosed) condition of Marfan's syndrome rather obvious.

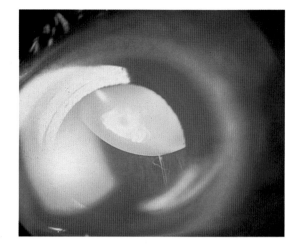

92. ACNE ROSACEA

This 50-year-old woman presented with recurrent unilateral and bilateral blepharokeratoconjunctivitis, dilated capillaries on skin, raised red papillae, and a congested nose tip (rhinophyma). Careful history indicated high alcohol intake and excess carbohydrate diet occasionally reported in acne rosacea patients.

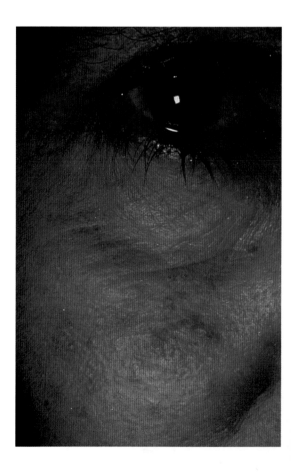

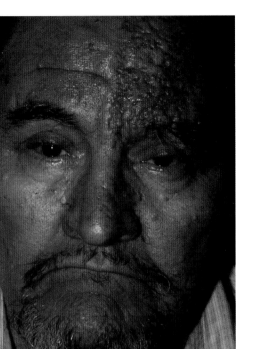

93. HERPES ZOSTER OPHTHALMICUS

This unfortunate patient is a 68-year-old white man who has had herpes zoster ophthalmicus since 1981 with severe post-herpetic neuralgia and "every possible" corneal complication (e.g., SPK, filaments, dendrites, infiltrates). With each complication; he generally produces an associated keratouveitis.

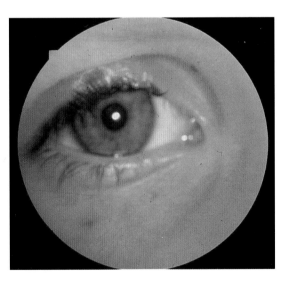

94. PSORIATIC LID LESION

This 19-year-old man had diagnosed psoriasis for 6 years. During eye examination, silvery scales were noted over a psoriatic lid plaque. Removal of the scales would cause multiple punctate bleeding points, called Auspitz sign.

95. BAND KERATOPATHY (HYPERPARATHYROIDISM)

Hypercalcemia produced in hyperparathyroidism frequently deposits calcium crystals in the intrapalpebral corneal zone at the level of Bowman's layer. Such a band keratopathy noted in a primary eye examination should raise suspicion and careful management.

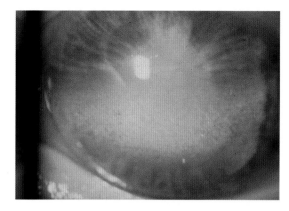

96. PORT-WINE STAIN (STURGE–WEBER SYNDROME)

Some systemic disorders produce distinct pigmented dermatitic lesions. This classic port-wine stain (hemangioma) in Sturge–Weber syndrome involves the superior lid, which produces a long-term high risk of glaucoma in this patient.

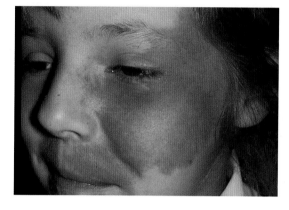

97. FOLDS IN DESCEMET'S MEMBRANE (STRIATE KERATITIS)

This 64-year-old black man with a history of diabetic retinopathy, 1 week post-lensectomy or vitrectomy, demonstrated 2–3+ folds in Descemet's membrane. Warm packs and self-resolution occurred over a 3-week period.

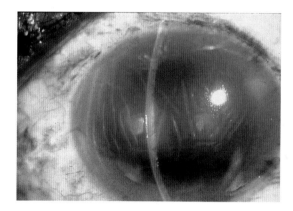

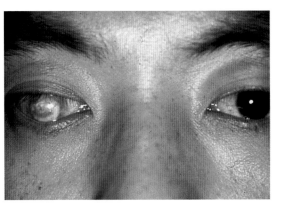

98. LEUKOMATOUS CORNEAL SCARRING

This 27-year-old patient had severe trauma resulting in a total retinal detachment and complete corneal decomposition with marked dense lipid infiltration. He was fit with a cosmetic (artificial) gel lens.

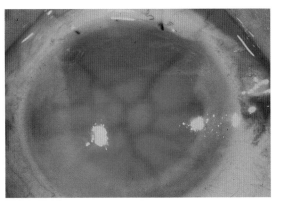

99. DENSE PHYSIOLOGICAL EDEMA

This 61-year-old white man with a history of diabetes and aphakia switched from spectacles to extended-wear lenses. Then, 25 hours postfit with a 55 percent soft extended-wear lens, he demonstrated 3–4+ edema. The mosiac pattern noted is from folds in Descemet's membrane.

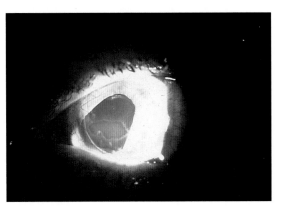

100. RECURRENT EROSION WITH BANDAGE SOFT CONTACT LENS

This severe epithelial abrasion on a grafted eye resulted in severe edema with epithelial breakdown. This patient is wearing a bandage contact lens to promote healing of the large epithelial defect. Bandage lenses are being used increasingly for RCE, EBMD, and even milder traumatic corneal abrasions.

II. Self-assessment Questions

For each color plate listed below, select the *most likely* subjective symptom:

1. For color plate 2:
   a. Itching
   b. AM syndrome
   c. Corneal irritation
   d. Burning irritation
2. For color plate 10:
   a. Itching
   b. AM syndrome
   c. Corneal irritation
   d. Patient concern
3. For color plate 28:
   a. Itching
   b. AM syndrome
   c. Corneal irritation
   d. Burning irritation
4. For color plate 36:
   a. Itching
   b. AM syndrome
   c. Patient concern
   d. Burning irritation
5. For color plate 43:
   a. Itching
   b. AM syndrome
   c. Late-day corneal irritation
   d. Burning irritation
6. For color plate 52:
   a. Itching
   b. AM syndrome
   c. Late-day corneal irritation
   d. Burning irritation
7. For color plate 56:
   a. Itching
   b. AM syndrome
   c. Late-day corneal irritation
   d. Burning irritation
8. For color plate 70:
   a. Itching
   b. AM syndrome
   c. Late-day corneal irritation
   d. Burning irritation
9. For color plate 80:
   a. Itching
   b. Burning irritation
   c. Corneal irritation
   d. Dull aching pain
10. For color plate 86:
    a. History of contusive injury
    b. History of lacerating injury
    c. Itching
    d. Burning irritation

For each color plate listed below, select the *least likely* associated objective sign:

11. For color plate 1:
    a. Edema
    b. Viral reaction
    c. Blowout fracture
    d. Crepitus
12. For color plate 8:
    a. Chemosis
    b. Dendrite
    c. Proptosis
    d. Systemic illness
13. For color plate 30:
    a. Subconjunctival hemorrhage
    b. Mucoid discharge
    c. Pseudoptosis
    d. Superior SPK
14. For color plate 40:
    a. Posterior embryotoxon
    b. Pupil abnormalities
    c. Kaiser–Fleischer ring
    d. Secondary glaucoma
15. For color plate 57:
    a. Straite keratitis
    b. Localized hyperemia
    c. Staphylococcal lid signs
    d. Peripheral "island" lesion(s)
16. For color plate 58:
    a. Deep infiltration
    b. Cells and flare
    c. Hypopyon
    d. Neovascurization
17. For color plate 68:
    a. Blepharoconjunctivitis
    b. Facial flush
    c. Peripheral SPK
    d. Orbital cellulitis
18. For color plate 69:
    a. Corridor hyperemia
    b. Hyperthyroidism
    c. Giant papillae
    d. Pseudodendrites
19. For color plate 82:
    a. Mutton fat KP
    b. Posterior synechiae
    c. Systemic disease
    d. Nongranulomatous disease
20. For color plate 91:
    a. Arachnodactylae
    b. Dwarfism
    c. Tall stature
    d. Congenital heart defects

For each color plate listed below, select the *least likely* differential diagnostic consideration:

21. For color plate 7:
    a. Marginal keratitis
    b. Blepharoconjunctivitis
    c. Allergic blepharitis
    d. Orbital cellulitis
22. For color plate 18:
    a. Sudoriferous cyst
    b. Basal cell carcinoma
    c. Sebaceous cyst
    d. Verruca
23. For color plate 26:
    a. Episcleritis
    b. Preseptal cellulitis
    c. Blepharoconjunctivitis
    d. Allergic reaction
24. For color plate 31:
    a. Corneal ulcer
    b. Chronic staph toxins
    c. Ultraviolet irritation
    d. Morax Axenfeld infection
25. For color plate 45:
    a. Keratitis sicca syndrome
    b. Superior limbic keratoconjunctivitis
    c. Anterior uveitis
    d. Vernal keratoconjunctivitis
26. For color plate 54:
    a. Viral keratitis
    b. Giant papillary conjunctivitis
    c. Staphylococcal toxic keratitis
    d. SPK of Thygeson
27. For color plate 61:
    a. Exposure keratitis
    b. Keratitis sicca syndrome
    c. Lagophthalmos
    d. Vernal keratoconjunctivitis
28. For color plate 67:
    a. Corneal penetration
    b. Corneal perforation
    c. Epithelial basement membrane disorder
    d. Intraocular foreign body
29. For color plate 81:
    a. Blepharoconjunctivitis
    b. Acute anterior uveitis
    c. Chronic uveitis
    d. Disseminated uveitis
30. For color plate 90:
    a. Diabetes
    b. Retinal vascular occlusive disease
    c. Neovascular glaucoma
    d. Acute anterior uveitis

For each color plate listed below, select the *most appropriate* treatment plan of first choice:

31. For color plate 5:
    a. Oral steroids
    b. Oral antibiotics
    c. Topical antistaphylococcal therapy
    d. No treatment indicated
32. For color plate 17:
    a. Incision and drainage
    b. Topical antibiotics
    c. Oral antibiotics
    d. Topical and oral steroids
33. For color plate 29:
    a. Oral steroids
    b. Fluorinated steroids
    c. Antibiotics
    d. Cold packs
34. For color plate 32:
    a. Oral steroids
    b. Antibiotics
    c. Topical steroids
    d. Cold packs
35. For color plate 44:
    a. Bandage soft contact lens
    b. Steroids
    c. Surgical repair
    d. Lubricants
36. For color plate 51:
    a. Lubricants
    b. Steroids
    c. Opticrom
    d. Hypertonic saline
37. For color plate 59:
    a. Garamycin
    b. Fortified aminoglycosides
    c. Bacitracin
    d. Sulfacetamide
38. For color plate 65:
    a. Stoxil
    b. Viroptic
    c. Vira A
    d. Oral acyclovir
39. For color plate 79:
    a. Pressure patching
    b. Topical vitamin A
    c. Oral vitamin A
    d. Steroids
40. For color plate 92:
    a. Oral acyclovir
    b. Oral gentamicin
    c. Oral tetracycline
    d. Oral cephalosporin

For answers, refer to Appendix 6

APPENDIX 1

Diagnostic Index of Subjective Symptoms

Subjective Symptoms Categories

A. Corneal irritation
B. Cosmetic concern (without pain)
C. Dull, aching ocular pain
D. Itching or burning irritation
E. Headache-type pain

F. Pain on palpation (or pressure) to eyelid or globe
G. Vision reduction (diminished visual acuity)
H. Visual loss (sudden or transient dimming or blindness)

A. CORNEAL IRRITATION*

Eyelids and Adnexa	ICD Number	Page Number
1. Chalazion (internal type)	373.2	32
2. Coloboma (large notch)	743.4	17
3. Ectropion	374.1	19
4. Entropion	374.00	19
5. Exophthalmos (exposure)	376.3	43
6. Foreign body on tarsus	374.86	19
7. Lagophthalmos (band region)	374.2	21
8. Marginal blepharitis (infectious types)	373.0	24
9. Molluscum contagiosum (at margin)	078.0	34
10. Subcutaneous cilia	374.54	22
11. Trichiasis	374.05	22
12. Verrucae (at margin)	078.1	37

Conjunctiva, sclera and episclera

	ICD Number	Page Number
1. Calcium concretions (severe on palpebral conjunctiva)	372.54	71
2. Conjunctivitis		
a. Bacterial (usually hyperacute forms)	372.03	49
b. Viral	077.9	55
c. Toxic or irritative (chronic)	372.10	64
d. Vernal	372.13	63
3. Episcleritis (severe)	379.00	66
4. Giant papillary conjunctivitis	372.14	62
5. Pinguecula (to pterygium)	372.51	73
6. Scleritis or sclerouveitis (advanced forms)	379.03	67

Cornea

	ICD Number	Page Number
1. Abrasion injuries	918.1	148
2. Band keratopathy	371.43	93
3. Bullous keratopathy	371.23	93
4. Burns		159
a. Chemical	940.4	159
b. Radiation	940.9	159
c. Thermal	940.0	159
5. Chlamydial keratoconjunctivitis	077.9	144
6. Cogan's microcystic degeneration	371.4	94

*Sandy, gritty, foreign-body sensation, or "something under my upper lid."

B. COSMETIC CONCERN (WITHOUT PAIN)

Eyelids and adnexa

	ICD Number	Page Number
Anterior chamber and iris ciliary body		
1. Acute anterior uveitis (severe)	364.0	185
2. Chronic anterior uveitis	364.1	200
3. Hyphema	364.41	206
4. Iris bombe	364.74	209
5. Pars planitis	363.21	204
6. Trauma	921.9	211

F. PAIN ON PALPATION (OR PRESSURE) TO EYELID OR GLOBE

Eyelids and adnexa

1. Blepharitis (acute forms)	373.8	24
2. Contusion (blunt) injuries	921.1	18
3. Dacryoadenitis	375.00	42
4. Dacryocystitis (acute and chronic)	375.30	38
5. Foreign bodies on tarsus	374.86	19
6. Hordeolum	373.1	33
7. Insect bites or stings	918.0	20
8. Meibomianitis (acute form)	373.12	26
9. Neoplasias (sometimes)	173.1	35
10. Orbital cellulitis	376.0	44
11. Preseptal cellulitis	373.9	25, 44

Conjunctiva, sclera and episclera

1. Episcleritis	379.00	66
2. Foreign bodies	918.6	77
3. Hyperacute conjunctivitis	372.00	54
4. Neoplasias (sometimes)	190.3	69, 73, 76
5. Parinaud's oculoglandular fever	372.02	59
6. Scleritis	379.03	66

Cornea

1. Blunt (concussion or contusion) injury	921.3	158
2. Epidemic keratoconjunctivitis (EKC)	077.1	130
3. Filamentary keratitis	370.23	111
4. Foreign bodies (embedded)	930.0	165
5. Herpes zoster ophthalmicus	053.2	139
6. Superior limbic keratoconjunctivitis (SLK)	370.32	145
7. Vernal keratoconjunctivitis	372.13	147

Anterior chamber and iris and ciliary body

1. Acute anterior uveitis	364.0	185
2. Chronic anterior uveitis (sometimes)	364.1	200
3. Hyphema	364.41	206
4. Neoplasias (sometimes)	190.0	210
5. Trauma (especially blunt)	921.9	211

G. VISION REDUCTION (DIMINISHED VISUAL ACUITY)

Eyelids and adnexa

1. Chalazion (irregular astigmatism)	373.30	32
2. Entropion	374.00	19
3. Lagophthalmos	374.2	21
4. Orbital tumors (diplopia)	190.1	45
5. Subcutaneous cilia	374.54	22
6. Trichiasis	374.05	22

APPENDIX 2

Diagnostic Index of Objective Signs

Eyelids and Adnexa	ICD Number	Page Number
1. Crepitus (emphysema or air in tissue), "crackling" sound on palpation		
a. Contusion (blunt) injuries	921.1	18
b. Ecchymosis	921.0	18
2. Drooping of upper lid (blepharoptosis)		
a. Chalasis (dermato- and/or blepharo-)	374.34	18
b. Congenital	743.61	15
c. Neurogenic (acquired)	364.31	16
d. Enophthalmos	376.50	84
e. Pseudoptosis (from multiple unrelated causes)	374.34	15
f. Syndrome related (congenital or acquired)	374.30	16
3. Edema or erythema		
a. Allergic or hypersensitivity (any type)	373.32	29
b. Cellulitis (preseptal or orbital)	376.0	44
c. Drug induced	692.3	29
d. Infection or inflammation (any cause)	373.0	25
e. Injury (any form)	921.0	18
f. Insect bites or stings	918.0	20
4. Loss of lashes (madarosis)		
a. Alopecia	704.0	21
b. *Staphylococcus* (chronic blepharitis or toxins)	373.4	24
c. Trichotillomania	300.3	23
5. Lumps and bumps		
a. Basal cell carcinoma	232.1	31
b. Chalazia	373.2	32
c. Dermoid	216.3	32
d. Hemangioma	228.01	32
e. Hordeolum	373.1	33
f. Keratoses	374.56	34
g. Molluscum contagiosum	078.0	34
h. Neoplasias (beyond basal cell)	173.1	35
i. Nevus (often flat)	216.3	35
j. Papilloma	216.1	36
k. Sebaceous cysts (superficial or deep)	374.84	36
l. Sudoriferous cysts	374.84	37
m. Verrucae	078.1	37
n. Xanthalasma	374.51	38
6. Marginal crusting or thickening		
a. Blepharoconjunctivitis (bacterial forms)	372.2	24
b. Chalazia (multiple)	373.2	32
c. Chronic staphylococcal blepharitis	373.0	24
d. Dacryocystitis	375.30	38
e. Demodicosis	373.0	30
f. Hordeolum (usually multiple forms)	373.1	33
g. Pediculosis	132.0	30
7. Misdirected lashes		
a. Entropion	374.0	19

Cornea (*cont.*)

Other objective signs (*cont.*)	ICD Number	Page Number
d. Cataract (usually mature or hypermature)	366.18	246
e. Congenital or familial	365.40	85
f. Dislocated lens	379.32	246
g. Drug induced (topical or systemic)	693.0	7
h. Essential iris atrophy	365.42	209
i. Glaucoma (all forms except "low tension" glaucoma)	365.0	7
j. Hyphema	364.41	206
k. Inflammation	365.62	192
l. Megalocornea	743.41	84
m. Microcornea	743.41	84
n. Neovascularization of angle	364.42	211
o. Plateau iris	364.75	210
p. Postsurgical (ocular)	365.65	367
q. Sclerocornea	365.40	85
r. Shallow chamber (narrow angle)	365.02	87
s. Steroid induced (topical or systemic)	365.03	8
t. Synechiae (anterior or posterior)	364.70	191
u. Systemic disease	365.9	200
v. Trauma (usually unilateral)	365.65	206
w. Tumors (intraocular or retrobulbar)	365.64	194
x. Uveitis	365.62	192
5. Lymphadenopathy or enlargement (preauricular)		
a. Adenovirus	077.9	57
b. Chlamydial (inclusion) infection	077.9	144
c. Dacryoadenitis	375.01	42
d. Epidemic keratoconjunctivitis (EKC)	077.1	131
e. Herpes simplex infection (primary and recurrent forms)	054.4	134, 135
f. Herpes zoster	053.2	141
g. Hyperacute conjunctivitis (bacterial or viral)	372.00	54, 57
h. Infectious keratitis (any advanced form)	370.0	118
i. Newcastle's disease	077.8	59
j. Orbital cellulitis	376.01	44
k. Parinaud's oculoglandular ("cat scratch") fever	372.02	59
l. Pharyngoconjunctival fever (PCF)	077.2	129
m. Preseptal cellulitis	373.9	25, 44
n. Trachoma	076.9	59
6. Mucoid discharge (nonpurulent)		
a. Allergic blepharitis and conjunctivitis	372.2	29, 60
b. Burns (to any lid or ocular tissue)	940.9	17, 159
c. Conjunctival laceration	918.2	78
d. Dacryostenosis	375.5	40
e. Drug induced	693.0	29, 60, 110
f. Dry eye–keratitis sicca-type syndromes	370.33	162
g. Filamentary keratitis	370.23	111
h. Giant papillary conjunctivitis (GPC)	372.14	62
i. Insect bites or stings	918.0	20
j. Pseudomembranous conjunctivitis (any cause)	372.04	131
k. Superior limbic keratoconjunctivitis (SLK)	370.32	146
l. Toxic causes (chemical, environmental, irritants)	692.9	29, 60, 110
m. Vernal keratoconjunctivitis	372.13	147
7. Purulent (or mucopurulent) discharge		
a. Bacterial blepharitis (usually *Streptococcus* or gram-negative)	372.20	25
b. Chlamydial infection	077.9	144
c. Dacryocystitis (acute or subacute)	375.30	39
d. Fungal infection (any tissue)	116.0	127
e. Hyperacute bacterial conjunctivitis (any type)	372.03	54
f. Infectious keratitis (bacterial or fungal)	370.0	125, 127
8. Rose bengal staining		
a. Chronic or toxic conjunctivitis	372.10	64

Index of Differential Diagnoses (Things to Rule Out)

Eyelids and adnexa (*cont.*)

	ICD Number	Page Number
b. Hyperlipidemia (especially hypercholesterolemia)	272.4	38
c. Neoplasia	173.1	35
d. Papilloma (amelanotic)	216.1	36
e. Sebaceous cyst(s) (superficial)	374.84	38
f. Systemic syndromes	374.9	244

Conjunctiva and sclera and episclera

	ICD Number	Page Number
1. Allergic conjunctivitis		
a. Adenovirus	077.3	57
b. Bacterial (all forms)	372.03	61
c. Blepharoconjunctivitis	372.20	54
d. Chlamydial	077.0	144
e. Dermatologically related	372.33	216
f. Drug induced	693.0	60
g. Dry eye syndrome	375.15	163
h. Epidemic keratoconjunctivitis	077.1	131
i. Episcleritis	379.0	66
j. Follicular types	372.02	55
k. Foreign-body (or contact lens) reaction	918.2	77
l. Giant papillary conjunctivitis (GPC)	372.14	61
m. Glaucoma (acute-angle closure)	365.22	192
n. Herpes simplex	054.40	28
o. Herpes zoster	053.2	29
p. Keratoconjunctivitis (all types)	370.3	128
q. Pharyngoconjunctival fever	077.2	129
r. Phlyctenular reaction	370.31	115
s. Pinguecula (inflamed)	372.51	73
t. Scleritis	379.03	66
u. Subconjunctival hemorrhage	372.72	70
v. Systemic related	372.9	244
w. Toxic or hypersensitivity	372.0	60
x. Uveitis (circumcorneal flush)	364.0	187
y. Venereal causes	091.0	224
z. Vernal keratoconjunctivitis	372.13	60, 147
2. Bacterial conjunctivitis		
a. Adenovirus	077.3	57
b. Allergic	372.03	60
c. Blepharoconjunctivitis	372.20	54
d. Chlamydial	077.0	144
e. Dermatologically related	372.33	216
f. Drug induced	693.0	60
g. Dry eye syndrome	375.15	163
h. Epidemic keratoconjunctivitis	077.1	131
i. Episcleritis	379.0	66
j. Follicular types	372.02	55
k. Foreign-body (or contact lens) reaction	918.2	77
l. Giant papillary conjunctivitis (GPC)	372.14	61
m. Glaucoma (acute-angle closure)	365.22	192
n. Herpes simplex	054.40	28
o. Herpes zoster	053.20	29
p. Keratoconjunctivitis (all types)	370.3	128
q. Pharyngoconjunctival fever	077.2	129
r. Phlyctenular reaction	370.31	115
s. Pinguecula (inflamed)	372.51	73
t. Scleritis	379.03	66
u. Subconjunctival hemorrhage	372.72	70
v. Systemic related	372.9	244
w. Toxic or hypersensitivity	372.0	60
x. Uveitis (circumcornel flush)	364.0	187

	ICD Number	Page Number
Cornea (*cont.*)		
7. Epithelial basement membrane disorder		
a. Acquired (trauma or irritation)	918.1	104
b. Cogan's degeneration	371.52	94
c. Degeneration (aging)	371.40	93
d. Diabetes	250.5	219
e. Dry eye–keratitis sicca-type syndrome	370.33	105, 164
f. Dystrophic	371.5	105
g. Fuchs' endothelial dystrophy	371.57	104
h. Meesman's dystrophy	371.51	88
i. Recurrent corneal erosion (RCE) syndrome	371.42	173
j. Superficial keratitis (any type)	370.2	107
8. Infectious keratitis		
a. *Acanthamoeba*	370.02	123
b. Bacterial (gram-positive or -negative)	370.03	124
c. Fungal	370.05	127
d. Herpes simplex	054.42	133
e. Herpes zoster	053.21	139
f. Sarcoidosis	135.0	205
g. Scleritis	379.03	67
h. Syphilis	090.3	205, 238
i. Tuberculosis	017.3	205, 238
9. Interstitial keratitis		
a. Burns (usually chemical)	940.4	159
b. Congenital (usually syphilis)	090.3	224
c. Herpes simplex (second most common cause)	054.43	133
d. Herpes zoster	053.29	139
e. Sarcoidosis	135.0	205
f. Syphilis (most common cause)	090.3	205, 238
g. Toxic (especially chemical poisons)	370.59	107
h. Tuberculosis	017.3	205, 238
10. Marginal furrow degeneration		
a. *Acanthamoeba* (ring ulcer)	370.02	123
b. Arcus senilis	371.41	93
c. Dellen	371.71	95
d. Drug induced (especially steroids)	693.0	112
e. Fungal ulcer	370.05	127
f. Marginal keratitis	370.01	112
g. Morren's ulcer	370.07	97
h. Pellucid marginal degeneration	371.48	97
i. Ring ulcers	370.02	123
j. Systemic disorders (especially rheumatoid)	371.9	97
k. Terrien's marginal degeneration	371.48	97
l. White limbal girdle of Vogt	371.15	98
11. Mooren's ulcer		
a. *Acanthamoeba* (ring ulcer)	370.02	123
b. Arcus senilis	371.41	93
c. Dellen	371.71	95
d. Drug induced (especially steroids)	693.0	112
e. Fungal ulcer	370.05	127
f. Marginal furrow degeneration	371.48	97
g. Marginal keratitis	370.01	112
h. Pellucid marginal degeneration	371.48	97
i. Ring ulcers	370.02	123
j. Systemic disorders (especially rheumatoid)	371.9	230
k. Terrien's marginal degeneration	371.48	97
l. White limbal girdle of Vogt	371.15	98
12. Ocular rosacea		
a. Atopic or allergic	370.32	110
b. Blepharoconjunctivitis (especially staphylococcal)	372.20	142

Common Clinical Diagnoses by Degree of Presentation

	Mild	Moderate	Severe
LIDS/ADNEXA			
Blepharitis, Allergic			
Etiology	Type 1/4/atopic	Type 1/4/atopic	Type 1/4
Subjective	Itching	Itching	Itching/irritation
Objective	Edema	Edema/erythema	Edema/erythema Excoriation
Assessment	R/O infectious	R/O infectious	R/O preseptal
Plan	Remove allergen	Remove allergen	Remove allergen
	Cold compresses	Cold compresses	Cold compresses
Drug	Antihist./Decong.	Antihistamine-decongestant	Antihistamine-decongestant
		Steroid (optional)	Steroid
Route	Topical drops	Topical drops/cream	Topical drops/cream
	Oral	Oral	Oral (both)
Dosage	Drops tid	Drops qid	Drops/cream qid
	Orals as directed	Orals per degree	Orals as directed
RTC	PRN	48–72 hr	24–48 hr
Complications	No response	Slow response	Systemic response
Blepharitis, Marginal			
Etiology	Seborrhea/*Staphylococcus*	*Staphylococcus*	*Staphylococcus/Streptococcus*
Subjective	Chronic	Chronic	Acute presentation
	Cosmetic	Sticking shut	Irritation/pain
Objective	"Granulated"	Tylosis/	Ulceration/excoriation
		Rosettes/	Edema/(bilateral)
		Red Mad./	
		Poliosis/	
		Trich.	
Assessment	R/O parasites	R/O strep	R/O preseptal
Plan	Staphyloccal prevention	Staphyloccal prevention	Heat
Drug	Polysporin (optional)	Combination (optional)	Erythromycin/ + ?
Route	Topical ointment	Topical ointment	Topical/oral
Dosage	hs	bid–tid	q4h
RTC	2–4 wk	1–2 wk	48 hr
Complications	Chronicity	Acute reactions	Preseptal
Dacryocystitis, Adult			
Etiology	Blockage	Acute/chronic	Stenosis
Subjective	Sudden onset	Pain (variable)	Chronic
			Painless
Objective	Tearing	Inner canthal erythema	Tearing
		Tearing	
Assessment	R/O infection	R/O stenosis	R/O neoplasia
Plan	D&l/heat/massage	Heat/delay D&l	Advise/refer (?)
Drug	Prophylactic (sulfacetamide)	Sulfacetamide	Prophylactic (PRN)
		Erythromycin	(sulfacetamide)
Route	Topical drops	Topical/oral	Topical drops
Dosage	tid × 1 wk	Topical qid	bid/tid
		Oral 250 mg qid	
RTC	PRN	48 hr	PRN
Complications	Recurrent	Preseptal	Chronicity

continued

	Mild	Moderate	Severe
LIDS/ADNEXA (*cont.*)			
Dacryocystitis, Congenital			
Etiology	Valve of Hasner	*Streptococcus*	*Streptococcus*/fungi
Subjective	Congenital history	Congenital (or infantile)	Pain
			Nonresponsive
Objective	Tearing (unilateral)	Purulence (unilateral)	Unilateral or bilateral
Assessment	R/O infectious	R/O noncompliance	R/O systemic foci
Plan	Heat/massage	Heat/massage/irrigation	Advise/refer
Drug		Sulfacetamide	Sulfa/penicillin
Route		Topical drops	Topical/oral
Dosage		tid/qid	By weight
RTC	PRN/6 wk	3–6 wk	1 wk/PRN
Complications	Infection (systemic)	9–12 months old	Strictures
Ecchymosis			
Etiology	Mild contusion	Contusion	Crepitus
Subjective	Cosmesis	Concern	Severe blow
		Mild pain	Palpable pain
Objective	Red blood	Black/purple	Dense blood
	Inferior lid	Superior/inferior lid	Crackling sound
Assessment	R/O eyeball	R/O crepitus	R/O blowout fracture
Plan	24 hr cold	24 hr cold	24 hr cold
	3–5 days hot	5–7 days hot	7 days hot
Drug		Benadryl	Benadryl
			Antistaphylococcal agent
Route		Oral	Oral
Dosage		tid–qid	250 mg qid
RTC	5 days	3–5 days	24–48 hr
Complications	Slow resolution	Sneezing	Blowout fracture
		Organized hematoma	Sneezing
			Orbital cellulitis
Hordeolum			
Etiology	Zeiss/Moll staphylococcal	Meibomian staphylococcal	Encapsulated
Subjective	Annoyance	Pain on palpation	Pain
Objective	External stye	Lump or edema	Abscess
Assessment	R/O sebaceous cyst	R/O chalazion	R/O dacryocystitis (inferonasal)
Plan	Heat/staphylococcal prevention	Heat/staphylococcal	Heat/drain?
Drug	Polysporin	Polysporin/gentamicin	Gentamicin/ + oral antibiotic
Route	External lid ointment	External lid ointment	Topical/oral
Dosage	bid–tid	qid	q4h/1g/day
RTC	3–5 days or PRN	48 hr	24–48 hr
Complications	Chalazion	Internal chalazion	Preseptal cellulitis
		Preseptal cellulitis	
Lash Problems			
Etiology	Madarosis	Poliosis	Trichiasis
Subjective	Cosmesis	Cosmesis/concern	Corneal pain
Objective	Sparse lashes	White lashes	In-turning lashes
	Lashes "falling out"		Corneal FBT
Assessment	R/O alopecia	R/O vitiligo	R/O entropion
Plan	Staphylococcal prevention	Staphylococcal prevention	Epilation
Drug	Bacitracin	Bacitracin	Lubricant
Route	Ointment on margins	Ointment on margins	Topical eye-drops
Dosage	hs/bid	hs/bid	q4h × 24hr
RTC	6 wk	6 wk	PRN
Complications	Permanent	Permanent	Corneal infection
Sudoriferous Cyst			
Etiology	Zeiss/Moll gland	Zeiss/Moll gland	Zeiss/Moll gland
Subjective	General examination	Cosmesis/concern	Concern
Objective	Small bubble in margin	Bigger bubble	"Balloon"
Assessment	R/O milia	R/O hordeolum	R/O granuloma

continued

	Mild	**Moderate**	**Severe**
LIDS/ADNEXA (*(cont.)*			
Plan	Lance/drain	Lance/drain	Lance/drain
Drug	Polysporin	Polysporin	Gentamicin
Route	Topical ointment	Topical ointment	Topical ointment
Dosage	1 ×	1 ×	tid
RTC	PRN	PRN	48 hr
Complications	Recurrence	Recurrence	Secondary infection
CONJUNCTIVA/EPLISCLERA			
Conjunctivitis, Allergic			
Etiology	Type 1/4	Type 1/4/contact	Type 1/4/contact
Subjective	Itching	Itching	Itching/irritation
Objective	Patchy chemosis	Chemosis	"Watch-glass" chemosis
			Hemorrhages
Assessment	R/O infectious	R/O infectious	R/O infectious
Plan	Remove allergen	Remove allergen	Remove allergen
	Cold	Cold	Cold
Drug	Opticrom 4% (optional)	Opticrom 4%	Antihistamine/decongestant
	Antihistamine/decongestant	Antihistamine/ decongestant	Steroid
		Steroid (optional)	
Route	Topical/oral	Topical/oral	Topical/oral
Dosage	Topical, qid	Topical, qid	Topical, q3–4h
	Oral, as directed	Oral, as directed	Oral, as directed
RTC	PRN	2–3 days	24–48 hr
Complications	No response	Slow response	Systemic reactions
Bacterial Conjunctivitis			
Etiology	*Staphylococcus*	*Staphylococcus/ Streptococcus*	*Streptococcus*/gram negative
Subjective	Awareness	Spread	Concern/irritation
Objective	Inferior hyperemia papillae	Meaty red/pus	Hyperacute
Assessment	R/O viral	R/O epithelial defect	R/O ulcer
Plan	Staphylococcal prevention	Heat/staphylococcal prevention	Culture
Drug	Polysporin (optional)	Polysporin/gentamicin	Erythromycin/Tobrex
Route	External lid ointment	Drops	Drops
	Drops		
Dosage	hs	qid (OU)	q3–4h
RTC	1–2 wk or PRN	2–3 days	24 hr
Complications	Chronicity/SPK	Pseudomembrane/marginal keratitis	Ulcer/scarring
Conjunctivitis, Chronic			
Etiology	Staph/drying/UV	Staph/drying/UV	*Moraxella*/drying
Subjective	Chronic/cosmesis	Chronic/cosmesis	Dry irritation
Objective	Inferior injection	Angular injection	Papillary palp.
	Angular conj. hyperemia	Papillary conj.	Angular conj.
	No discharge	No discharge	Xerosis
Assessment	R/O cornea	R/O infection	R/O cornea/infection
Plan	Lubrication/UV protection	Lubrications/UV tints	Lubrications/UV tints
Drug	Antistaphylococcal	Antistaphylococcal	Gentamicin/zinc
Route	Topical ointment	Topical drops and ointments	Topical drops and ointments
Dosage	bid–tid	tid	tid–qid
RTC	3–4 wk	2–3 wk	1–2 wk
Complications	No improvement	Increasing	Corneal involvement
Conjunctivitis, Viral			
Etiology	Nonspecific	PCF/EKC	EKC
Subjective	Burning	Burning/irritation	Irritation
Objective	Pink, follicles	Preauricular nodes	Hyperacute
	Inner canthal involvement	Pseudomembrane	Hemorrhagic
	BUT		
Assessment	R/O *Staphylococcus*/HSV	R/O *Chlamydia*/HSV	R/O gram-negative/HSV

continued

	Mild	Moderate	Severe
CONJUNCTIVA/EPLISCLERA (*cont.*)			
Plan	Advise/cold	Advise/cold	Culture
Drug	Lubrications/decongestant	Antibiotics/lubrications	Antibiotics/steroid (?)
Route	Topical eyedrops	Topical eyedrops	Topical eyedrops
Dosage	q4h	q4h	q2–3h
RTC	7th–8th day	7th–8th day	48 hr
Complications	Contagious	Secondary bacterial	EKC
		EKC	Preseptal
Conjunctival Laceration			
Etiology	Laceration	Laceration to Tenon's	Laceration to sclera
Subjective	Awareness	Concern	Irritation
	Concern	Mild irritation	Foreign-body sensation
Objective	Small conjunctival rent	Conjunctival break	Tenon's capsule rent
		Subconjunctival hemorrhage	Bare sclera
Assessment	R/O foreign matter	R/O Tenon's rent	R/O perforation
Plan	Irrigate/reassure	Irrigate reassure	Irrigate/dilate/examine
Drug	Polysporin	Polysporin	Gentamicin
Route	Topical ointment	Topical ointment	Topical ointment
Dosage	1 × or hs	hs	tid–qid
RTC	PRN	1 wk	3–5 days
Complications	Subconjunctival hemorrhage	Slow resolution	Lid traction
Episcleritis			
Etiology	Unknown	Collagen vascular (?)	Systemic (?)
Subjective	Awareness	Pain on palpation	Pain (on movement)
Objective	Sector injection	Deep injection/diffuse infiltration	Nodular formation
Assessment	R/O inflamed pinguecula	R/O angular conjunctivitis	R/O anterior uveitis
Plan	Heat	Heat	Heat
Drug	Ibuprofen (optional)	Steroid/ibuprofen	Steroid/ibuprofen
Route	Oral	Topical/oral	Topical (oral?)/oral
Dosage	800–1200 mg/day	400 mg/qid	400 mg/q3–4h
RTC	1 wk	3–5 days	48 hr
Complications	Chronic	Nodular	Scleritis
GPC			
Etiology	Mechanical trauma (chronic irritation)	Protein on SLs	Mast cell reaction
Subjective	Mild irritation	Lens/corneal irritation	Severe irritation
Objective	1–2+ GPC	2–3+ GPC	3–4+ GPC
	Lens slippage	Discharge	Heavy mucoid
Assessment	R/O lens surfaces	R/O acute inflammation	R/O vernal, SLK, etc.
Plan	Clean SLs	Temporary D/C SLs	D/C Sls
Drug	Opticrom (optical)	Opticrom 4%	Prednisolone drops Opticrom
Route	Topical	Topical	Topical
Dosage	qid	qid (without SLs)	Prednisolone qid 1 wk Opticrom qid, 6 wk
RTC	2 wk	2–4 wk	1 wk
Complications	Lingering	Persistent	Objective signs persist
CORNEA			
Abrasion, Epithelial			
Etiology	Squamous epithelium	To basement membrane	50% involvement Diabetes
Subjective	Hx	Trauma or spontaneous	Trauma or spontaneous Recurrent erosion
Objective	Superficial straining	NaFl pooling	NaFl stromal seepage Loose edges
Assessment	R/O foreign body	R/O foreign body, penetration	R/O foreign body, perforation

continued

	Mild	Moderate	Severe
CORNEA (cont.)			
Plan	Irrigate	Irrigate/patch or SL	Irrigate/patch or SL
Drug	Polysporin	Cyclo-Dil/gentamicin/ hypertonics (ibuprofen/ aspirin)	Same + SL on recurrence
Route	Top oint	Topical (oral)	Topical (oral)
Dosage	tid	1×	Lubricant ⎫ 8–12 wk SL ⎭
RTC	PRN or 24 h	24 hr	24 hr/weekly with prophylaxis
Complications	Secondary infection	Re-erosion	Secondary infection
Burns, Chemical			
Etiology	Acid/aromatic	Acid/aromatic/alkaline	Acid/aromatic/alkaline
Subjective	When, What, How much? Foreign-body sensation	Same	Same
Objective	SPK, visible iris Hyperemia	SPK, hazy iris Chemosis	SPK, obscure iris Ischemic patches
Assessment	R/O alkaline	R/O stroma	R/O collagenolysis
Plan	H₂O irrigation 20–30 min	H₂O irrigation 30–60 min Swab cul-de-sac	H₂O irrigation 30–60 min pH tears
Drug	Cyclo/dilate/Tobrex Steroid (if secondary uveitis)	Cyclo/dilate/Tobrex Steroid after 3–5 days	Cyclo/dilate/Tobrex/Mucomyst Steroid after 5 days
Route	Topical drops	Topical drops	Topical drops and ointment
Dosage	qid	q4h	q2h
RTC	48–72 hr	24–48 hr	24 hr
Complications	Persistent injection	Symblepharon Scarring	Scarring Corneal melt
Burns, Radiation			
Etiology	Diffuse UV	Concentrated UV	Thermal (Eschar)
Subjective	Dry eye feeling Sunlight hx	Corneal pain Hx of UV exposure	Foreign-body sensation Hx of hot particle
Objective	Mild SPK (band) 1–2+ hyperemia	Dense SPK	Focal white charred epithelium
Assessment	R/O keratitis sicca	R/O uveitis	R/O particle(s) embedded
Plan	Lubricate	Patch(?)	Remove as foreign body
Drug	Polysporin (optional)	Polysporin/gentamicin Cyclo/dilate	Gentamicin Cyclo/dilate
Route	Topical ointment	Topical ointment	Topical ointment/drops
Dosage	tid	qid	qid
RTC	PRN	24 hr	24 hr
Complications	Secondary infection	Secondary infection	*Pseudomonas*
Dellen			
Etiology	Drying area	Raised conjunctival lesion	Focal dry spot
Subjective	Asymptomatic General examination	Asymptomatic	Asymptomatic
Objective	Hazy epithelium	Depression	Deep peripheral corneal cup with sharp edges
Assessment	R/O marginal degenerations	R/O marginal ulcer	R/O penetrating lesion (very rare)
Plan	Advise	Anti-UV lenses (if pinguecula the cause)	
Drug	Lubricate	Patch	Patch/SL
Route	Topical		
Dosage	q2–4h	Constant wear	Extended wear for 3–5 days
RTC	3–5 days	1–2 days	24 hr
Complications	Tear disruption	Recurrence	Secondary infection
Dry Eye/Keratitis Sicca Syndromes			
Etiology	Squamous metaplasia	Mucin deficiency	Aqueous deficiency
Subjective	Late-day irritation	Advancing sxs	Pain (> late-day) VA problems
Objective	Hyperemia/band SPK/BUT/ Papillae/Mucus/rose bengal	Advancing signs Epithelial breakdown	Complications Filaments

continued

	Mild	Moderate	Severe
CORNEA (cont.)			
Assessment	R/O EBMD or bacterial/ viral/irritation	R/O same	R/O secondary bacterial/viral
Plan	Advise on chronicity	Check compliance	Punctal occlusion
			Gel tears, Healon, Vitamin A ointment/drops
Drug	Lubricate	Lubricants or SL (DW) Vitamin A drops	Low water SL with lubricants and prophylaxis
Route	Topical	Topical	Topical
Dosage	ad lib	q1–2h or SL	q3–4h/hs
RTC	2 wk	2 wk	1 wk
Complications	Compliance	Complications (e.g., infection/filaments)	Secondary infection
EBMD			
Etiology	Degeneration	Degeneration/acquired dystrophy	Acquired/dystrophy
Subjective	Asymptomatic	AM syndrome reduced visual acuity	AM syndrome Spontaneous erosion
Objective	Maps/dots Negative staining	Maps–dots–fingerprint Negative (positive) stain	Anterior stromal haze Brawny edema
Assessment	R/O dry eye	R/O infection	R/O other corneal disorders
Plan	Advise	Advise	Advise
Drug	Hypertonic saline	Hypotonic solution gtts/ oint/extended-wear SL	Extended-wear SL + prophylactic antibiotics
Route	Topical drops/oint	Topical	Topical drops
Dosage	ad lib/PRN	q3–4h/hs or SL	Extended-wear + bid drops
RTC	Routine/PRN	3–4 wk or extended-wear schedule	Extended-wear schedule for 8– 12 wk
Complications	AM syndrome Spontaneous erosion	VA reduction Spontaneous erosion	1–3 yr duration Patient despair
Foreign Body			
Etiology	Superficial	Penetration	Perforation
Subjective	Hx Corneal pain Uveitic pain	Hx Corneal pain Uveitic pain	Hx Corneal pain Uveitic pain
Objective	Epithelial	Stroma	Full-thickness corneal signs
Assessment	R/O penetration	R/O perforation	R/O intraocular foreign body
Plan	Irrigate and remove	Refer to corneal specialist	Refer to corneal specialist
Drug	Treat as moderate abrasion	Cyanoacrylic glue and SL bandage	Radiography
Route			Ultrasound Dilated fundus examination Oral cephalosporin Cyanoacrylic glue and SL bandage
Dosage			
RTC		Per consultant	
Complications	Hemosiderosis	Scarring	Scarring Panophthalmitis
Fuchs' Dystrophy			
Etiology	Endothelial dystrophy	Edema	Advancing edema
Subjective	Asymptomatic Menopausal females	AM syndrome	Bullous Pain
Objective	Guttata Pigment dusting	Epithelial and stromal edema	Bedewing Bullous keratitis
Assessment	R/O other dystrophy	R/O EBMD/bacterial	R/O degeneration
Plan	Advise	Advise Antiedema measures	Advise Possible keratoplasty
Drug	Hypertonic solution	Hypertonic solution/heat/ Rxs	Extended-wear SL
Route	Top gtts/oint	Topical gtts/oint	Topical gtts/ointment
Dosage	PRN	3–4 ×/hs	bid
RTC	6 mo/PRN	3 mo	Extended-wear schedule q6–12wk
Complications	AM syndrome	Bullous	Fibrosis

continued

	Mild	Moderate	Severe
CORNEA (cont.)			
Inclusion KC			
Etiology	Maternal *Chlamydia*	Acquired *Chlamydia*	Prolonged *Chlamydia*
Subjective	Inclusion blenorrhea	Sexually active adult	Recurrent
		Recurrent	Prolonged therapy
Objective	Bacterial/viral	Bacterial/viral	Bacterial/viral
	keratoconjunctivitis	keratoconjunctivitis	keratoconjunctivitis infiltrates
Assessment	R/O gram-negative (GC or	R/O bacterial/viral causes	R/O other keratites
	H. flu)		
Plan	Advise mother	Advise patient	Advise patient
		Inclusion bodies (?)	Inclusion bodies (?)
Drug	Erythromycin	Tetracycline or	Tetracycline/erythromycin
		erythromycin	(topical steroid +/−)
Route	Topical/oral	Topical/oral	Topical/oral
Dosage	qid (by wt.)	1–2 g/day	1–2 g/day
RTC	3–5 days	10 days	3–5 days
Complications	Dacryo./otitis	Corneal infiltrates	Scarring
Keratitis, Adenoviral			
Etiology	Nonspecific	PCF/EKC	EKC
Subjective	Mild burning	Burning/irritation	Corneal irritation
			Reduced VA
Objective	Diffuse SPK	Diffuse SPK (2+)	SPK/SEI (3–4+)
	Follicles	Follicles	Pseudomembrane
Assessment	R/O PCF/EKC Herpes	R/O Herpes	R/O herpes, bacterial
		Thygeson's	
Plan	Advise	Advise	Advise
Drug	Lubricants/decongestant	Antistaphylococcal/	Cyclo/dil
	(optional)	lubricants	+ steroids
Route	Topical drops	Topical drops	Topical drops
Dosage	q3–4h	q4h	q4h
RTC	7th to 8th day	7th to 8th day or 3–5	48–72 hr
Complications	Secondary bacterial/toxic	Secondary bacterial/toxic	Infiltrative scarring
	Contagious	Contagious	
Keratitis, HSV Epithelial			
Etiology	Recurrent HSV	Primary HSV	Postinfection (metaherpetic)
Subjective	Mild or no corneal irritation	Malaise	Resistant HSV
		Corneal pain	
Objective	Dendrite (>75%)	Lymphadenopathy	Anterior stromal involvement
		Epithelial	Indolent epithelial ulcer
			BM involvement
Assessment	R/O infiltrative dendrite	R/O HSV-2 (genital)	R/O deep stroma
Plan	Gentamicin qid	Gentamicin qid	Denude ulcer
Drug	Viroptic drops	Viroptic drops	Viroptic drops
	Vira A or IDU ointment	Vira A or IDU ointment	Vira A or IDU ointment
		Acyclovir ointment (skin)	Prednisolone drops
Route	Topical	Topical	Topical
Dosage	Drops q2h	Drops q3–4h	Viroptic qh
	Ointment-hs	IDU ointment-hs	Vira A, hs
		Acyclovir (on skin) qid	Prednisolone drops ~tid
RTC	48 hr	48–72 hr	48 hr
Complications	Resistant strain (>14 days)	Recurrence	Scarring
		Metaherpetica	Stromal keratitis
Keratitis, HSV, Stromal			
Etiology	Immune response	Unknown etiology	Virulent strain
Subjective	Multiple recurrences	With or without HSVEK	Multiple recurrences
	Uveitic pain		Uveitic pain
Objective	Deep stromal infiltration	Disciform stromal edema	Interstitial keratitis
Assessment	R/O interstitial keratitis	R/O bacterial ulcer	R/O melting
Plan	Refer to corneal specialist	Monitor epithelium	Refer to corneal specialist
Drug	Steroids	Steroids	Steroids
		Antiedema	Penetrating keratoplasty
Route	Topical	Topical	
Dosage	Variable	qid–q4h	
RTC	Per consultant	48–72 hr	

continued

	Mild	Moderate	Severe
CORNEA (*cont.*)			
Complications	Scarring Wessley ring	No response Scarring	Pthisis bulbi
Keratitis, Staphylococcal			
Etiology	Diffuse toxic/irritative Sterile SPK	Focal toxic/hypersensitive infiltrative	Bacterial invasion
Subjective	Lid hx. Cornea (AM) irritation	AM syndrome	Hot eye/pain
Objective	Inferior or diffuse SPK Staph lid signs	Peripheral infiltrate Edema-Island lesion(s) Superficial-leash of vessels	Congestion-deep stromal Chemosis-post. cornea 360° violet anterior chamber Depressed pus
Assessment	R/O other infection/KCS	R/O ulcer	R/O endophthalmitis
Plan	Antistaphylococcal (lids)	Antistaphylococcal (lids)	Hospitalize Refer to corneal specialist
Drug	Lubricants	Combo	Triple aminoglycosides
Route	Topical drops	Topical drops	Topical drops/injectables
Dosage	6–10 × daily	qid q4h	q30min
RTC	7–10 days	48–72 hr	24 hr
Complications	Marginal K	Secondary infection	Scarring/perforation
Ocular Rosacea			
Etiology	Dermatoblepharitis	Dermatoblepharacon- junctivitis	Dermatoblepharokeratocon- junctivitis
Subjective	Dermatologic history (+/−) (30–60 age range)	Chronic/nonresponsive Dermatologic hx (+/−)	Recurrent Dermatologic (+/−)
Objective	Blepharitis with or without dermatitis	Blepharoconjunctivitis with or without dermatitis	Peripheral corneal involvement (360°)
Assessment	R/O *Staphylococcus* seborrhea	R/O bacterial/viral	R/O bacterial/viral
Plan	Lid scrubs Hot packs	Oral tetracycline 250 mg qid × 15 days Achromycin suspension	Oral tetracycline 250 mg qid × 30 days Achromycin suspension
Drug	Tetracycline ointment (Achromycin)		Prednisolone drops
Route	Topical	Topical	Topical
Dosage	qid	qid	q4h
RTC	1–2 wk	1 wk	3–5 days
Complications	Nonresponsive	Corneal involvement	Corneal complications
SLK			
Etiology	Hyperthyroid (?)	Unknown/hyperthyroid	SLs/Thimerosal
Subjective	Mild irritation	Corneal irritation	SL irritation
Objective	Superior injection Superior SPK Mild tarsal reaction	Pseudodendrites Anterior stromal haze Tarsal involvement	Superior infection Superior SPK, SEI Mild tarsal reaction
Assessment	R/O SLs/Thimerosal	R/O Vernal	R/O Theodore SLK
Plan	Lubricants	Silver nitrate (+/−) Prophylax	D/C SLs/Thimerosal
Drug	Opticrom (?) Prednisolone (?)	Steroid (first) Opticrom (?)	Silver nitrate Steroid (first) Opticrom (?)
Route	Topical	Topical	Topical
Dosage	tid–qid	q4h	q4h
RTC	1 wk	1 wk	1 wk
Complications	Recurrence	Secondary infection	Deep stromal
SPK of Thygeson			
Etiology	Unknown	Viral (?)	Herpes zoster (?)
Subjective	Asymptomatic (white eye)	↓ BVA (white eye)	Severe discomfort
Objective	Fine SPK "No company"	Dense SPK/epith. infiltrates "No company"	Bilateral, dense "No company"
Assessment	R/O bacterial/viral	R/O bacterial/viral	R/O bacterial/viral
Plan	Don't D/C SLs	Viroptic (?)	Viroptic (?)
Drug	Lubricants/steroids (?)	Lubricants/steroids (?)/SLs	Steroids/SLs
Route	Topical drops	Topical drops	Topical drops
Dosage	qid	q3–4h	q2h
RTC	1–2 wk	1 wk	3 days
Complications	Inc. SPK/infiltrates	Exacerbations	Chronicity

continued

	Mild	Moderate	Severe
CORNEA ((cont.)			
Vernal KC			
Etiology	Type 1, Mild	Seasonal	Eosinophilic
Subjective	Corneal irritation	Itching	Severe discomfort
		Discomfort	Persistent
Objective	Limbal (vernal)	Giant papillae	Psuedodendrites
	Mild edema	Superior SPK	Tranta's dots
			Mucoid discharge
Assessment	R/O staphylococcal marginal keratoconjunctivitis	R/O other immune keratoconjunctivitis	R/O infection
Plan	Prophylax tid	Antihistamines/ decongestants	Oral steroids (?)
Drug	Prednisolone drops (to Opticrom)	Prednisolone drops (to Opticrom)	Prednisolone drops
Route	Topical	Topical	Topical
Dosage	qid	q4h	q2–3h
RTC	3–5 days	2–3 days	48 hr
Complications	Recurrence	Maintenance	Recurrence
ANTERIOR CHAMBER			
Anterior Uveitis			
Etiology	Trauma/unknown	Trauma/unknown/systemic	Unknown/systemic
Subjective	Mild aching	Moderate–severe aching	Mild to no pain
Objective	Circumcorneal/cells/ FI/KP/↓ intraocular pressure	Pseudoptosis/plasmoid/ ↓ visual acuity	Mutton fats/synechiae
Assessment	R/O vitreous	R/O posterior/systemic	R/O active systemic disease
Plan	Heat/shades	Heat/shades/plus (add)	Medical consultation
Drug	Cyclo/steroid(?)/ibuprofen	Cyclo/steroid/ibuprofen	Cyclo/steroid (topical/oral)
Route	Drops/oral	Drops/oral/depot (?)	Drops (drops/oral)
Dosage	qid/drops/800–1600 mg/ day	q4h drops/1600 md/day	q2h drops 30–50 mg/day
RTC	2–3 days	48 hr	48 hr
Complications	Keratic precipitates	Synechiae	Multiple anterior and posterior

Postoperative Complications (by Time) in Aphakic and Pseudophakic Intraocular Lens Care

Possible Complication	In Operating Room	First 24 Hours	First 2 Weeks	Third Week to Years
Astigmatism				
Continuous sutures			Spherical equivalent	Cut suture(s)
Interrupted sutures			Spherical equivalent	Remove suture(s)
Loose sutures		Tighten or add	Reduce IOP	Wedge resection
Bullous keratopathy			High H_2O soft lens	High H_2O soft lens
Capsular fibrosis				YAG laser
Choroidal effusion		Retinal consultation		
Corneal clouding	Superior 1/3	Follow	Monitor IOP	Corneal consult
Corneal edema	Superior 1/3	Follow	5% NaCl	High H_2O soft lens
Cystoid macular edema				Fluorescein angiography
Diplopia		Follow		Check neurologist
Displaced IOL			Consider VA	Consider VA
Endophthalmitis		Emergent care	Emergent care	Emergent care
Foreign-body sensation			Check sutures	Trim sutures
Hyphema		Follow	R/O sickle cell	
Hypotony	Check sutures	Resuture	Reconstruct	
Increased IOP		Timoptic or Diamox	Switch to FML	Avoid epinephrine drugs
Infection	Antibiotics	Antibiotics	R/O Hypopyon	
Iris prolapse		Surgical repair	Surgical repair (and Cyl/dilate)	
Iritis	Steroids	Steroids	Steroids and Cyl/dilate	Standard therapy (1–3 mo)
Posterior vitreous detachment (PVD)			Visual fields	R/O retinal detachment
Pseudofibrosis				Scrub or YAG
Ptosis		Follow		Check neurologist
Pupillary entrapment			Dilate to reposition	Attempt repositioning
Reduced VA	Follow	Follow	Determine cause	
Retinal detachment		Retinal consultation	Retinal consultation	BIO examination
Seidel test +		Add suture(s)	Tighten or add	
Vitreal hemorrhage		Retinal consultation	Retinal consultation	BIO examination

APPENDIX 6

Answers to Self-assessment Questions

I. CHAPTER ONE

1. d	11. d	21. a	31. c
2. a	12. c	22. a	32. a
3. c	13. d	23. c	33. d
4. b	14. b	24. b	34. b
5. c	15. c	25. c	35. d
6. d	16. d	26. d	36. b
7. a	17. b	27. b	37. b
8. b	18. a	28. c	38. b
9. b	19. b	29. b	39. d
10. a	20. d	30. a	40. b

II. CHAPTER TWO

1. c	11. d
2. b	12. c
3. d	13. b
4. a	14. b
5. a	15. d
6. c	16. c
7. b	17. a
8. b	18. d
9. d	19. d
10. a	20. a

V. CHAPTER FIVE

1. c	11. e
2. a	12. j
3. b	13. b
4. d	14. f
5. a	15. i
6. b	16. h
7. d	17. a
8. a	18. c
9. d	19. g
10. c	20. d

III. CHAPTER THREE

1. c	11. d
2. a	12. b
3. a	13. b
4. a	14. a
5. b	15. c
6. d	16. a
7. d	17. d
8. b	18. c
9. c	19. b
10. a	20. a

VI. CHAPTER SIX

1. i	11. d
2. g	12. h
3. h	13. b
4. f	14. j
5. c	15. c
6. j	16. a
7. b	17. f
8. e	18. i
9. d	19. e
10. a	20. g

IV. CHAPTER FOUR

1. b	11. b
2. c	12. c
3. a	13. c
4. c	14. b
5. c	15. c
6. d	16. a
7. d	17. d
8. a	18. d
9. b	19. a
10. a	20. c

VII. CHAPTER SEVEN

1. c	11. b
2. b	12. b
3. d	13. a
4. c	14. c
5. a	15. c
6. b	16. d
7. d	17. d
8. c	18. a
9. c	19. b
10. b	20. a

VIII. CASE REPORTS WITH COLOR PLATES

1.	c	21.	a
2.	a	22.	b
3.	d	23.	a
4.	c	24.	a
5.	b	25.	c
6.	b	26.	b
7.	b	27.	d
8.	c	28.	c
9.	d	29.	a
10.	a	30.	d
11.	b	31.	c
12.	b	32.	a
13.	a	33.	d
14.	c	34.	c
15.	a	35.	a
16.	d	36.	d
17.	d	37.	b
18.	c	38.	b
19.	d	39.	a
20.	b	40.	c

Index